Mariacarla Gadebusch Bondio (ed.)
Medical Ethics

AURORA

Schriften der Villa Vigoni

Gegründet von Gregor Vogt-Spira,

herausgegeben von Immacolata Amodeo

Band 2

Mariacarla Gadebusch Bondio (ed.)

Medical Ethics

Premodern Negotiations between Medicine and Philosophy

Franz Steiner Verlag

Gedruckt mit freundlicher Unterstützung der Deutschen Forschungsgemeinschaft (DFG)
und der Medizinischen Fakultät der Universität Greifswald

Bibliografische Information der Deutschen Nationalbibliothek:
Die Deutsche Nationalbibliothek verzeichnet diese Publikation in der Deutschen Nationalbibliografie; detaillierte bibliografische Daten sind im Internet über <http://dnb.d-nb.de> abrufbar.

Druck: AZ Druck und Datentechnik, Kempten
Gedruckt auf säurefreiem, alterungsbeständigem Papier.
Printed in Germany.
ISBN 978-3-515-09835-9 (Print)
ISBN 978-3-515-10819-5 (E-Book)

CONTENTS

INTRODUCTION

Mariacarla Gadebusch Bondio

> Matters concerned with conduct and questions of what is good for us have no fixity, any more than matters of health. The general account being of this nature, the account of particular cases is yet more lacking in exactness; for they do not fall under any art or precept but the agents themselves must in each case consider what is appropriate to the occasion, as happens also in the art of medicine or of navigation.
>
> Aristotle, *Nicomachean Ethics*, II, 2: 1104a[1]

In the long period which comprises the pre-modern era, medicine had always worked on the development of a definition of its professional ethos. The legacy of this ethical awareness is the evidence of reflection on the possibilities, boundaries and the dangers of medical science, and the moral profile of its representatives. Although the efforts towards a codification of medical practices through the establishment of moral standards document the desire for self regulation and self-criticism, this tradition has so far only been explored in a fragmentary way.[2] Seen from the *longue durée* perspective, medico-ethical traditions show that despite the broad spectrum of positions, in addition to performing successful treatment doctors have always endeavoured to obtain their patients' trust and to safeguard the reputation of their profession.

1 Aristotle, *The Nicomachean Ethics*, tr. by D. W. Ross, ed. by L. Brown, Oxford 2009.

2 After the editors of *Doctors and Ethics* 1993 declared the history of medical ethics to be a desideratum of research, a number of studies have appeared. See: A. Wear – J. Geyer-Kordesch – R. French (eds.), *Doctors and Ethics. The Earlier Historical Setting of Medical Ethics*, Amsterdam / Atlanta 1993; R. Baker, "The History of Medical Ethics", in: W.F. Bynum – R. Porter (eds.), *Companion of the History of Medicine*, vol. 2, London / New York 1993, pp. 852-887; W. Schleiner, *Medical Ethics in the Renaissance*, Washington, 1995; E. Seidler, *Ethics in Medicine. Historical Aspects of the Present Debate*, Sheffield 1996; K. Bergdolt, *Das Gewissen der Medizin. Ärztliche Moral von der Antike bis heute*, München. 2004. Still fundamental for medical ethics in antiquity: K. Deichgräber, "Die ärztliche Standesethik des hippokratischen Eides", *Quellen und Studien zur Geschichte der Wissenschaften und der Medizin* 3 (1932), 97-8. K. Deichgräber, *'Medicus gratiosus': Untersuchungen zu einem griechischen Arztbild* (Akademie der Wissenschaften und der Literatur, Abhandlungen der geistes- und sozialwissenschaftlichen Klasse), Mainz 1970; P.Cordes, *Iatros. Das Bild des Arztes in der Griechischen Literatur von Homer bis Aristoteles*, Stuttgart 1991.

For a doctor, the treatment of sick and vulnerable persons represents a great responsibility which does not just end with indicated measures of a diagnostic, therapeutic or palliative nature. If indecision exists, then the risk of acting badly or incorrectly inevitably increases. Thus since antiquity we can find deliberations on the uncertainty, dangers and consequences in medical literature which are associated with medical practice. The expectations of patients and their families can easily lead doctors to make commitments or promises which when disappointed will demonstrate the boundaries of medical knowledge and ability. Such testimonies of critical and self-critical reflection always have pragmatic drawbacks. They reveal dimensions of medical practice and indicate the sphere of action of premodern physicians who, as a rule, had to treat and advise patients from many different social classes: rich, poor, influential, educated or simple people, men and women of all ages and of various backgrounds. Sometimes it might also be simulators, criminals or even enemies who sought the help of doctors. This variety of patients has always demanded that doctors have a strong social awareness, a degree of flexibility, and above all a good knowledge of human nature.

Up until and into the early modern era, moral orientation was still being sought in the philosophical and theological foundations of humanist influenced medicine. This search pertained to the question, for example, of whether and how a doctor should approach a patient with no chance of recovery. Connected to this was the much debated question of whether a doctor may lie or be obliged to tell the truth. These are examples for timeless problem areas of medicine which even today arouse lively discussion.

In times when medical ethics has tended towards adopting the research style and publication culture of biomedicine, a concern with past traditions may seem to be an anachronistic task. However, as Robert B. Baker and Laurence B. McCullough, editors of *The Cambridge World History of Medical Ethics*, stressed in their foreword in 2009, a historical foundation and cultural embedding are today more necessary than ever.[3] In their argumentation they refer to the new generation in bioethics: "old" medical ethicists were an extremely interdisciplinary group with a broad humanist education in history, philosophy, theology and/or jurisprudence, medicine and nursing science. Thanks to this humanist background it was, for example, possible to support the ethical challenges which the development of medical technologies led to in the 1970s, initiating successful negotiations in a pluralistic society. Baker and McCullough's statement that the original broad knowledge base of established bioethics – to which its success is largely due – "is atrophying" provides food for thought.[4] Whilst the tripartite department "History, Theory and Ethics of Medicine" can be found in German universities as an interdisciplinary package or cross-section, the potential of this diversity of disciplines, however, is frequently surrendered in favour of a one-sided focus.

3 R. B. Baker – L. B. McCullough (eds.), *The Cambridge World History of Medical Ethics*, Cambridge 2009, XV-XVIII.

4 Baker – McCullough, *The Cambridge World History*, XV.

Today, in professionalised bioethics a pragmatic, problem-orientated approach can be observed as well as a growing tendency towards the empiricism and production of evidence-based data. In bioethics the expression "empirical turn" is used: through the application of methods of empirical and sociological sciences, the traditional philosophical and normative way of thinking should be both complemented and sustained.[5] In this trend, experimental ethics laboratories ("ethics labs") have emerged with the declared aim of 'objectively' determining the ethical competence or moral values with individuals and groups. Under the slightly confusing label "Ethics in the Laboratory", "experimental examinations of ethically relevant decision-making processes" are aimed at.[6] In the course of this change in the direction of medical thinking, it is not surprising that there is intense debate as to whether and how the performance of ethics committees and ethics councils should be evaluated.[7] Welcome though the establishment of medical ethics and bioethics[8] may be as an integral part of the curriculum of medical training, and as promoter of a culture of discussion and reflection in daily clinical practice, its one-sided "application-orientated" development affecting those who are convinced of the potential of a humanist-oriented ethics is all the more sobering. The cultural and humanistic substance of medical ethics as a perpetual part of a self-reflecting medicine succumbs to the impulse towards assimilation in a biomedical approach to thinking and working: but moral philosophy and medicine – and thus medical ethics – will, as stated in the opening quotation, always have to decide in each individual case what contributes to the 'good' in specific situations.

A concern with the genesis and development of medico-ethical discussions facilitates the understanding of the diversity of discourses from the changing contexts from which they arise, and the ability to deal with the manifold sources in which they were expressed and handed down. This approach to the prime developmental stages of a pre-modern medical ethics which defines its profiles not only within medicine, but also in dialogue with literature, philosophy and theology, shows the cultural and historical specificity of ethical discourse. This ideational

5 S. Salloch – J. Schildmann – J. Vollmann, "Empirical research in medical ethics: How conceptual accounts on normative-empirical collaboration may improve research practice", *Medical Ethics* 13:5 (2012), pp. 1-7. [http://www.biomedcentral.com/1472-6939/13/5 (19.01.14)].

6 This burgeoning tendency in economic ethics is also indicated in medicine [http://www.wirtschaftsethik.edu.tum.de/forschung/ (19.01.14)].

7 The position held by Meinolfus Strätling, who pleads for evidence-based, "measurable" evaluations of the results of the activities of clinical ethics committees, is the cause of discussions in the bioethical community: M. W. M. Strätling – B. Sedemund Adib, "Ethikberatung: Ethische Kernkompetenzen in die Medizin zurückholen", *Deutsches Ärzteblatt* 110/17 (2013), A-825 / B-713 / C-713. For a critical reaction to this see: C. Wiesemann, "Ethikberatung: Heiße Luft", *Deutsches Ärzteblatt* 110/26 (2013), A-1321 / B-1157 / C-1144.

8 The term bioethics, as with biomedicine, has increasingly established itself in recent years as the so-called life sciences have flourished, and is often used as a synonym for medical ethics. Bioethics has, however, a broader meaning than medical ethics and includes the ethics of life and the disciplines which deal closely with life. I am using "medical ethics" here as the older and more traditional term, whilst I use bioethics as the modern term for "ethics in biomedicine", which also includes medical ethics.

realization can and should serve as a corrective to the operationalising of bioethics.

One further reason for the return of bioethics to its cultural heritage is its so far only fragmentarily explored relationship to philosophy. The thesis supported by Daniel Fox in 1979 of a "segregation" of medical ethics which would have resulted as a consequence of the "curious disconnection" of medical ethics and moral philosophy since the mid 18th century, could be put into perspective, above all on the basis of historical examinations. [9] Hans Jonas[10] and Georg Gadamer[11] can be considered as examples for the emerging "involvement" of philosophy in discussions on the ethical responsibility of medicine.[12]

The influence of philosophy on medicine took place over time. This is apparent from the effects of Platonic and Aristotelian philosophy on pre-modern medico-ethical debate on, for instance, the obligation of a doctor to truthfulness. Ideas and concepts which have proven fruitful in medical ethics, for example the Kantian idea of autonomy had to be adapted so that they might be applied to concrete examples. In order to understand this delayed influence, historical reconstruction work is necessary. The historical analysis of texts which deal with questions of medical ethics shows their philosophical substrates. It allows dialogue between doctors and philosophers, where traces of both the Old and the New Testament can be recognised, to blossom across time.

The 15 articles collected here originated largely as part of a colloquium which took place at Villa Vigoni in November 2010. They place emphasis on different topics and cover the long period from antiquity to the early modern period, together with their reception.

How a doctor should act in hopeless cases and with poor prognoses is a classic question of medical ethics. It is examined and treated differently in Hippocratic and Galenic texts, as well as in the works of authors such as Celsus. The discussion allows us to visualise medicine on the ancient Greco-Roman cultural horizon. The prejudices, platitudes and clichés against medicine which circulated in this

9 D. M. Fox, "The Segregation of Medical Ethics: a Problem in Modern Intellectual History", *Journal of Medicine and Philosophy* 4 (1979), pp. 81-97; For critical comments see: R. B. Baker – L. B. McCullough, "The Discourses of Philosophical Medical Ethics" in: id., *The Cambridge World History*, pp. 281-309; R. M. Veach, *Disrupted Dialogue: Medical Ethics and the Collapse of Physicians-Humanist Communication (1770-1980)*, New York 2005.

10 H. Jonas, *Technik, Medizin und Ethik. Praxis des Prinzips Verantwortung*, Frankfurt am Main 1985, p. 12: in medicine's "completely new instruments of power", which constitute its contributions to scientific and technical progress, Jonas sees the loss of its never questioned "beneficence". Medical "feasibilities", which affect above all the beginning and end of life, raise questions which revolve around the idea of humanity: "these are real questions for philosophers".

11 H.-G. Gadamer, *Über die Verborgenheit der Gesundheit. Aufsätze und Vorträge*, Frankfurt am Main 1993.

12 Habermas speaks about "the interfering" of philosophy in medical ethical matters in his foreword to: J. Habermas: *Die Zukunft der menschlichen Natur. Auf dem Weg zu einer liberalen Eugenik?*, Frankfurt am Main 2001, p. 9.

context nurtured the permanent scepticism of patients and the extreme caution of the attending physicians. This found expression, amongst other things, in the doctor's fear of making mistakes. The decision not to treat the seriously injured belongs in this context to the precautions taken to protect both reputation and profession. (CHRISTIAN SCHULZE)

From late antiquity to early humanism, medicine and philosophy struggled initially to define and demarcate their individual areas of responsibility, and then – with the emergence of universities – to achieve a higher position in the hierarchy of the arts. Testimonies of this rivalry are works such as the *Conciliator differentiarum quae inter philosophos et medicos versantur* by Pietro d'Abano. The situation changed between the 14th and 15th centuries. With invigorated self-confidence, medicine now concerned itself with an increasingly broad range of themes in order to style itself a divine science. (CHIARA CRISCIANI)

A closer look at medical practice in the Middle Ages reveals areas of action in which tension between medicine and Christian morality was unavoidable. Thus a poor prognosis and the notification of impending death belong to the most difficult tasks of a physician. In this context mistakes are considered especially serious and defamatory. Here a doctor must arm himself with virtues. The armamentarium of codes of behaviour and moral attributes, above all prudence and temperance, which physicians such as Pietro d'Abano and Jacques Despars have compiled, were perceived as a remedy for mistakes. (DANIELLE JACQUART)

Compared to Petrarch's brutal criticism of doctors, even the most solid efforts towards good medicine seem predestined to fail. What the well-know *Invectivae* of an apparently somewhat arrogant poet indicate is his "campaign" for those areas of knowledge which today are considered humanities, and which Coluccio Salutati termed *studia humanitatis*. (KLAUS BERGDOLT)

In the second half of the 14th century, learned physicians felt the necessity to clarify the value and benefit of good and true medicine. Such endeavours towards professionalising the discipline pursued, at the same time, the aim of strengthening the image and reputation of the medical profession in years when critical voices had been raised against the supposed ignorance, arrogance, crudeness and bad practice of doctors. They were reflected in translations of classical writings and in their compilation in hand-written codices. One anonymous manuscript from Montpellier, with texts which are devoted to the behaviour and the duties of a physician, reveals precisely this intention (*De lege*, *De commendatione*, *Tabula Arnaldi*). The text *De commendatione medicine*, contained in a codex in the Vatican archives, is edited and made accessible here for the first time. (MICHAEL MCVAUGH)

More than half a century later, in the kingdom of Naples, the correspondence between Ippolita Sforza and her brother Galeazzo Maria attests the concern felt by the duchess for her sick husband Alfonso. Her secretary, the humanist Giovanni Pontano, reports precisely the symptoms of the duke's illness. If we focus on the views of the family, those close to him and of the patient himself regarding his illness, then a completely different picture of humanistic medicine emerges. The doctor-patient relationship in its insurmountable asymmetry can also be seen as a dynamic interaction between laymen and experts. Mistrust, but also a sense of responsibility and critical potential are the particular weapons of the patient, should he possesses a certain authority and be able to display "cautela" when dealing with his physician. The poet and secretary Pontano was able to write critically about his experiences and (in his *Charon*) allowed topoi of classical and humanistic criticism of physicians – from Pliny to Petrarch – to interact. The genre must have been in great demand as Ariosto also wrote a satire (*Erbolato*) in which ultimately the patient is advised to be prudent and heedful when dealing with a doctor. (MATTIAS ROICK)

As a humanist, doctor, philosopher, astrologist, translator and commentator on Plato, Marsilio Ficino embodied the applied fusion of medicine and philosophy. In platonic philosophy, as well as in hermetic tradition, he recognised the necessary conditions of a medicine which, as "queen of the arts", addressed the body and soul of a person. In his remarks on the plague, Ficino translates his holistic approach into a therapeutic and preventative programme in which moderation and modest luck are declared the most effective medical means of combating epidemics. At the core of this moral lifestyle, the example of Socrates points the direction towards physical and mental equilibrium and to health. (TEODORO KATINIS)

What was really new in medical ethics in the age of Humanism? The question results from an attentive reading of Gabriele Zerbi's *De cautelis medicorum* (1495). The ambivalence of this text shows the author's clinging to standard medieval points of view, as well as his efforts to introduce original reflexions. The novelties of Zerbi's ethical approach are underlined by his explanations concerning a physician's practical experience, and by the way he incorporates the concepts of *humanitas* and *misericordia*. Although Zerbi abundantly copies passages from the works of other authors, his treatise contains a number of his own visions when it comes to stressing the duty to search for new theories, and lastly when he remarks how the plurality of physicians treating the same case under the guidance of a principal doctor contributes to the avoidance of medical errors. (JOSEPH ZIEGLER)

However, Gabriele Zerbi's short treatise not only reflects contemporary conceptions of medical ethics, but also reveals certain aspects of the author's personality and his living environment at the time when he composed his book. Traces of Zerbi's direct encounter with the impact of the Spanish Inquisition on the Iberian Jews, and the beginning of the great European witch-hunt during the time of his service at the Papal court in Rome, can be identified in several passages in which the physician's religious ideas seem to meld with his visions of medical ethics. By taking his turbulent socio-cultural background into consideration, light is shed on new and so far unknown aspects of Zerbi's *medicus cautus* and his negative counterparts. (KAY PETER JANKRIFT)

Man's place in nature and his interaction with other living beings, above all with animals, is one of the core problems of religion and philosophy. Ancient ideas provide the material for a hitherto rarely considered discussion on vegetarianism in the first half of the 16th century. The fascinating, even "polymorphous" reception history of Porphyry's text *De abstinentia* demonstrates a blossoming interest in the relationship between man and beast, as well as between body and soul in the Renaissance period. Linked to this is not only the topic of meat-based nutrition, but also the ritual sacrifice of animals and violence against animals. This is an excellent example for the fertile interrelationship of philosophical, religious, ethical and medical and hygiene interests in the Renaissance. (CECILIA MURATORI)

Following Galen, the theory commonly held since antiquity that the control of the emotions and their balanced relationship are characteristics of a good, virtuous and healthy person is systematically discussed in the 16th century by the doctor and philosopher Luigi Lusini, and placed upon a (patho-)physiological foundation. In his treatise *De compescendis animi affectibus per moralem philosophiam et medendi artem* published in 1562 and divided into three books, Luisini is able to reveal the integral interconnection of the theories the soul and the emotions, moral philosophy and medicine. This allows two complementary approaches to therapy to be developed which from today's perspective appear almost prophetic: a complete cure for the soul is only possible through the combination of philosophy and medicine. (ROBERTO POMA)

On first sight, humour and laughter appear to have no real claim to medical relevance. However, the French doctor Laurent Joubert dealt with this topic in a monography *Le traité du ris* (1579), and recommended laughter as a proven remedy. This type of humour – the term should be understood explicitly in the modern and not in the humoral pathological sense – results in particular from the mainly asymmetrically connoted doctor-patient communication which might contain both pure situational comedy, as well as ingenious and amusing play with gender, religious or group-specific prejudices. From our present point of view it is obvious that this takes place at the expense of political correctness; the early modern period appears, however, to have regarded hearty laughter at the sickbed to have been healing and liberating – both for the patient and the doctor. (WINFRIED SCHLEINER)

In early modernity, as well as the *optimus medicus*, the ideal of the *optimus chirurgus*, was also developed. The catalogue of the characteristics of such a surgeon had already been developed in antiquity and in the Middle Ages. These included: universal education, longstanding expertise, ingenuity and moral integrity. The numerous early modern descriptions of appalling *errores* provide ample evidence that by no means all surgical activities met the demands of these strict professional ethics – thus it is not surprising that in German surgical literature the ideal of a fully-qualified and experienced surgeon is invoked, although sometimes with a strong focus on surgical practice. Their general tenor, however, is not compatible with the ideals of universities: the best protection against mistakes is offered by medical and surgical competence. (KLARA VANEK)

In difficult times when public health and morals were under threat from epidemics such as the plague, the adoption of security measures came under the jurisdiction of lawyers. The selection of a city doctor, a good Christian with enough experience, moral stature and good character to be able to work effectively in exceptional situations, is vital. The correct behaviour (*condotta*) of a physician in difficult times is described in texts written by legal scholars directed at their colleagues. In these recommendations the concept of a 'proper' physician is reflected, and prejudices circulated (for example against Jewish doctors). The treatises show the willingness to compromise of those officials responsible for order in the city during times of crisis who were prepared to abandon their ideals when men, or indeed doctors, were needed: then even simple surgeons or Jewish doctors were good enough to provide medical aid. These forerunners of the "medical police", or of modern public health, show clearly that medicine cannot be reduced to a patient-doctor relationship. As early as the 16th and 17th centuries, officials of the state or of the city felt responsible for health care and its organisation. (VIVIAN NUTTON)

In pre-modern medicine, just as in countries like Japan or Italy today, the doctor's responsibility for honest, accurate disclosure of a hopeless prognosis is far from self-evident. The option of the mild lie produces, however, a sphere for reflection in which philosophical and theological positions are already being discussed. In medicine, sick-bed truth becomes an issue both in view of its consequences for the sick, and in terms of the moral attitude of the doctor. As early as the decades around 1500, the dialogue between doctor and patient in medical texts which deals with professional ethos and medical conduct becomes the subject of normative endeavours. The results of the spreading or withholding of information on the part of the patient or the doctor can be of either therapeutic, moral and religious, or a legal and forensic nature. The increasing sensitivity for the social dimensions of the medical profession – especially in delicate situations when the patient is incurable – characterizes the works of Rodrigo de Castro and Paolo Zacchia. Karl Jaspers' deliberations on the possibility of a doctor being both truthful and maintaining hope show just how this option was and remains a constant challenge to doctors and patients. (MARIACARLA GADEBUSCH BONDIO)

The authors and their works which are presented and analysed, or indeed edited here open up a wide spectrum of problems and questions which have concerned doctors, patients, philosophers and intellectuals over the centuries. Some of these discussions have lost nothing of their fascination even today. The constant search for methods of approach, decision-making procedures and strategies for action, form the core of historical analysis. Centuries-old medical and ethical problems with the traditional discourses which they have triggered can be seen as focal points of critical and self-critical reflection. The ethical concepts of Plato and Aristotle, which do not harmonise well together, are the most striking example for the plight in which physicians interested in ethical questions found themselves. The position of the authorities had continually to be renegotiated and, in view of the casuistic wealth of experience, to be put to the test. The purpose of historical work with old sources and testimonies of medical culture lies in the reconstruction of these negotiations.

For the opportunity of holding the conference in the German-Italian Centre for European Excellence Villa Vigoni (Menaggio), my thanks go to Gregor Vogt-Spira, then (November 2010) secretary-general of that *locus amoenus*, as well as

to the German Research Foundation for their generous financial support of the event.
Furthermore I would like to thank the Medical Faculty of the University of Greifswald who have subsidised the printing costs of this publication.
Finally my thanks go to Jenny Linek and Martin Neutmann for their assistance with the editorial work which began in Greifswald, as well as to Leo Maier who gave this book the final editorial finishing touches in Munich.

‚UNTERLASSENE HILFELEISTUNG' IN DER ANTIKE

Christian Schulze

In Deutschland wie auch mit vielerlei Abwandlungen in anderen Staaten existiert eine gesetzlich festgeschriebene Pflicht zur Hilfe bei Unglücksfällen, gemeiner Gefahr oder Not; zu den Unglücksfällen gehören auch Straftaten gegen Leib und Leben. Wer der Pflicht zur Hilfeleistung nicht nachkommt, obwohl sie erforderlich und den Umständen nach zuzumuten ist, insbesondere ohne erhebliche eigene Gefahr und ohne Verletzung anderer wichtiger Pflichten, dem droht Freiheitsstrafe bis zu einem Jahr oder eine Geldstrafe gemäß § 323c StGB. Natürlich besitzt diese Reglung ebenfalls Geltung für professionelle Kräfte wie Rettungssanitäter oder Ärzte. Wer sich der ‚unterlassenen Hilfeleistung' schuldig macht, sieht sich in der Regel aber nicht nur strafrechtlich belangt, sondern wird unter Umständen auch mit einem moralischen Makel belegt.

Den Fachausdruck ‚unterlassene Hilfeleistung' gab es in der griechisch-römischen Antike nicht: Weder formulieren ihn die zahlreichen juristischen Fachschriftsteller als eigenen, fest umrissenen Straftatbestand aus, noch begegnet ein entsprechende Bezeichnung bei den medizinischen Autoren. Die deutschsprachige Forschungsliteratur benutzt daher neben ‚unterlassene Hilfeleistung' verbreitet das eher beschreibende Wort des ‚Behandlungsverzichts'.[1] So sei mit diesen Begriffen lediglich ein allgemeiner Verständnisrahmen abgesteckt, in dem sich die nachfolgenden Ausführungen bewegen werden; wir können den § 323 StGB nicht auf die vergangene Epoche übertragen.

Der folgende Beitrag möchte zunächst darstellen, inwiefern ‚Hilfeleistung' eine in der Antike selbstverständliche Verpflichtung des Arztes war, anschließend fragen, welche abweichenden Haltungen sich in der medizinischen Fachliteratur finden lassen, danach kurz aus antiker Patientensicht auf das Problem blicken, und in einem vierten Schritt nach den Gründen für unterlassene Hilfeleistung fragen.

1. HILFELEISTUNG ALS GRUNDSATZ ANTIKEN MEDIZINISCHEN HANDELNS

Die Verpflichtung, anderen in Notlagen zu helfen, ist nicht erst ein Novum christlicher Zeit, die den *caritas*- und *misericordia*-Gedanken im Römischen Reich verankerte und damit Spätantike und Mittelalter prägte. Zwar schärfte man hier den

1 Siehe beispielsweise M. Stamatu, „Behandlungsverzicht", in: K.-H. Leven (Hg.), *Antike Medizin. Ein Lexikon*, München 2005, S. 140f.

Aspekt der unentgeltlichen Behandlung – dies war im Rahmen der ärztlichen Tätigkeit bislang ungewöhnlich –, aber auch der heidnische Medizinbetrieb hatte schon lange zuvor Selbstverpflichtungen für den Arzt entwickelt. Am bekanntesten sind heute entsprechende Aussagen des Hippokratischen Eides, so vor allem die, in denen der Arzt schwört:

> Meine Verordnungen werde ich treffen zu Nutz der Kranken, nach bestem Vermögen und Urteil; ich werde sie bewahren vor Schaden und willkürlichem Unrecht.
> [...]
> Heilig und rein werde ich mein Leben und meine Kunst bewahren.
> [...]
> Welche Häuser ich betreten werde, so will ich zu Nutz der Kranken eintreten, mich enthalten jedes willkürlichen Unrechtes und jeder anderer Schädigung [...].[2]

Der Autor – es war sicherlich nicht Hippokrates selbst – formulierte im *Ius iurandum* also eine Reihe von Selbstverpflichtungen des Arztes. Als oberstes Ziel des ärztlichen Handelns gilt der Nutzen des Kranken. Gemäß einer nicht weniger bekannten Stelle aus dem ersten Buch der *Epidemien* sollte, dem Nutzen nachrangig, zumindest der Schaden vermieden werden.[3] Freilich hatte der Eid in klassischer Zeit nicht die Bedeutung und Umsetzung erfahren wie später im byzantinischen und arabischen Mittelalter oder in der Frühen Neuzeit. So blieb, wie wir der *Clavis commentariorum* von Sibylle Ihm entnehmen können, auch die Zahl der Kommentare zum ‚Eid' bis zum Beginn der Kommentartätigkeit der Schule von Salerno erstaunlich klein (ganz im Gegensatz z. B. zu den *Aphorismen* und anderen Hippokrates-Opera) – nur Galen erläuterte ihn, außerdem kennen wir einige Fragmente bei arabischen Autoren.[4] Das noch heute beeindruckende deontologische Prinzip der hippokratischen Medizin besaß also in antiker Zeit allein wegen seiner mangelnden Präsenz keine Allgemeingültigkeit.

Dass freilich die Hilfeleistung im Arzt-Patienten-Verhältnis eine grundlegende Verpflichtung war, belegt neben zahlreichen Textstellen nicht zuletzt auch eine griechische Bezeichnung für den Patienten. So hieß der Kranke nicht nur *nos*(*e*)*on* (also eigtl. „krank Seiender") oder *pathon* (also „Leidender"), sondern wurde auch mit dem Partizip Präsens Passiv *boethoumenos* (wörtlich: „einer, dem geholfen wird") bezeichnet. Das Wort *boetheo* ist eine Zusammensetzung und bedeutet ursprünglich „auf einen Hilfeschrei hin herbeilaufen". Wenn also der Patient auch so bezeichnet wird, spiegelt sich hierin zweifellos die grundsätzliche Situation von Hilfesuchen und Hilfeleistung wider.

2 Hippocrates, *Iusiurandum*, 3, 5, 7, in: Ders., *Hippocrates*, Bd. 1 (The Loeb Classical Library; 147), übers. von W. H. S. Jones, London / Cambridge (Mass.) 1923 (Nachdruck 1972), S. 289–301.

3 Siehe Hippocrates, *Epidemien*, 1, 11, in: Ders., *Hippocrates*, Bd. 1, S. 146–287.

4 Siehe S. Ihm, *Clavis commentariorum der antiken medizinischen Texte* (Clavis commentariorum antiquitatis et medii aevi; 1), Leiden u. a. 2002, S. 263 (mit entsprechenden Verweisen).

2. DER RAT ZUM BEHANDLUNGSVERZICHT

Eine für den modernen Rezipienten besonders irritierende Verhaltensweise des antiken Arztes soll im Folgenden näher beleuchtet werden: der Umgang mit Schwerkranken und Schwerverletzten. Bereits in der hippokratischen Schriftensammlung finden sich an mehreren Stellen deutliche Fingerzeige. So heißt es in der chirurgischen Fachschrift *De fracturis* („Über die Knochenbrüche") über das Vorgehen bei komplizierten Oberschenkel- bzw. Oberarmbrüchen, der Arzt solle bei derartigen Fällen versuchen, sich einer Behandlung zu entziehen, so gut es gehe.[5] Er solle lieber eine gute Ausrede vorbringen. Es gebe nämlich in solch schweren Fällen nur wenig Hoffnung, aber große Gefahren, und wenn man die Einrichtung des Knochenbruches nicht vornehme, könnte man den Eindruck erwecken, nichts von der Kunst zu verstehen. Umgekehrt führe der Versuch einer Einrichtung den Patienten eher zum Tode als zur Heilung.[6]

Es ist dies ein für den heutigen Betrachter befremdlicher Schluss: Mit Hilfe von Ausreden soll sich der überforderte Arzt aus dem Staube machen und den Verletzten erst gar nicht zu behandeln versuchen. Textstellen vergleichbarer Art finden sich nicht selten in dem unter Hippokrates' Namen laufenden Werk. Die Zwangslage der Behandlungssituationen ist dabei meist vergleichbar: Eine infauste Prognose lässt es den Autoren dieser Schriften angeraten scheinen, dem Arzt eine Art ‚Behandlungsverweigerung' anzuraten – oder, wie wir heute sagen würden, ihn zur ‚unterlassenen Hilfeleistung' aufzufordern. Die Möglichkeiten der Medizin seien überschritten.[7]

Solche Empfehlungen sind nicht nur mit dem Namen Hippokrates verknüpft. In der frühen Kaiserzeit schrieb die Portalfigur der römischen Medizin, Aulus Cornelius Celsus, acht Bücher über die Medizin. Celsus, der als Person nicht näher bekannt ist, hat uns damit einen kenntnisreichen, isagogisch angelegten Gesamtüberblick über die Medizin seiner Zeit hinterlassen. Sein Interesse galt neben Diätetik und Pharmazeutik auch der Chirurgie. Was man dort liest, lässt staunen: Der Autor stellt schwierige und sehr gefährliche Operationen vor, zum Beispiel den Blasensteinschnitt (Lithotomie), die Trepanation des Schädels oder Eingriffe, die heute bei der plastischen Chirurgie einzuordnen wären. Es handelt sich um überaus anspruchsvolle Operationen und Techniken. Zudem wird manche Behandlung überhaupt zum ersten Mal bei Celsus erwähnt, so beispielsweise bestimmte Operationsschnitte und -nähte.[8]

5 Siehe Hippocrates, *De fracturis*, 36, in: Ders., *Hippocrates*, Bd. 3 (The Loeb Classical Library; 149), übers. von E. T. Withington, London / Cambridge (Mass.) 1928, S. 94–199.

6 Grundlegung zu Textstellen und ethischer Problematik: R. Wittern, „Die Unterlassung ärztlicher Hilfeleistung in der griechischen Medizin der klassischen Zeit", *Münchner Medizinische Wochenschau* 121 (1979), S. 731–734.

7 Siehe Hippocrates, *De arte*, 3, 13, in: *Hippocratis opera* (Corpus Medicorum Graecorum; 1,1), hg. von I. L. Heiberg u. a., Leipzig / Berlin 1927, S. 9–19.

8 Die folgenden Überlegungen nach C. Schulze, *Aulus Cornelius Celsus – Arzt oder Laie?* (Bochumer Altertumswissenschaftliches Colloquium; 42), Trier 1999, S. 73–80.

Umso irritierender mag erscheinen, gerade im Zusammenhang mit der Chirurgie, folgende Passage aus dem fünften Buch zu lesen:

> Incipiam a vulneribus. In his autem ante omnia scire medicus debet, quae insanabilia sint, quae difficilem curationem habeant, quae promptiorem. Est enim prudentis hominis primum eum, qui servari non potest, non adtingere (nec subire speciem eius, ut occisi, quem sors ipsíus interemit).
>
> Ich will mit den Wunden beginnen. Diesbezüglich aber muss der Arzt vor allen anderen Dingen zunächst wissen, welche Wunden unheilbar, welche schwer und welche leichter zu heilen sind. Denn es spricht für einen klugen Menschen, denjenigen, der nicht gerettet werden kann, erst gar nicht in Behandlung zu nehmen [...].[9]

Ein kluger Arzt soll einen Schwerstverletzten also erst gar nicht zu behandeln versuchen. Dafür mag es durchaus gute Gründe geben. Es wäre ja beispielsweise vorstellbar, dass man bei einer größeren Katastrophe zuerst einmal andere, leichter Verwundete behandelt, die eine mutmaßlich bessere Überlebenschance haben – Hinweise zur Triage also? Vielleicht möchte er auch bestimmten Patienten eine unnötige Leidensverlängerung ersparen. Aber Celsus formuliert seine Anweisung verdächtig allgemein. Es sei noch einmal beim letzten Satz des Zitates eingesetzt. Es hieß dort:

> Est enim prudentis hominis primum eum, qui servari non potest, non adtingere nec subire speciem eius, ut occisi, quem sors ipsius interemit.
>
> Denn es spricht für einen klugen Menschen, denjenigen, der nicht gerettet werden kann, erst gar nicht in Behandlung zu nehmen, um nicht den Anschein zu erwecken, er, der Arzt, sei für dessen Tod verantwortlich, den doch sein eigenes Schicksal dahingerafft hat.[10]

Es ist offenbar nicht die eben gemutmaßte Versorgungseffizienz oder eine unnötige Leidensverlängerung, die unseren Autor inspiriert hat. Nein – Schwerstverletzte sollen allein deshalb nicht behandelt werden, damit dem Arzt der wahrscheinlich sowieso eintretende Tod des Patienten nicht angelastet werden kann. Der Ratschlag schützt also, wie schon in den hippokratischen Vorgängerschriften, nicht den Patienten, sondern den Ruf des Arztes. Im gleichen Tenor führt Celsus seine Ratschläge fort. Betrachten wir den nächsten Absatz:

> [...] deinde, ubi gravis metus sine certa tamen desperatione est, indicare necessariis periclitantis in difficili spem esse, ne, si victa ars malo fuerit, vel ignorasse vel fefellisse videatur.
>
> [...] ferner muss der Arzt, sobald große Furcht, aber keine vollkommene Verzweiflung besteht, den Angehörigen des Kranken mitteilen, dass die Erwartung höchst bedenklich sei, damit er, der Arzt, nicht als jemand erscheint, der sich getäuscht habe oder die Angehörigen betrogen habe, wenn seine Kunst von der Krankheit besiegt wird.[11]

Bei einem Verwundeten, dessen Überlebenschancen zwar klein, aber immerhin gegeben sind, seien also die Angehörigen vorzuwarnen. Doch auch dieser Rat

9 Celsus, *De re medica*, 5, 26, 1B–C, in: *A. Cornelii Celsi quae supersunt* (Corpus Medicorum Latinorum; 1), hg. von F. Marx, Leipzig / Berlin 1915 (eigene Übersetzung).

10 Ebd.

11 Celsus, 5, 26, 1C.

sorgt sich nicht mit hehren Zielen um die bangende Verwandtschaft, sondern dient wieder allein der Absicherung des Arztes vor eventuellen Vorwürfen. Im Anschluss daran wird Celsus sogar ausführliche Diagnoselisten mitteilen, anhand derer der Arzt abschätzen kann, welchen Behandlungen er besser aus dem Weg geht. Ein Beispiel:

> Servari non potest, cui basis cerebri, cui cor, cui stomachus, cui iocineris portae, cui in spina medulla percussa est; cuique aut pulmo medius aut ieiunum aut tenuius intestinum aut ventriculus aut renes vulnerati sunt; cuive circa fauces grandes venae vel arteriae praecisae sunt.

> Es kann derjenige nicht gerettet werden, bei dem die Basis des Gehirns, das Herz, die Speiseröhre, die Leberpforte, das Rückenmark, der Mittelteil der Lunge, der Leerdarm, Dünndarm, Magen oder die Nieren verletzt wurden, oder bei dem die großen Venen oder Arterien zu beiden Seiten der Luftröhre durchtrennt worden sind.[12]

Bei solchen Verletzungen also soll der Arzt gleich ganz von einem Behandlungsversuch absehen. Und wie es der didaktisch klugen, ineinandergreifenden Geschlossenheit des Werkes entspricht, folgen im nächsten Kapitel sogleich die entsprechenden Beschreibungen zum zweiten Ratschlag. Bei welchen nicht völlig aussichtslosen Fällen sei nun die Verwandtschaft vorzuwarnen?

> Vix autem ad sanitatem perveniunt, quibus ulla parte aut pulmo aut iocineris crassum aut membrana, quae continet cerebrum, aut lienis aut vulva aut vesica aut ullum intestinum aut saeptum transversum vulneratum est. Ii quoque in praecipiti sunt, in quibus usque ad grandes intusque conditas venas in alis vel poplitibus mucro desedit. Periculosa etiam vulnera sunt, ubicumque venae maiores sunt, quoniam exhaurire hominem profusione sanguinis possunt.

> Kaum aber erlangen diejenigen ihre Gesundheit wieder, bei denen an irgendeiner Stelle entweder die Lunge oder die dicken Teile der Leber, die Hirnhaut, Milz, Gebärmutter, Blase, irgendein Darmteil oder das Zwerchfell verwundet wurde. Es schweben auch die in höchster Gefahr, bei denen ein Dolch bis zu den großen, innenliegenden Adern in den Achselhöhlen oder Kniekehlen durchdringt. Gefährlich sind auch Wunden immer dort, wo größere Gefäße liegen, weil sie den Menschen durch Blutverlust schwächen können.[13]

Wir sehen: Celsus hat seine Aufforderung zum Behandlungsverzicht nicht nur einfach in den Raum gestellt, sondern er flankiert sie mit detaillierten Symptom- oder Diagnoselisten, er gibt exakte, ausführliche Hinweise. Mit ihrer Hilfe soll der Arzt in die Lage versetzt werden, genau zu wissen, wann er wie vorzugehen habe.

Insbesondere schwerste Verletzungen waren ein wichtiges Thema. Es sei etwa an die vielen Gladiatorenkämpfe erinnert. Auch Wanderer wurden bei Überfällen oft übel zugerichtet. Solche Verletzungen müssen immerhin so häufig vorgekommen sein, dass die Medizinschule der Empiriker empfohlen hatte, der angehende Arzt solle seine anatomischen Kenntnisse hauptsächlich an den klaffenden Wunden verletzter Gladiatoren oder an überfallenen Wanderern schulen. Leichenöffnungen brauche man zu Ausbildungszwecken gar nicht.[14] Ein anderer Punkt: Unfälle geschahen nicht weniger oft als in der Moderne, beispielsweise im Bergbau oder im Handwerk, und sie gingen bei vergleichbaren Tätigkeiten oft weniger

12 Celsus, 5, 26, 2F.
13 Celsus, 5, 26, 3A–B.
14 Siehe Celsus, 1, prooem. passim.

glimpflich aus als heute, weil die Antike keine wirksamen Sicherheitsstandards kannte.

Besonders häufig aber begegnen schwere Kriegsverletzungen. Celsus geht detailliert auf verschiedene Geschoßarten ein: Pfeile, die zudem mit Widerhaken versehen sein konnten, kleine Geschosse, breite Geschosse, Wurfbleie, Steine usw. Ausführlich werden die daraus resultierenden Verletzungen besprochen, so die Weichteil-, Ader-, Sehnen-, Knochen- oder Gelenkverletzungen.[15] Unter Kaiser Augustus war ein geordnetes Militärsanitätswesen eingeführt worden, nämlich im Zuge der Heeres-Neuorganisation nach der Schlacht bei Actium (31 v. Chr.). Es überrascht daher nicht, dass Celsus, dessen Werk nur wenige Jahre nach Augustus' Tod entstand, nun auch auf diese neuen Aufgabengebiete des Arztes eingeht. Jetzt, wo Ärzte offenbar erstmalig eine geregelte Laufbahn beim Militär einschlagen konnten, durften auch kriegschirurgische Aspekte in der Lehre nicht fehlen.

Die Sorge um den Ruf des Arztes begegnet – zumindest implizit – immer wieder. Man achte beispielsweise einmal genau auf folgende Anweisung: „Nachdem man nun untersucht hat, wo jemand, der noch gerettet werden kann, getroffen worden ist, müssen sogleich zwei Dinge beachtet werden: Dass den Patienten weder Blutverlust noch Entzündung töte."[16]

Nicht das Stillen der Blutungen ist hier die wirklich primäre Aufgabe des Arztes, sondern ganz bewusst schickt unser Autor die Einschränkung vorweg *qui servari potest* – „wer (überhaupt) gerettet werden kann". Nicht mit der Überlegung „wie?", sondern mit der Frage „wer?" beginnt die Erstversorgung. Es verwundert daher nicht, wenn Seneca in *De beneficiis* sich einen Arzt wünscht, der ihm nicht nur wie einem Auftraggeber (*imperator*), sondern als einem Freund (*amicus*) einen Krankenbesuch abstattet, wobei die ärztliche Sorge nur dem Patienten gelten solle, und nicht dem eigenen Ruf.[17]

Wir müssen uns fragen, ob Ratschläge solcher Couleur nicht eine Art ‚Insidertipp' waren, egal, ob Hippokrates, Celsus oder andere Fachschriftsteller sie geäußert haben. Es wäre ja – so denkt der moderne, unvoreingenommene Leser – geradezu fatal, wenn ein Außenstehender derartige Anleitungen zum Umgang mit Verwundeten oder mit Schwerverletzten zu Gesicht bekäme, besonders mit der nicht ganz unwahrscheinlichen Vorstellung vor Augen, irgendwann selbst einmal Patient werden zu können. Die antiken Aufforderungen zur ‚unterlassenen Hilfeleistung' entbehren nicht einer gewissen Brisanz, und es ist leicht vorstellbar, dass das Vertrauensverhältnis zwischen Patient und Arzt nachhaltig erschüttert würde, wenn solche Hinweise für jedermann publik würden.

Zu Anfang war bereits der Hippokratische Eid als ein Gegenpol vorgeführt worden, und in der Tat soll nicht der Eindruck erweckt werden, fragwürdige Ratschläge der referierten Art hätten monolithisch die ärztliche Ethik der Antike be-

15 Siehe Celsus, 7, 5, 1–5.

16 Celsus, 5, 26, 21A.

17 Siehe Seneca, *De beneficiis*, 6, 16, 1–5, in: Ders., *Philosophische Schriften*, Bd. 5, hg. und übers. von M. Rosenbach, lat. Text von F. Préchac, Darmstadt 1989, S. 95–593.

stimmt. Es lassen sich nicht nur aus dem *Eid*, sondern auch aus anderen Texten der griechischen Fachliteratur durchaus Gegenmeinungen finden. So heißt es im hippokratischen *De morbis*:

> Fachgerecht aber ist es, [...] bei der Behandlung diejenigen Krankheiten, die heilbar sind, bis zur Heilung zu behandeln, von den unheilbaren aber zu wissen, weshalb sie unheilbar sind, und bei der Behandlung derjenigen Patienten, die an einer unheilbaren Krankheit leiden, Hilfe zu geben, indem man deren Behandlung nach der Heilbarkeit ausrichtet.[18]

Hier also haben wir ein eindeutiges Bekenntnis dazu, auch unheilbar Kranke zu behandeln. Der Arzt darf sie nicht außen vor lassen, die ethische Richtlinie ist klar erkennbar und verbindlich formuliert. Das war übrigens auch die außerhalb der medizinischen Fachliteratur zu findende Aufforderung: Aristoteles etwa sah auch die Behandlung Unheilbarer als eine Aufgabe der Medizin.[19]

3. EIN PATIENTENZEUGNIS

Bislang haben wir ausschließlich Statements aus der Feder von Ärzten bzw. medizinischen Fachschriftstellern kennengelernt. Es wäre nun wünschenswert, dies mit dem Bericht eines antiken Patienten zu vergleichen, um die Behandlung bzw. Nichtbehandlung von Schwerkranken auch aus dessen Blickwinkel kennenzulernen und ein von der ärztlichen Fachdiskussion unabhängiges Urteil abgleichend anzufügen. Sieht man freilich von den üblichen Polemiken gegen die Ärzte ab, wie beispielsweise Seneca, Plinius maior oder Martial sie zum Besten geben, müssen wir feststellen, dass nur äußerst wenige Patientenberichte aus griechisch-römischer Zeit existieren. Am bekanntesten sind vielleicht die Beschreibungen des Redners Aelius Aristides, dem die Nachwelt mannigfaltige Einblicke in den Kult und Heilbetrieb eines Asklepiostempels verdankt.

Für unsere spezielle Frage nach der Behandlung von Schwerkranken mag nun ein bislang wenig bekannter Papyrus zumindest indirekt Auskunft geben. Der Papyrus, dessen genauer Fund- bzw. Entstehungsort unbekannt ist, stammt aus dem dritten Jahrhundert n. Chr. Es handelt sich um einen Privatbrief eines Unbekannten an seinen Bruder mit folgender Nachricht:

> [...] Wir sind nach Deiner Abreise von schwerer Krankheit heimgesucht worden, ich und [...] (*Name unleserlich*) [...] (und) ihre Kinder. Der kleine Mimos ist gestorben, ich selbst habe nach überstandener Krankheit ein Fußleiden zurückbehalten. [...] bislang war ich noch nicht recht wieder munter. Aber ich habe auf meinen Namen des Arztes wegen Geld zusammengeborgt und an ihn bis 20 Drachmen bezahlt. Darum bitte ich Dich, lieber Bruder, wenn Du et-

18 Hippocrates, *Die hippokratische Schrift „De morbis I"*, 1, 6 (Altertumswissenschaftliche Texte und Studien; 3), hg., übers. und komm. von R. Wittern, Heidelberg / New York 1974, S. 150f.

19 Aristoteles, *Ars rhetorica*, 1, 1, 1355 b12f (Oxford Classical Texts), hg. von W. D. Ross, Oxford 1959.

> was für mich tun willst, sende mir (Geld) auf das Schiff, und von der Gerste, die du nun empfangen hast, sende mir zum Lebensunterhalt [...] (*Abbruch des Textes*).[20]

Trotz vieler Unsicherheiten bezüglich des Schreibers, Adressaten oder der genauen Krankheitsumstände lassen sich immerhin folgende Informationen aus dem Text gewinnen:[21]

1. Der unbekannte Briefschreiber und mehrere, wohl der Familie angehörige Personen seines Umfeldes waren an einem uns unbekannten Leiden erkrankt.
2. Wir erfahren ausdrücklich von der Schwere der Krankheit, die sogar ein Todesopfer gefordert und beim Schreiber gravierende Folgeschäden hinterlassen hat.
3. Ein Arzt hat die Kranken behandelt und dafür auch Geld bekommen. Ob er die Behandlung widerwillig und voller Bedenken durchgeführt hat, erfahren wir nicht ausdrücklich.

Offenbar also ist hier ein antiker Arzt tätig geworden, obwohl die Situation der Patienten sehr ernst gewesen sein muss. Und obwohl es diesem Arzt nicht gelungen ist, Tod und schwere Folgeschäden zu verhindern, bekam er seinen Lohn; auch beschwert sich der Briefschreiber in den erhaltenen Passagen nicht über die Leistung oder ein Zögern des Arztes, wofür in der privaten Briefsituation ohne weiteres Platz gewesen wäre. Indirekt belegt dieser Papyrus also, dass eine Behandlungsverweigerung schwerer Fälle keineswegs generell praktiziert worden ist. Jener unbekannte Arzt aus dem dritten nachchristlichen Jahrhundert hat sich augenscheinlich nicht der ‚unterlassenen Hilfeleistung' schuldig gemacht. Mehr als ein Anhaltspunkt in diesem Sinne kann der Papyrus allerdings nicht sein. Diese seltene Primärquelle belegt aber immerhin, dass ein Arzt auch in der Antike häufig mit schweren Erkrankungen konfrontiert wurde, dass er sich immer wieder einer Situation ausgesetzt sah, in der er über eine mögliche Behandlungsverweigerung hätte nachdenken können.

Es wurde ausgeführt, dass antike Medizinautoren in zahlreichen Einzelfällen den Ratschlag aussprechen, die Behandlung von Schwerkranken bzw. Schwerverletzten zu unterlassen. Umfangreiche Diagnosehilfen werden gleich mit an die Hand gegeben. Man ahnt, dass es sich hier um ‚Insidertipps' handelt, welche von Arzt zu Arzt bzw. innerhalb der reinen Fachliteratur weitergegeben worden sein mögen. Relativierend verraten anderslautende Textstellen aus dem *Corpus Hippocraticum* wie auch aus dem exemplarisch zitierten Straßburger Papyrus, dass es in der Ärzteschaft offenbar keine Einheitsmeinung zu diesem heiklen Thema gab

20 Pap. Straßburg gr. 1531, in: F. Preisigke, *Griechische Papyrus der klassischen Universitäts- und Landesbibliothek zu Strassburg*, Bd. 1: Urkunden Nr. 1–80, Leipzig 1912 (Nachdruck 1969), S. 210–212.

21 Siehe C. Schulze, „Angst um die eigene Gesundheit. Patientenzeugnisse aus der Antike", in: W. Geerlings – A. Mügge (Hgg.), *Gesundheit. Geisteswissenschaftliche und Medizinische Aspekte* (Religiösität – Spiritualität – Gesundheit; 4), Berlin 2009, S. 11–24.

und zumindest einzelne Ärztegruppen auch schwere Fälle nach allen Möglichkeiten der Kunst therapierten.

4. BEGRÜNDUNGEN DES BEHANDLUNGSVERZICHTS

Nach diesem Blick auf die antiken Zeugnisse gilt es nun zu fragen, aus welchen Beweggründen antike Ärzte den grundsätzlich offenbar ja vorhandenen Konsens zur Hilfeleistung gebrochen haben. Welche gesellschaftshistorischen Rahmenbedingungen führten zum Rat auf den Behandlungsverzicht?

Grundsätzlich ist zunächst festzustellen, dass die hippokratischen Autoren wie auch der Römer Celsus in fast allen anderen Fragen hervorragende Medizinschriftsteller, vorbildliche Vertreter ihrer Kunst auf dem jeweiligen Stand ihrer Zeit waren. Schon deshalb dürfte es unwahrscheinlich sein, dass unsere Autoren ausgerechnet beim Thema ‚unterlassene Hilfeleistung‘ und ‚Ruf des Arztes‘ gleichsam einem ‚ethischen Kurzschluss‘ erlegen seien.

Die Medizin war seit hippokratischer Zeit eine Kunst zwischen den Werturteilen: Sie zählte weder zu den ‚schmutzigen Künsten‘ (zu den *Artes sordidae*) noch schaffte sie es auf der anderen Seite, unter die ‚freien Künste‘ (also in die *Artes liberales*) aufgenommen zu werden. Dies spiegelt sich im Personal wider: Viele Sklaven und Freigelassene tummelten sich in der Medizin; es gab, wie vor allem der kaiserliche Leibarzt Galen aus Pergamon berichtet, auch eine Menge Scharlatane. Auf der anderen Seite aber entstammte mancher Arzt angesehenen römischen Familien, *gentes*, die sogar Konsuln und Inhaber anderer hoher Ämter stellten. Man konnte als Arzt außerordentlich viel Geld verdienen, ein hohes Ansehen erwerben und bis in höchste Gesellschaftskreise vordringen.[22] Pauschal darf man hinzufügen, dass die Medizin und der Arzt bei den Griechen eher höher, bei den Römern dagegen eher niedriger eingestuft wurden.

Der Arztberuf bot also durchaus Chancen. Man lief aber auf der anderen Seite ständig Gefahr, beispielsweise durch einen Kunstfehler seine Existenzgrundlage zu riskieren. Diese Gefahr wurde noch dadurch erhöht, dass zumindest in Rom viele Klischees, viele Vorurteile gegenüber Ärzten im Umlauf waren. Besonders polemisch tat sich Plinius der Ältere in seiner *Naturalis historia* hervor: Plinius schimpft über astronomische Einkommen; Beredsamkeit sei für den Erfolg wichtiger als fachliches Können, und mit der Kaiserin ins Bett gegangen zu sein, habe durchaus das Ansehen eines Arztes heben können. Insbesondere sei es aber einzig und allein den Ärzten möglich, vollkommen straflos einen Menschen umzubringen.[23]

22 Siehe F. Kudlien, Die Stellung des Arztes in der römischen Gesellschaft. Freigeborene Römer, Eingewanderte, Peregrine, Sklaven, Freigelassene als Ärzte (Forschungen zur antiken Sklaverei; 18), Stuttgart 1986.

23 Plinius, *Naturalis historiae*, 29, 18, hg. von L. Jan und C. Mayhoff, Leipzig 1892–1909, 7 Bde. (Nachdruck Stuttgart 1967–1970).

Solche teils grotesken Urteile hatten eine lange Tradition. Schon über 200 Jahre vor Plinius schrieb der ältere Cato an seinen Sohn:

> Ich werde dir über diese Griechen an der rechten Stelle sagen, mein Sohn Marcus, was ich in Athen erkundet habe, und dass es gut ist, ihre Schriften anzusehen, nicht aber auswendig zu lernen. Ich werde erhärten, dass ihre Art nichtsnutzig und unbelehrbar ist. Und dies, glaube mir, hat ein Seher gesagt: Wenn einmal dieses Volk uns seine Schriften gibt, wird es alles verderben, dann aber noch mehr, wenn es seine Ärzte hierhin schickt. Sie haben sich untereinander verschworen, alle Barbaren durch ihre Medizin zu verderben, aber selbst dies werden sie für Bezahlung tun, damit ihnen Vertrauen entgegengebracht wird und sie leichter töten können. Auch uns nennen sie immer wieder Barbaren, und noch unflätiger als andere beschimpfen sie uns mit der Bezeichnung ‚Opiker' (= „Dummköpfe", C.S.). Ich habe dir die Ärzte untersagt.[24]

Zwar muss bezweifelt werden, dass die hier ausgesprochene Missachtung eine allgemein übliche Einschätzung des fremdländischen Ärztestandes widerspiegelt. Catos Worte haben gewiss etwas von Überkompensation an sich. Aber immerhin, es gab offenbar Tendenzen, es gab Stimmen und Gruppen, die ein solches Negativ-Bild pflegten. Bezeichnend scheint auch, was der Philosoph Seneca zum Besten gibt. Er will Marcia, die Tochter des umgekommenen Geschichtsschreibers Cremutius Cordus, trösten, indem er ihr die Härten dieser Welt aufzählt. Es heißt dort:

> Füge noch hinzu Feuersbrünste, Verwüstungen, Schiffbrüche und die Metzeleien der Ärzte, die Knochen aus lebenden Körpern herausoperieren, ihre Hände komplett in Eingeweide hineinsenken und Geschlechtsteile unter nicht leichten Schmerzen behandeln [...].[25]

Man erkennt also: Der Arzt hatte es vor allem zur Zeit des Celsus nicht leicht. Er und seine Kunst standen leicht unter Pauschalverdacht. Der Arzt wurde gebraucht, aber auch gefürchtet und verhöhnt. Wehe ihm also, wenn der bedauernswerte *medicus* tatsächlich einmal die Klischees bestätigte. Die zitierten Äußerungen scheinen besonders drastisch zu sein, hängen natürlich auch mit den Konventionen ihrer literarischen Gattungen zusammen, spiegeln aber durchaus die Polemiken der nichtärztlichen Literaten pointiert wider, insbesondere, wenn sie aus dem Genus des Epigramms, der Satire, aber auch, wie bei Seneca, aus der Trostliteratur stammen.

Der seriöse Arzt war nun gewiss nicht so schlecht, wie man ihn hier gemacht hat. Vivian Nutton schätzt sogar, dass ein antiker Meister der Diagnose mindestens ebenso erfolgreich gewesen sein wird wie ein Arzt in der ersten Hälfte des 20. Jahrhunderts.[26] Das übergeordnete Medizinkonzept, in dem sich Heiler wie Kranker bewegten, scheint also einen Therapieerfolg positiv messbar gemacht zu haben und im jeweiligen Zeit- und Kulturhorizont Erfolge formulierbar gemacht

24 Cato, *Librorum ad filium et ceterorum reliquiae: Praeter librum de re rustica quae exstant*, 1, hg. von H. Jordan, Stuttgart 1860 (Nachdruck 1967), S. 75–93.

25 Seneca, *Dialogorum libri duodecim*, 6, 22 (Oxford Classical Texts), hg. von L. D. Reynolds, Oxford 1977.

26 Siehe V. Nutton, „Medizin", in: H. Cancik – H. Schneider (Hgg.), *Der Neue Pauly* 7 (1999), Sp. 1107–1117.

zu haben. Dennoch: Vor dem Hintergrund der Klischees, der Vorurteile und der Vorverurteilungen, vor dem Hintergrund der in ihren faktischen, vor allem operativen Möglichkeiten beschränkten Medizin ohne Narkose und Antisepsis, ging der Arzt natürlich ein besonderes Risiko ein, wenn er seine Kunst an Schwerstverletzten erprobte. Nur zu leicht drohte ihm der Misserfolg, nur zu leicht sahen sich die nicht zimperlichen Angehörigen in ihren Vorurteilen bestätigt – gerade eben die Angehörigen, die Nichtmediziner, vor deren ungerechtem Urteil die hippokratischen Autoren wie auch Celsus mehrfach warnen. Zudem stand zu befürchten, dass man Schadensersatzforderungen an ihn stellte.[27] Der Rat zum Behandlungsverzicht hatte also auch eine juristische Komponente, freilich sind wir über konkrete Fälle von Schadensersatzforderungen aufgrund von Kunstfehlern oder Tod des (schwerverletzten) Patienten schlecht informiert.

Der antike, speziell der römische Arzt steckte also in einer Zwickmühle. Außerdem erschöpfte sich die Gefahr nicht darin, dass die zornige Verwandtschaft sich in Klischeebestätigung übt. Vielmehr konnten solche Misserfolge für den Arzt auch mittel- und langfristige Folgen haben, unabhängig davon, ob wirklich er für den Misserfolg, d. h. für den Tod des schwerverletzten Patienten verantwortlich war oder nicht. Für die Meinung des klischeegeleiteten Kundenkreises war das meist unerheblich. Catos, Plinius' oder Senecas Statements zeichnen sich eben nicht gerade durch Differenziertheit und sachlicher Fairness gegenüber den Ärzten aus.

Für den Arzt stand also viel auf dem Spiel: Heidnische, zuweilen aber auch christliche Medizin war ein üblicherweise bezahltes Handwerk, ähnlich den Bäkkern oder Steinmetzen, und wie andere Handwerker arbeitete auch der Arzt normalerweise in Konkurrenz zu seinen Mitbewerbern. Gebietszuteilungen, staatliche Beschränkungen der Ärztezahl, zentrale Befähigungsnachweise wie die Approbation oder eine Arbeitslosenunterstützung für Gescheiterte gab es in der Antike nicht. Wenn nun der Tod eines schwerstverletzten Patienten den Ruf des Arztes zu Unrecht ruinierte, dann sah sich der Arzt zuweilen gar seiner Existenzgrundlage entzogen. Genau davor warnt Celsus, nur vor diesem Hintergrund sind seine Ratschläge verständlich, jedenfalls ein wenig besser nachzuvollziehen als in einer vorschnellen Verurteilung, die nur ethische Bedenken gelten lässt und die die historische Situation weitgehend außer Acht lässt. Der Grat zwischen ethischen Ansprüchen und existenzvernichtender, ungerechtfertigter Rufschädigung war schmal, und nirgendwo sonst kulminierte dieses Problem derart stark für den griechisch-römischen Arzt wie bei der Behandlung Schwerverletzter.

27 Siehe K.-H. Below, *Der Arzt im römischen Recht*, München 1953.

MEDICINE AND PHILOSOPHY IN THE MIDDLE AGES. SISTERS, COMPANIONS, RIVALS*

Chiara Crisciani

The links between medicine and philosophy in the medieval millennium are constant but variable, to a greater or lesser degree. Their detailed examination is not a task which can be covered exhaustively in one paper,[1] yet it is possible to identify some particularly significant phases in these relations, which are more evident and varied from the 12th century onwards. It is also useful, however, to concentrate briefly on the situation prior to this period in order to have a better understanding of the radical transformation which took place in certain areas, and to point out their latent presence as active elements, even against a greatly modified social and cultural background.

I

All through the High Middle Ages – a period we consider as being the first phase in the ideal chronological scheme we followed – patients, disease, recovery and therapy seem to have been organized not by scientific coordinates in a rational scheme, but primarily by the foundations of a Christian religious anthropology.[2] Indeed in the High Middle Ages we notice how with regard to both collective representations and material reality (at best poor, and where the fine line between health and disease is in fact weak) disease, or rather, *infirmitas*, is perceived not as an occasional, awkward moment of imbalance in comparison with the rule of health, but as 'the' rule, that is to say as the natural condition for man or *viator*

* Translation by Gionata Liboni (University of Ferrara).

1 A shorter work on this theme, resulted from a lecture held for the doctorate course at the University of Ferrara, was published in a less complex version and without notes in *I castelli di Yale* 9 (2007/2008).

2 See J. Agrimi – C. Crisciani, *Malato, medico e malattia nel medioevo*, Turin 1978; eaed., "Carità e assistenza nella civiltà cristiana medievale", in: M. D. Grmek (ed.), *Storia del pensiero medico occidentale,* I: *Antichità e medioevo*, Rome / Bari 1993, pp. 217–259; W. J. Sheils (ed.), *The Church and Healing*, Oxford 1982; Y. Violé O'Neill, "Il corpo dello spirito. Medicina e Cristianesimo", *Kos* 14 (1985), pp. 18–32; C. Crisciani, "Religione e medicina", in: *Storia della scienza Treccani*, vol. II.A, cap. 28, Roma 2001; see also P. Biller – A. J. Minnis (eds.), *Medieval Theology and Natural Body*, Woodbridge (Suffolk) 1997; P. Biller – J. Ziegler (eds.), *Religion and Medicine in the Middle Ages*, Woodbridge (Suffolk) 2001; J. Le Goff – N. Truong, *Une histoire du corps au Moyen Age*, Paris 2003.

after the Fall. In fact, disease, weakness, physical vulnerability is one of the *tria mala* which entered the world, time and history as a consequence of Adam's Sin. It was Adam who lost – both for himself and his descendants – the image and likeness of God, as well as the integrity of his body, enjoyed in the Earthly Paradise and which the blessed will enjoy again, but only at the end of time at the Last Judgment. This 'normality' of disease/*infirmitas*, in a manner of speaking, is 'natural' for man in his condition as *viator*, whereas in the classical world it is conceived as an imbalance and deviation from the rule of health and nature.

Disease, then is, normal. It is considered man's real nature, or perhaps in a sense his second nature. Disease and all that is related to it seems to take on a religious aspect, which is radical but at the same time ambivalent. So the patient is a living image of sin (which is the cause of his suffering and in his suffering reveals itself), but is also a personified expression of the paternal but harsh justice of a God who smites the body in order to 'treat' the soul. Finally, and maybe above all, he is the image, perpetually reproduced, of the suffering Christ, wretched and in need of assistance.

As can be seen, such a religious appreciation appeals to the polarity between health (of the body) and salvation (of the soul), which is itself rooted in the hierarchy between the inferior needs of the body and the primary values of the soul. This interconnection of plans and values leads to a real 'pedagogy of suffering' and to a 'healthful' use of disease, as well as to forms of 'spiritual therapy' for both sick and healthy people. All solicitations are directed at the health of the soul and supported by specific virtues: for the sick, the virtue of patience is of primary importance: patience enables the sick to suffer in silence, like Christ and Job before them. Malaise and pain are 'healthful' in that they 'treat' the evils/sins of the soul. For the healthy, the virtue of charity is all important, because through it they are able to relieve the patient's suffering. Through these act of mercy the donor is seeking benefits for his own soul rather than looking to relieve the suffering of the sick person. This overall representation, together with its ambivalence, has its origins in the figure of Christ on the cross. In Christ's image patience, disease, therapy and recovery are made sacred in the unity of a symbol, and that is also why such a representation is so substantial and lasting. Christ is indeed a physician, because he provides true health for mankind which has lost its way. At the same time he is also a patient, since in the Incarnation and the Passion he takes on himself the weakness of the human body and, with his death, he takes all its fragilities and sufferings to the limit. He therefore becomes ill (that is to say human) in order to become both medicine and physician (for the whole mankind). Moreover, with the Resurrection of his body, he pre-announces and promises everybody the final glorification of the body.

II

This overall perspective is primarily aimed at the health of the soul. It does not express itself in stereotyped formulas but is wholly theologically founded. It is also deeply rooted in the material conditions of an extremely precarious ecosystem. Finally, symbols play a fundamental role in its structure, their function being to stimulate and guide behaviour and judgment. Set in this context, of course, the pursuit of a healthy body through technical means cannot be looked upon favourably, namely with slow and uncertain procedures like those seen in medicine, a profane science of body health. Medicine, even though it is impoverished in its doctrinal contents, still subsists even in the High Middle Ages, but it hardly shows the independent features of a legitimate body of knowledge or useful techniques. Therefore, what is the relationship between medicine and philosophy, and, first and foremost, the role of philosophy in this context? I shall confine myself to a few schematic considerations. 1) For this period it is not appropriate to refer to theology and philosophy as articulate disciplines: it is better to refer to the elaboration of a Christian *sapientia*, where reason, enlightenment and faith coordinate themselves in order to detect, illustrate and finally contemplate God's mysteries and therefore help mankind on its way to salvation. Moreover, in the foreground – especially in the modest teaching programmes actually offered – it is not so much philosophy, as the seven liberal arts, which are meant to be a preliminary instrument for philosophy (identified as Christian knowledge), or a constituent part of it, considered as the whole profane knowledge that the Christian can and has to utilize. It is, however, to these liberal arts that a propaedeutical, auxiliary, instrumental role is essentially attributed. 2) Philosophy, together with its many different potential meanings in such a context, is neither therapeutical nor consolatory for the soul. That said, the period does start with just such a work – Boethius' *De consolation philosophiae* – in which Lady Philosophy introduces herself as a therapist who doses those remedies best suited to relieve Boethius from his spiritual prostration-illness.[3] Generally, then, philosophy is not medicine of the soul, and it cannot be considered as such in relation to medicine of the body. 3) If there is a connection between medicine and philosophy, it takes rather the shape – at least until the 12th century – of an exclusion and a refusal. As Martianus Capella specified in his Neoplatonic background, medicine must not be included among the seven liberal arts, because it works with and on the body, that is to say it concerns that part of man which is not free, which does not elevate itself, as it is imprisoned and conditioned by earthly and concrete needs.[4]

Of course a number of voices have been raised against this disdainful exclusion. Firstly, they include physicians', in the modest but extant centres of medical training in Alexandria and Ravenna between the 5th and 9th century.[5] Here we see

3 This work, though very influent all through the Middle Ages, did not represent a vehicle for the image of philosophy as medicine of soul, a role that – as we have seen – is rather held by Christ.

4 Up to all the 12th century (at least as regards some monastic currents), the reflections on the statute of medicine grow generally in the broader context of the discussion about the role of the *artes mechanicae*.

5 See A. Beccaria, *I codici di medicina del periodo presalernitano secoli IX, X e XI*, Rome 1956; id., "Sulle tracce di un antico canone d'Ippocrate e Galeno", *Italia medievale e umanistica* 2 (1959); 4 (1961); 14 (1971).

the idea of philosophy as medicine of the soul circulating, thus raising medicine to a higher level. In the prologues of their scanty didactical commentaries these physicians – for example John of Alexandria[6] and Agnellus of Ravenna,– invented and attributed to Aristotle a double definition. No such definitions, however, are to be found in such terms in Aristotle's works. Philosophy – they remark – is the mother of all the arts, and so medicine is one of its daughters. Medicine, however, resembles more closely the mother as it involves various skills and expertise and also because of the excellence of its object, the human body. It is better to define it as the sister of philosophy: as philosophy treats the passions of soul and is medicine for the soul, so medicine is rational inquiry, namely philosophy, of the body. These voices and definitions are at the moment isolated and not used to the advantage of the physicians, though they are taken up again in the most famous encyclopedia of the High Middle Ages, that is Isidore of Seville's *Etymologiae*.[7]

III

Now, focusing on the 12th and 13th centuries, we find a completely different viewpoint, the result of the extraordinary effervescence which the West – particularly in the 12th century – experienced in every field, from demography and economy to philosophy and general culture. With regard to this tumultuous period, I shall underline here just three interesting aspects for our theme which operate in a kind of synergy. Firstly, in this period the entire Aristotelian *corpus* is being progressively translated, thereby enriching the medical textual heritage out of all proportion both in quantity and quality.[8] In any case, medicine is no longer definable as fragile knowledge, theoretically insubstantial or of uncertain practical success, nor can it be considered as the practice of a vain and undue curiosity. Moreover, authorized centres, including those for medicine, are being set up first for translation purposes, then go on to be centres of learning and training (such as the Schools of Salerno and Montpellier). These schools are able to reformulate and hand down

6 See *Johannis Alexandrini Commentaria in librum De sectis Galeni*, ed. by C. D. Pritchet, Leiden 1982, pp. 4, 5, 14–15; N. Palmieri, *L'antica versione latina del 'De sectis' di Galeno*, Pisa 1989; Agnellus of Ravenna, *Lectures on Galen's 'De sectis'*, Buffalo 1981; A. Z. Iskandar, "An attempted Reconstruction of Late Alexandrian Medical Curriculum", *Medical History* 20 (1976), pp. 235–258; O. Temkin, "Studies on Late Alexandrian Medicine. I. Alexandrian Commentaries on Galen's De sectis ad introducendos", in: id., *The Double Face of Janus and Other Essays in the History of Medicine*, Baltimore / London 1977, pp. 178–197.

7 See Isidore of Seville, *Etymologiarum sive originum Libri XX*, ed. by W. M. Lindsay, Oxford 1962, I, IV, xiii, 5: medicine "secunda philosophia dicitur. Utraque enim disciplina totum nomine sibi vindicat. Nam sicut per illam anima, ita per hanc corpus curatur".

8 See at least D. Jacquart, "Principales étapes dans la transmission des textes de médecine (XIe–XIVe siècles)", in: J. Hamesse – M. Fattori (eds.), *Rencontres de cultures dans la philosophie médiévale*, Louvain-la-Neuve-Cassino 1990; ead., "Aristotelian Thought in Salerno", in: P. Dronke (ed.), *A History of Twelfth-Century Western Philosophy*, Cambridge 1988.

the new doctrinarian contributions.[9] Here the physician is educated and becomes a *peritus*: he is now a fully fledged professional figure for health. Finally, this development is also the effect of the new concept of nature, which in turn is favoured by the new philosophic-scientific culture, and by the medical one in particular.[10] The new philosophic-naturalistic relationship between man, God and nature, between the Creator and his creation is both mediate and regular and can be questioned by human reason. This also means that health, illness and recovery are no longer considered as merely the instantaneous, unpredictable expression of God's will in the form of punishment or miracle, or as an effect directly associated with the events of the soul, but as instances that depend on natural occurences, which in turn can then be studied solely by the physician, the *peritus* of the bodies. The human body itself – still inferior and bound to material needs – becomes a thing of value, not only because it represents one of the most elevated manifestations of God's creative rationality, but also because it is his means of operating in the world, and its efficiency is necessary to carry out those now diversified tasks which man, still *viator*, has to accomplish as a moral duty throughout his earthly journey.Thus the polarity between health and salvation, the hierarchy between soul and body are still fundamental, but they acquire more articulated characteristics, a closer rapport. So health is considered important, and now has its own specialist, the physician. In the same way the treatment of the soul has its own specialist, a qualified *peritus*, who also has a specific position: the priest or the theologian, not the philosopher.[11]

The relationships between medicine and philosophy are still very fluid during this transition. In general, the overall context of the philosophical-naturalistic inquiry is rich and offers many possibilities of exchange. Science is not yet rigidly compartmentalized into disciplines (medicine, alchemy, astronomy, etc.),[12] so

9 See P. O. Kristeller, "Bartolomeo, Musandino, Mauro da Salerno e altri antichi commentatori dell' *Articella*", in: id., *Studi sulla scuola medica salernitana*, Naples 1986, pp. 97–151; see also the volumes (editions of works and proceedings) recently published within the national edition of Salernitan works coordinated by D. Jacquart and A. Paravicini Bagliani. With regard to Montpellier see D. Le Blévec, (ed.), *L'Université de Médecine de Montpellier et son rayonnement (XIIIe–XVe siècles)*, Turnhout 2004; L. Dulieu, *La médecine à Montpellier,* I: *Le Moyen Age*, Avignon 1975.

10 This kind of integration between philosophy and scientific-naturalistic knowledge develops, for example, in the School of Chartres.

11 See J. Agrimi – C. Crisciani, *Medicina del corpo e medicina dell'anima. Note sul sapere del medico fino all'inizio del sec. XIII*, Milan 1978, in particular chapter III (Medici e sacerdoti) for an outline of the various exchanges and interactions between the two 'healers' in the 12th century; see also, for instance, the work attributed to Archimatthaeus (Anonymous Salernitan or Archimatthaeus of Salern), *De instructione medici*, published in S. De Renzi (ed.), *Collectio Salernitana*, Naples 1852–1859, vol. II, pp. 74–75, vol. V, pp. 333–349, where it is stated that, in a Christian house with a person lying ill, the place of honour is given to the physician and to the priest.

12 See C. Burnett's introduction to his edition of Hermann of Carinthia's *De essentiis*, Leiden 1982, where he underlines that "the dividing line between alchemical works and other works of natural science is difficult to draw at this period"; this remark is referable also to such works as Constantine of Pisa, *The book of Secrets of alchemy*, ed. by B. Obrist, Leiden 1990,

philosophers, physician-philosophers, theologians, alchemists can all speak about and discuss the elements, humours and astral influences.

In any case, the 12th century – which we may define as the second phase in our scheme – is probably the one that registers the most diverse range of positions of this relationship, simply because *philosophia* has so many diverse meanings. At the same time, the 'schools' which elaborate these different philosophical trends differentiate as well: from the Victorine school, to the cathedral school of Chartres, to the free city schools where the different meanings of the terms *phisica*[13] or *medicina* are discussed and utilized. These subjects require a more detailed study; whereas I prefer to concentrate more on the characteristics of medical knowledge during the 13th and 14th centuries, an era that for medicine can be defined as a period of standardization, an institutional and in particular an epistemological settlement, and its moment of greatest doctrinal elaboration.

IV

In this period medicine is taught in one of the four faculties of the newly created universities. It therefore appears as a discipline, namely as a consistent and organic body of texts – first and foremost – which are explained using defined teaching methods, set out in a graduated order into a *curriculum*, articulated in stages, and marked by examinations. Henceforth in Europe, only students who follow this institutional and (comparatively) homogeneous course, are considered true physicians and can legitimately teach and practise the profession.

To understand this defining process better, it is useful to remember that translations of medical works are being carried out at the same time as the entire Aristotelian *corpus* is spreading and entering the teaching programmes.[14] Indeed, some medical works were the first to adopt Aristotelian issues and discussion methods.[15] Broadly speaking, this Aristotelian background is the main feature in 13th century medicine, by now a defined entity with a uniform terminology. The Aristotelian *corpus*, in fact, shows a pattern of rationally ordered relationships between different sciences, in which medicine also has its own proper place. Moreover, it provides a set of data, theories and general biological-naturalistic

or the *Quaestiones Nicolai peripatetici*, ed. by S. Wielgus, *Mediaevalia Philosophica Polonorum* 17 (1973), pp. 57–155 (especially pp. 60–63).

13 See J. J. Bylebyl, "The Medical Meaning of *Physica*", *Osiris*, second series, 6 (1990), pp. 16–41.

14 Among the large number of studies regarding this matter, see the first two chapters of the collection of studies edited by L. Bianchi, *La filosofia nelle Università*, Florence 1997, pp. 1–23.

15 See S. Wingate, *The Mediaeval Latin Versions of the Aristotelian Scientific Corpus, with Special Reference to the Biological works*, London 1931; A. L. Birkenmajer, "Le role joué par les médecins et les naturalistes dans la réception d'Aristote au XIIe et XIIIe siècles", in: id., *Études d'histoire des Sciences et de la philosophie du Moyen Age*, Wroclaw 1970, pp. 73–87.

doctrines which turn out to be valuable for the general background of more specialized, medical knowledge. Finally and most importantly, it delivers a uniform scientific lexicon and a repertoire of conceptual tools and methods (reading, teaching and research) to be shared. Medicine is now inserted into a well-structured scientific system. It is equipped with articulated, conceptual instruments and a terminology that make it consistent with other forms of naturalistic knowledge which it joins or on which it depends. Now greatly enriched in terms of texts, medicine becomes a 'scholastic' discipline within the universities (and this therefore is the third part of my study).[16] In Padua[17] and Bologna,[18] the Faculties of Theology will only later be established, whereas the Faculties of Arts and Medicine become centres for philosophical and naturalistic-medical learning. It is considered almost to be the highest point in scientific research. In other words, here the study of logic and natural philosophy is not aimed at the study of theology, but is the basis of a physician's training.[19]

In this institutional, normalized and normalizing framework, against a background of the whole of Aristotelianism, there is an essential problem to be tackled which also concerns philosophy, and that is the definition and placement of medical knowledge. From this epistemological standpoint, the main problem (not easy to solve, so much so, that physicians worked on it for over a century) is to ensure that such knowledge has scientific status, operative effectiveness and relative autonomy. The solution – which I discuss here in a very schematic form – is to characterize medicine as a specialist science, where theory and practice – both essential in the physician's overall skills – are coordinated in such a way as to give medicine all the requirements of a science, but defined and limited (and therefore specialist). It is aimed at certain kinds of interventions and on a particular *subiectum* (not the human body in general, but the body in so far as it is suscepti-

16 See D. Jacquart, "La scolastica medica", in: *Storia del pensiero medico occidentale*, cit., pp. 261–322; J. Agrimi – C. Crisciani, *'Edocere medicos'. Medicina scolastica nei secoli XIII–XV*, Milan / Naples 1988; eaed., "La medicina scolastica. Dalla scuola di Salerno alle Facoltà universitarie", in: G. P. Brizzi – J. Verger (eds.), *Le Università dell'Europa – Le scuole e i maestri, Il medioevo*, Milan 1994; P. G. Ottosson, *Scholastic Medicine and Philosophy. A Study of Commentaries on Galen's 'Tegni' (ca. 1300–1450)*, Naples 1984; A. Paravicini Bagliani, *Medicina e scienze della natura alla corte dei Papi nel Duecento*, Spoleto 1991; C. O'Boyle et al. (eds.), *El aprendizaje de la medicina en el mundo medieval. Las fronteras de la enseñanza universitaria*, Granada 2000; C. Crisciani, "Curricula e contenuti dell'insegnamento. La medicina dalle origini al sec. XV", in: P. Brizzi (ed.), *Storia delle Università in Italia*, Messina 2007, pp. 182–204.

17 In regard to Padua, N. G. Siraisi, *Arts and Sciences at Padua. The 'Studium' of Padua before 1350*, Toronto 1973 is still indispensable.

18 See N. G. Siraisi, *Taddeo Alderotti and His Pupils. Two Generations of Italian Medical Learning*, Princeton 1981; ead., Medicine and the Italian Universities, 1250–1600, Leiden 2001; ead., Medieval and Early Renaissance Medicine, Chicago / London 1990; T. Pesenti, "Arti e medicina. La formazione del curriculum medico", in: L. Gargan – O. Limone (eds.), *Luoghi e metodi di insegnamento nell'Italia medioevale (secoli XII–XIV)*, Galatina 1989, pp. 153–177.

19 See C. Crisciani, "La formazione del medico nel medioevo. Dottrina ed etica", in: M. Ferrari – P. Mazzarello (eds.), *Formare alle professioni. Figure della sanità*, Milan 2010, pp. 36–57.

ble to change, from health to illness and *vice versa*). The definition of this specialism – which puts together both effective interventions, in so far as they are guided by appropriate theories, and appropriate theories, in so far as they are aimed at specific interventions – is not at all uniform and has shades and variations depending on the seat of learning and its residing principal.[20] In all its manifestations, however, the problem involves a careful definition of boundaries. Upwards: medicine depends on the theoretical views of natural philosophy, but it does not mix with them because it determines them, it deepens them within its narrower field of investigation and directs them all towards action (a theory does not have this aim)[21]; and downwards: the physician's work is not 'empirical' (a term which here has a disparaging meaning)[22] because it is guided by *rationes* and *regulae*, and is effective for this reason and this reason only. It therefore has nothing to do with blind practicalism, which is repetitive and has no theoretical explanation, peculiar to 'empirics', or with healers, to those, in short, who do not have a theoretical grounding behind them to explain what they do.[23] Finally, at the end of a centuries-old debate, and despite a remarkable variety of trends, medical knowledge is presented to us as unitary, but flexibly organized into interconnected

20 Referring to the Italian area, for instance, Taddeo Alderotti's, Peter of Abano's and Gentile of Foligno's positions are diversified: see R. French, *Canonical Medicine. Gentile da Foligno and Scholasticism*, Leiden 2001; id., "Gentile da Foligno and the 'via medicorum'", in: J. D. North – J. J. Roche (eds.), *The Light of Nature*, Boston 1985, pp. 21–34; J. Chandelier, *Gentile da Foligno, médecin et universitaire du XIVe siècle. Etude et édition critique du commentaire au 'Canon' d'Avicenne (3,11,1)*, Paris 2002; N. G. Siraisi, "Pietro d'Abano and Taddeo Alderotti. Two Models of Medical Culture", *Medioevo* 11 (1985), pp. 139–162.

21 See C. Crisciani, "'Experientia' e 'opus' in medicina ed alchimia. Forme e problemi di esperienza nel tardo Medioevo", *Quaestio* 4 (2004), pp. 149–173.

22 See P. Kibre, "The Faculty of Medicine at Paris. Charlatanism and Unlicensed Medical Practices in the Later Middle Ages", *Bulletin of the History of Medicine* 27 (1953), pp. 1–20; V. L. Bullough, *The Development of Medicine as a Profession*, New York 1966; T. Pesenti, "'Professores chirurgie', 'medici ciroici' e 'barbitonsores' a Padova nell'età di Leonardo Buffi da Bertapaglia († dopo il 1448)", *Quaderni per la storia dell'Università di Padova* 11 (1978), pp. 1–38; W. Eamon – G. Keil, "'Plebsamat empirica'. Nicholas of Poland and his Critique of the Medieval Medical Establishment", *Sudhoffs Archiv* 71 (1987), pp. 180–196; J. Agrimi – C. Crisciani, "Immagini e ruoli della 'vetula' tra sapere medico e antropologia religiosa (secoli XIII–XV)", in: A. Paravicini Bagliani – A. Vauchez (eds.), *Poteri carismatici e informali. Chiesa e società medievali*, Palermo 1992, pp. 224–261; F. Collard – E. Samama (eds.), *Mires, Physiciens, barbiers et charlatans. Les marges de la médecine de l'Antiquité au XVIe siècle*, Langres 2004.

23 In regard to the difference between empirica and experimenta see J. Agrimi – C. Crisciani, "Per una ricerca su 'experimentum-experimenta'. Riflessione epistemologica e tradizione medica (secoli XIII–XIV)", in: P. Janni – I. Mazzini (eds.), *Presenze del lessico greco e latino nelle lingue contemporanee*, Macerata 1990, pp. 9–49 (especially the second part); C. Crisciani, "Fatti, teorie, 'narratio' e i malati a corte. Note su empirismo e medicina nel tardo medioevo", *Quaderni storici* 36 (2001), pp. 695–718. Now see also T. Bénatouil – I. Draelantes (eds.), *'Expertus sum'. L'expérience par les sens dans la philosophie naturelle médiévale*, Florence 2011.

levels:[24] the theoretical-scientific part, the practical-scientific part, the trade and its operating rules, and accurate intervention. While the first level connects medicine to natural philosophy (and ensures the scientific quality of it), the final scope, the intervention, ensures the specialism of it and therefore its relative autonomy. Also significant is the way in which the levels are formulated and the position of medicine itself which is laid out in a more popular and less sophisticated form in Vincenzo of Beauvais' encyclopedia. In the *Speculum doctrinale*[25], medicine as well should have a place within the *artes mechanicae*; this, however, "non tantum in operatione manuum consistit sicut cetere, sedetiam in mentis speculation consistit, videlicet quantum ad causarum considerationem, unde quasi media inter practica et theoricam [...]." Medicine, therefore, appears here as intermediate and an intermediary between mechanical arts and theoretical disciplines: it is the most theoretical of the arts, and the most practical of the sciences; its theoretical part "videtur esse potissima naturalis philosophie pars quia de tota fere hominis natura disserit".

The overall context of knowledge in which this arrangement takes place is that of a hierarchical structure of disciplines, strengthened by the institutional organization of the universities. They are connected by relationships of vertical dependency (*subalternatio*), in which each disciplinary level (and the inner levels of each of them) can develop – within its own limits – horizontally in an indefinite way, according to each one's specific rules and methods.

V

The relationship between medicine and philosophy, therefore, has to be investigated within a context which takes into account the polarity between health and salvation, still an underlying force, and a style of rationality – concerning the precise definition of its relevance – common to all areas of university knowledge. The Christian plan of salvation, which continues to be of primary importance now has its own specialists – neither philosophers nor physicians, but theologians and shepherds of souls. The result is that any possible relationship (of antagonism, cooperation, competition) between medicine and philosophy is flattened, that is to say neither of them is of primary importance to the *salus animae*, and, in any case, is placed at the level of secular and doctrinal knowledge, which is any how argumentative and textual.

In this context, the simultaneous presence of at least two forms of relationships between medicine and philosophy, corresponding to two different meanings

24 This is the scheme outlined by the Florentine physician Nicolò Falcucci (†1412), in his widely-circulated *Sermones medicinales*, Papiae 1481–1484, Sermo I.

25 *Speculum doctrinale*, Duaci 1624, l. 12.105, 13.1, 14.1, 16.1. See S. Schuler, "'Medicina secunda philosophia'. Die Einordnung der Medizin als Hauptdisziplin und die Zusammenstellung ihrer Quellen im 'Speculum maius' des Vinzenz von Beauvais", *Frühmittelalterliche Studien* 33 (1999), pp. 169–251.

of philosophy, which do not fully coincide should also be noted.[26] First of all, we can see an epistemological relationship – that refers to the famous and equally equivocal passage of Aristotle's *De sensu*[27] – where medicine is subordinate to natural philosophy, the general theories of which constitute the principles (and therefore do not need to be proved) and the theoretical basis of the more specific doctrines worked out by physicians. In this case the emphasis is on a theoretical dominance of philosophy over medicine, and we have seen how carefully physicians restrict and weigh such a principle, claiming the specialism of their investigation. This philosophical grounding is therefore considered necessary for the most part, provided, however, it is not too invasive.[28] Secondly, we can see a utilitarian relationship, closer perhaps to the institutional one, which concerns both natural philosophy and philosophy as the seven liberal arts as a whole. Physicians interpret the contributions of the liberal arts as an aid (they call them indeed *subservientes* disciplines) which they use because the unity and complexity of their object – the human body – requires the merging of different skills into medical expertise, which the physician alone knows how to coordinate and put into practice in order to achieve good health. Such a relationship is expressed very clearly in Peter of Abano's *Conciliator*.[29] So a relationship of theoretical prominence (of philosophy over medicine) is possible as long as they are useful to each other. Finally, it should not be forgotten that the authorities, e. g. Aristotle, Galen, and mainly Avicenna, whose works provide knowledge for the physician, are also and sometimes above all philosophers, and that their views do not always coincide even in biology and physiology – fields which are of most interest to the physician. It is not easy in these cases to establish a hierarchy of values, or to put aside definitively such authoritative foundations, or even to simply use the term 'error' in a tradition which is such because it conveys truth.

The difficult approach towards the occurrence of different conceptions in prestigious and indispensable *auctores*, and the dual role of dominion and service that philosophy seems to assume or, more generally, the definition of a proper relationship between medicine and philosophy, are made feasible – at least in principle – by that style of scholastic inquiry definable as 'semantic'. It means that, as regards a theme, the first question that must be asked is: who can speak about it, and in what sense can we talk about? That is to say, from which perspective and according to what criteria should it be investigated? In the case of scholastic medicine, this procedure is set out explicitly and leads to a typical result, the *conciliatio*. This does not mean concordism, or eclecticism, or rhetorical pacification of contrast, rather it expresses that it is not different truths but different points

26 See C. Schmitt, "Aristotle among the Physicians", in: A. Wear et al. (eds.), *The Medical Renaissance of the Sixteenth Century*, Cambridge 1985, pp. 1–15.

27 Aristotle, *De sensu et sensato*, 1.436a17–21.

28 See M. R. McVaugh, "The Nature and Limits of Medical Certitude at Early Fourteenth-Century Montpellier", *Osiris*, second series, 6 (1990), pp. 62–84.

29 Peter of Abano, *Conciliator controversiarum quae inter philosophos et medicos versantur*, Venice 1565 (anastatic reprint Padua 1985).

of view and different approaches, all of them legitimate, which have the right to coexist.

VI

Two examples illustrate how physicians proceed in this conciliated-scholastic process. I have choosen two well-known figures, Peter of Abano and Arnold of Villanova, who both worked between the 13th and 14th centuries. In all other respects, these two physicians have little in common in that they come from two very different schools and work in different contexts. Their ideas on the relationship between medicine and philosophy differ. When discussing precise medical doctrines their results are often very different. On the relationship between medicine and philosophy, however, they share the same formal approach.

The title of Peter of Abano's major work alone – *Conciliator differentiarum* or *controversiarum quae inter philosophos et medicos versantur* – leads us straight to the heart of the problem: medical texts express different opinions on many points, as opposed to philosophers, who, on the other hand, should be providing the foundations and principles of medical doctrines. For Peter it is not a problem but only an outward contrast, not based on an absolute value of truth (otherwise one of the two contenders would be in error), but rather depends on the level of research carried out by each one, on the standards it requires, and to the type of truth (or rather of sense) that is appropriate and achievable at such a level. This sense is not in conflict with the other 'truths', but has equal legitimacy and can be, in any case, more or less general, more or less specific, more or less useful for the intervention. So that in the concept of *sanitas*, for instance, Peter distinguishes between what the word means for a natural philosopher and a physician, before specifying the precise meanings that are peculiar to the physician such as *speculans* or *practicus*.[30] The result is a separation of levels, a semantic distinction, sometimes an epistemological hierarchy between generality and specialism, but hardly ever conflict.

Even clearer is Arnold's argument, discussed in his various works, and in particular in his *De intentione medicorum*[31] (this is also a meaningful title). Arnold's case is actually very interesting because we can see how such a system of permeable but independent levels and boundaries also works on a larger scale. In his eventful career, in fact, Arnold also wishes to be a philosopher and expressed himself in the theological field as well. In *De intentione* Arnold explains his views on the relationship between medicine and philosophy, and reasserts that the former is defined in a specialist sense by its own peculiar finality (*intentio*). Physicians' arguments have to be rooted in this epistemological level of *scientia operativa* and are regulated by its own peculiar criteria of truth and effectiveness. Such

30 See *Conciliator*, ff. 109 Gb–111 Cb.

31 See Arnold of Villanova, *De intentione medicorum*, in: *Arnaldi de Villanova Opera Medica Omnia*, V.1, ed. by M. R. McVaugh, Barcelona 2000.

criteria are not always opposite, but of course they are different from a natural philosopher's point of view, whose theoretical horizon does not include these ends. So, for instance, Galen's *Sermones* have to be interpreted in the medical field "secundum quod medicinali speculation conveniunt"[32], in order to satisfy their medical purpose. If then, in another instance, Isaac and Galen seem to be in contrast – about a particular case proposed by Arnold, on the definition of heat and fevers – the physician commentator, puzzled, will finally acknowledge that the truth is just one if he considers the different platforms from which each one is speaking. Galen, as a natural philosopher and *universaliter*, aims at perfect knowledge; Isaac speaks as a physician, and specifies the same remarks in a therapeutic and specialist sense, which is less at one with universal truth, but more useful in giving instructions to those in the medical field. As for Arnold, he has no qualms about expressing himself at the philosopher's level. He places himself on this level in various works, such as *Aphorismi de gradibus*, *De intentione medicorum*, and *Tractatus de humido radicali*. From the very beginning of these works, however, he always specifies that he is speaking as a natural philosopher, and his aim is therefore to attain, in that specific matter (for instance the nature and restoration of radical moisture), the *veritas perficiens intellectum*. But then, when Arnold turns to the religious field in Spiritual Franciscans' favour and writes theological-prophetic works, he of course arouses suspicion and is criticized, not only for of the contents, but above all because – as he himself states – as a physician he is talking about a subject which is not his. He has no expertise on the matter and knows nothing about its rules. Arnold does not refute this objection, remembering his even modest theological background, nor does he claim this right unduly, because, as a physician, he acknowledges he has none. Rather he declares that every Christian must intervene in what concerns the salvation of the soul. He himself took a stand on the matter of Franciscan poverty and the imminent end of the world not as a physician, but as a simple Christian.[33] We can see then how far Arnold transgresses the rules of the game, as deeply as he obeys them, and how he uses the call to salvation strategically, in order to cross every precise specialistic boundary, thereby maintaining, when necessary, all its radicality.

Apart from Arnold's singular but very significant position, in the 14th century a delicate but stable balance between medicine and philosophy is indeed noticable, where each of them has its own place and specific function, and the hierarchy of the whole does not prevent independent elaboration on various levels.

32 Arnold of Villanova, *Tractatus de humido radicali*, II.3, in: *Arnaldi de Villanova Opera Medica Omnia*, V.2, ed. by M. R. McVaugh, Barcelona 2010, fol. 41rb.

33 See J. Ziegler, *Medicine and Religion c. 1300. The Case of Arnau de Vilanova*, Oxford 1998; C. Crisciani, "'Exemplum Christi' e sapere. Sull'epistemologia di Arnaldo da Villanova", *Archives Internationales d'Histoire des Sciences* 28 (1978), pp. 245–92; see *De intentione medicorum*, cit., pp. 101–03, 106–11.

VII

Actually, this system which now includes medicine paves the way for the occurrence of totalizing tendencies with various justifications, at each doctrinal-epistemological level. Such an outcome may seem paradoxical, but it is really the obvious result of a system where the disciplinary levels are so precise and rigid, it almost makes them self-consisting and even impervious. Between the14th and the first half of the 15th century, especially in Italy, medicine tends in fact to have an all pervasive approach in every field, which not only attracts and makes use of the *subservientes* liberal arts, but intends also to make use of the most varied fields of knowledge (in addition to astronomy/astrology, also oneiromancy, eugenics, physiognomy, alchemy, balneotherapy, meteorology, gastronomy), or rather in certain cases stimulates these sciences, and anyhow takes possession of them and gathers them around itself for its doctrinal and practical purposes. Medicine, as we have seen, remains a specialist *scientia operativa* concerning the curable body. This object, however, is so complex and is the hard core of so many relations as to require – in the opinion of many physicians at the end of the 14th century – a very broad approach, so much so that it can attract many different sciences, and claim therefore a doctrinal solidity, equal or even superior to philosophy. In Iacopo of Forlì's *oratio in laudem medicine*,[34] at the beginning of the 15th century, we read not only that medicine is the sister of philosophy, but also that, as man is the most 'divine' being in the whole of creation, the learned man who works with it – the *medicus gratiosus* – is closer than anybody else to the divine science. Reasons are many: the solidity of his knowledge, the moral gifts necessarily related to it, and the fact that he must investigate the remotest and deepest issues concerning his subject.

I have included this speech because, if the noble image drawn by scholastic physicians about their knowledge is clearly stated in the epistemological debate, it is even more evident in the acts of university rhetoric[35] – such as funeral orations for famous, deceased masters, course-opening and graduation speeches – or in sections of texts (prologues, introductions, dedications) where the *commendation artis* is often expressed, that is the examination of qualities and merits which de-

34 Iacopo of Forlì, *Medicina artium preclarissima* [...] (Città del Vaticano, Biblioteca Apostolica Vaticana, ms. Vat. Lat, 5223), published in Agrimi – Crisciani, *'Edocere medicos'*, cit., pp. 263–273.

35 This theme is still largely unexplored in medicine. Clémence Revest is working; see a Gentile of Foligno's graduation speech published in Agrimi – Crisciani, *'Edocere medicos'*, cit. (where in the appendix is published also Iacopo of Forlì's *oratio* in praise of medicine: see here n. 33); another Gentile's speech is published in C. C. Schlam, "Graduation Speeches of Gentile da Foligno", *Medieval Studies* 40 (1978), pp. 96–119. See anyway G. Fioravanti, *Università e città. Cultura umanistica e cultura scolastica a Siena nel' 400*, Florence 1981; G. Fransen – D. Maffei, "Haragues universitaires du XIVe siècle", *Studi Senesi* 83 (1971), pp. 7–22; L. Bertalot, "Eine Sammlung Paduaner Reden des XV. Jahrhunderts", *Quellen und Forschungen aus italienischen Archiven und Bibliotheken* 26 (1936), pp. 245–267; K. Müllner, *Reden und Briefe italienischer Humanisten*, Munich 1970.

fine the excellence of medicine. In these judgments two main aspects stand out. Firstly, we notice the emphasis on the doctrinal lucidity of medicine, expressed in the firmness of the methodical procedures, through which it achieves the knowledge of causes, and also in the richness, antiquity and prestige of its texts and venerable *auctores*. Secondly, and no less important, the quantity and variety of purposes coordinated by medicine, the effectiveness of its applications and usefulness of its practical results. The usefulness of the purposes of medicine involves not only the individual patient but society, or rather mankind as a whole, to whose constitutive *necessitas* medicine comes to the rescue through the providential will of God. Its aims concern the body and its health, now of primary importance to man, at least from a certain point of view, because without health no activity, no possession, no honour could actually exist. Such an idea is common not only to physicians, but also to philosophers and theologians. In the 13th century it had already been concisely exposed by the Dominican Master General Humbert of Romans[36] in his sermon to medical students, and it was taken up again many times, for example in 1396 by Henry of Langenstein, the organizer of the new University of Vienna, in his *Sermo de Sancta Katharina*, the saint protectress of the Faculty of Arts. He explains the prerogatives of the different disciplines and the reciprocal relationships between the various faculties: in regard to medicine he points out that it is the *sciencia regitiva* of man's faculties and natural occurrences, and therefore:

> [...] hec est sciencia, sine cuius auxilio et beneficio irruente morbo grammatica tacet, rhetorice eloquentia silet, loyca non sillogissat, dyalectica disputare nescit, iurista iudicium perdit, theologia non predicat, miles non pugnat, sacerdos non orat, rusticus non laborat.[37]

This is not his only remark. He also declares that medicine, in its entirety and articulation, is a science which has a theoretical, doctrinal foundation and such useful applications, that it is close to God.[38] In fact, while in general true knowledge can only be achieved provided that it stimulates the strengthening of good morals and the elimination of sordid vices, in the case of medicine, the scholar deals with the human body. This is at the top of the creation pyramid, and is the best possible place from which to witness the power and rationality of the Creator and discover the most secret and profound structures in his plan of the creation. In addition, the physician, more than any other scientist or practitioner, will certainly be gratified by his knowledge, but will also in all humility recognize his limits. Being so aware of the many health-related conditions which are not always controllable, there is no one who knows better than he does how essential it is to implore divine

36 Humbert of Romans, *De eruditione praedicatorum libri duo*, II (Maxima Bibliotheca Veterum Patrum; 25), Lugduni 1677, pp. 488–489.

37 See A. Lang, "Die Katharinenpredigt Heinrichs von Langenstein", *Divus Thomas* 26 (1948), pp.123–159, 233–249. It will be noticed that here are enumerated the activities related to the seven liberal arts and the three orders of the Christian society.

38 In an anonymous *sermo* in praise of medicine we are told that: "[...] ita quod ipsa (medicina) inter artes maxime appropinquat scientie divine" (*Sermo de operatione medicine a Deo*, Città del Vaticano, Biblioteca Apostolica Vaticana, ms.Vat. Lat, 4464, ff. 71vb–73ra).

help and grace in undertaking a therapy. In addition to this, Henry of Langenstein does not fail to remind us that, firstly, the deontological dictates that physicians must respect bring his profession even closer to the priesthood and its vows (as Cassiodorus had already remarked centuries earlier)[39]. Secondly, that the physician's knowledge, more than any other, brings him into contact with *res sacrae*. Finally, it is actually thanks to his knowledge, which is also practical, that the physician-surgeon – best expressed by the surgeon Henri de Mondeville in the 14th century – appeases the salvation of his own soul. In fact, he can help man in what is essential, his physical health, without which any other aid (work and sustenance, clothing, food, various works of mercy, the *viator*'s own journey to salvation) does not even have the necessary support to accomplish its aims. So Henri reminds his students and future surgeons that without pilgrimages, other devotions and alms "ex scientia vestra potestis salvare animas vestras"[40] (provided, obviously, that this *scientia* is true science). Scholastic physicians, then, frequently acknowledge that – no matter whether the physicians are grounded in subtle and close epistemological examinations or express themselves in smooth rhetorical texts, in commentaries on the *auctores*' works or in manuals of *practica* – there is a sort of ethical, as well as specifically philosophical hegemony of medicine in the field of naturalistic knowledge.

VIII

As may be seen, all these claims and prerogatives are rooted in a constant and growing appreciation of the theoretical and doctrinal character of medicine. At the beginning of the 15th century this is clearly pointed out by the Chancellor John Gerson in his *oratio* for medical student graduates, namely in an official speech given at the end of the course of studies and addressed to the learned and expert physicians educated at the university.[41] The *oratio* defines three prerogatives or characteristics of medicine: *vigor*, *splendor*, *valor*. These terms express the dignity of the origin of medical knowledge (*vigor*); the illustriousness of the doctrine it produces (*splendor*); the effectiveness of the practice which emanates from it (*valor*). It is up to physicians, Gerson concludes, not to stain this science with scant grounding, poor updating, operative negligence, temptation and attraction towards magic. In his opinion, besides being *donum*, or rather *verbum Dei*, medicine is – coming back to our theme – a *Philosophiae pars preclara*.

39 See Cassiodorus, *Variarum libri XII*, ed. by A. J. Fridh, CCSL XCVI, Tournhout1973, pp. 248–250.

40 J. L. Pagel (ed.), *Die Chirurgie des Heinrich von Mondeville nach Berliner, Erfurter und Pariser Codices*, Berlin 1892, p. 135. In this regard see M. C. Pouchelle, *Corps et chirurgie à l'apogée du Moyen Age*, Paris 1983; M. R. McVaugh, *The Rational Surgery of the Middle Ages*, Florence 2006.

41 See *Joannis Gersonii Doctoris et Cancellari Parisiensis Oratio pro licentiandis in medicina*, in: Joannis Gersonii... Opera Omnia, IV, Antverpiae 1706, coll.210–219.

These claims on medicine can also be made because even in this phase – which is the fourth on our agenda – philosophy does not heal the soul or console man: it aims at and leads – at least in some Aristotelian currents – to 'mental happiness', the full realization of the intellect in the contemplation of truth. Scholastic physicians, however, do not have any difficulty in showing that the theoretical side of medicine is a part of natural philosophy, and even coincides with it, and that consequently physicians too, or rather the physician-philosopher, attains a happy and bright union with the truth: a divine *consortium*.[42] Furthermore, as we have seen, with his medical knowledge he is also closer to God: he is his minister, the essential mediator in giving the gift of health. These claims of priority, however, do not modify the system of epistemological relationships that we have seen between medicine and philosophy, where both seem to have their own place and task. The hierarchy that may be determined between them does not prevent independent elaboration, and experts in every field are aware that they share the same rules to produce knowledge.

We note then that in the late Middle Ages the greatest distinction between medicine and philosophy takes place both from a formal and from an epistemological point of view. At the same time – especially in important institutions such as Italian universities[43] – a sort of identification and superimposition occurs. This is particularly emphasized in the rhetorical speeches of certain physicians, but actually seems to be verified by facts as well, especially when philosophy is reduced to being just logic and natural philosophy – as is revealed by the usual bitter Petrarchan sarcasm. If philosophy is reduced to this, then the identification is almost automatic, so much so that Petrarch, in his *Invectives contra medicum*, looks upon medicine as the prototype of natural philosophy and offends two identical targets: the philosopher/physician. In other words, Petrarch, among others, complains about the latency of a different form of philosophy.[44]

So the self-image projected by medicine in the mid 14th century is that of a strong, 'scientistic' knowledge, which requires nothing more than natural foundations and purpose, but at the same time can reach, in its own way, the divine. This image, however, is not a little bruised by an epochal event, the plague of 1348. Faced with this catastrophe the theoretical equipment of scholastic medicine is perfectly able to put forward explanations which are almost too comprehensive, but these do not turn into effective therapeutic weapons. "And not physicians nor medicines were of use – observes a chronicler with outspoken criticism, offending only the physicians' doctrinarian and 'scientistic' pride –, either because those

42 This theme is considerably developed in Gentile of Foligno's *orationes*.

43 Their specificity, which we have frequently referred to, is first of all that arts and medicine are together in the same faculty, where it is possible to set out on different *curricula*: the most frequent is actually the one of arts and medicine. In this way the naturalistic knowledge (peculiar to the arts after Aristotle's entry in the universities) becomes propaedeutic and oriented to the height of the faculty, that is medicine.

44 In this regard see M. Bertè et al. (eds.), *Petrarca e la medicina*, Messina 2006.

diseases were as yet unknown, or because physicians had not yet studied them."[45] The plague continues and becomes endemic, but the prestige of medicine does not crumble, its methodical, doctrinarian background is too ductile, flexible and rich in resources.[46] The following events in medical knowledge, however (the emergence of uncertainty about the relationship between theory and practice; the alliances that it sometimes interweaves with other practices;[47] the opening of new research strategies based on the importance of practice and 'particulars';[48] the analyses on the plurality of methods), are mostly to be read as innovative anxieties caused or at least influenced by the continuing failure in the face of the epidemic.

On the other hand, new questions arise concerning not only the physical structure of the world and the human body's place in it, but also man's destiny – going back to Augustinian anxiety of the restless *viator* and the questions "where are we going, where have we come from". They are directed at a philosophy that is absent, or does not always know the answer, but – as claimed by many, including Petrarch – that must be redefined and, most of all, must find a new role and renewed enthusiasm to deal with the task of *renovatio*.

All these elements enter into the wider crisis – or renewal – of the Renaissance. On the one hand, there is the contribution that this new philosophy will provide to such a *renovation* (thanks to it, for example, Plato[49] and Hermes are reintroduced into the philosophical circulation), and the uncertainty of medicine, which is no longer even sure of the complete correctness of its own textual tradition and methodological criteria. On the other hand, there is the interweaving of these two perspectives which together will actually reorganize and reestablish relationships between the various disciplines in the early modern age. Paracelsus' work is actually emblematic of the new philosophical, medical trends, but before

45 See Marchionne di Coppo Stefani, *Historia fiorentina*, Florence 1776, rubric 634, pp. 230–232.

46 A number of essays (those for example collected in A. Wear et al. (eds.), *The Medical Renaissance of the Sixteenth Century*) point out that, also for its flexible and plural methodological structure, for the fruitful interweaving among Galenism, Avicennianism and Aristotelianism, medicine does not bring about, in the transition between medieval and early modern period, catastrophic failure or massive 'revolutions', but rather adjustments, corrections and additions: in short, there is an 'evolution of a tradition', as says the subtitle of the important collection of essays M. R. McVaugh – N. G. Siraisi (eds.), *Renaissance Medical Learning. Evolution of a Tradition* (*Osiris*, second series; 6), Philadelphia 1990.

47 See for instance C. Crisciani – A. Paravicini Bagliani (eds.), *Alchimia e medicina nel medioevo*, Florence 2003; J. Agrimi, *Ingeniosa scientia nature. Studi sulla fisiognomica medievale*, Florence 2002.

48 See D. Jacquart, "Theory, Everyday Practice and Three Fifteenth-Century Physicians", *Osiris*, second series, 6 (1990), pp. 140–160; C. Crisciani, *Fatti, teorie*, cit.; M. R. McVaugh, "The 'Experience-Based Medicine' of the Thirteenth Century", *Early Science and Medicine* 14 (2009), pp. 105–130.

49 In regard to the link between medicine and philosophy in Plato, see M. Vegetti, *La medicina in Platone*, Venice 1995; Ficino takes up this approach again (see T. Katinis' works quoted in the next note).

him there is Marsilio Ficino,[50] physician and priest, who often describes himself as a philosopher who can heal the soul and the body. In his work *De vita*[51], for instance, he is able to create new perspectives by integrating the contributions of Hermes' *prisca theologia* and Ps. Arnold of Villanova's research on the prolongation of life,[52] with the findings of late-scholastic physicians on vital spirits[53] and *spiritus*.

50 See here T. Katinis' contribution, and id., *Medicina e filosofia in Marsilio Ficino. Il 'Consilio' contro la pestilenza*, Rome 2007.

51 See Marsilio Ficino, *De vita libri tres (Three Books on Life). A critical Edition and Translation with Introduction and Notes*, ed. by J. R. Clark, New York 1989.

52 See C. Crisciani – L. Repici – P. B. Rossi (eds.), *Vita longa. Durata della vita, vecchiaia e 'prolongatio vite' nella tradizione aristotelica e medica tra Antichità e Rinascimento*, Firenze 2009; C. Crisciani – G. Ferrari, "Introduzione to Arnold of Villanova, Tractatus de humido radicali", in: *Arnaldi de Villanova Opera Medica Omnia*, V.2, ed. by M. R. McVaugh, Barcelona 2010.

53 Cfr. D. Jacquart, *La médecine médiévale dans le cadre parisien (XIVe–XVe siècle)*, Paris 1998; E. R. Harvey, *The Inward Wits*, London 1975; D. P. Walker, *Spiritual and Demonic Magic from Ficino to Campanella*, London 1958; H. Hirai, *Le concept de semence dans les théories de la matière à la Renaissance*, Turnhout 2005.

LE MEDECIN MEDIEVAL ET LES BONNES MŒURS

Danielle Jacquart

Les occasions de tension entre médecine et morale chrétienne au Moyen Âge furent nombreuses, mais elles furent rarement explicitées par les médecins.[1] S'offrent plutôt au regard de l'historien, en lui ouvrant un vaste domaine de recherche, les manières dont ils surent adapter leur discours aux exigences morales du temps et les contourner au besoin. Dans le domaine de la sexualité, par exemple, ils firent entendre leur voix sans se livrer à des transgressions qui auraient été jugées inacceptables et que, d'ailleurs, pour la plupart ils jugeaient peut-être eux-mêmes inacceptables, étant donné le cadre social et religieux de leur activité. Sur ce sujet, comme sur d'autres, ils s'en tinrent à prescrire mesure et modération, à préconiser un juste milieu où morale et médecine trouvaient leur point d'entente.[2] En ce sens, ils furent des sortes de moralistes, dont la vogue des régimes de santé fut l'une des manifestations à la fin du Moyen Âge.[3] Un autre type de tensions, également rarement explicité, touchait à l'art du pronostic. Le médecin devait-il dire la vérité au malade et à son entourage, lorsque s'annonçait une issue fatale?[4] Cette question prenait toute son acuité en contexte chrétien, puisque l'approche de la mort devait inciter à faire venir le prêtre et à prendre des disposi-

1 Sur le problème plus général des tensions et accords entre médecine, science du corps, religion et théologie, on se reportera à: P. Biller – A. J. Minnis (éds.), *Medieval Theology and the Natural Body*, Woodbridge (Suffolk) 1997; P. Biller – J. Ziegler (éds.), *Religion and Medicine in the Middle Ages*, Woodbridge (Suffolk) 2001.

2 Le ton est donné dès le *De coitu* de Constantin l'Africain à la fin du XIe siècle, qui tout en prenant en compte les bienfaits de l'activité sexuelle, y compris en dehors de sa finalité procréatrice, oriente vers la modération, cf. D. Jacquart, «Sexualité et maladie durant le haut Moyen Âge», in: *Comportamenti e immaginario della sessualità nell'alto medioevo* (Settimane di studio della Fondazione Centro Italiano di Studi sull'Alto Medioevo; 53), Spolète 2006, pp. 323–343. Les pratiques homosexuelles firent partie de l'inacceptable pour un médecin médiéval, à part de rares transgresseurs, comme Pietro d'Abano: D. Jacquart – C. Thomasset, *Sexuality and Medicine in the Middle Ages*, Cambridge / Princeton 1988, pp. 139–167; J. Cadden, «Nothing Natural is Shameful. Vestiges of a Debate About Sex and Science in a Group of Late-Medieval Manuscripts», *Speculum* 76 (2001), pp. 66–89.

3 M. Nicoud, *Les régimes de santé au Moyen Âge. Naissance et diffusion d'une écriture médicale (XIIIe–XVe siècle)* (Bibliothèque des Ecoles françaises d'Athènes et de Rome; 333), Rome 2007.

4 Sur cette question je me permets de renvoyer à une précédente étude: D. Jacquart, «Le difficile pronostic de mort (XIVe–XVe siècles)», in: *Éthique et pratiques médicales aux derniers siècles du Moyen Âge* (Médiévales; 46) Saint Denis 2004, dossier coord. par L. Moulinier-Brogi et M. Nicoud, pp. 11–21; voir aussi l'article de Michael McVaugh dans le présent volume.

tions pour le salut de l'âme de celui qui allait rendre son dernier souffle. Les médecins ne furent pas tout à fait clairs sur ce sujet. D'une part, maintenir l'espoir, la confiance du patient était considéré comme une partie intégrante du traitement que justifiait la théorie médicale. D'autre part, comme l'écrivait subtilement le montpelliérain Bernard de Gordon dans les toutes dernières années du XIIIe siècle, les signes d'une mort annoncée pouvaient être trompeurs: «Il faut comprendre cependant qu'une issue fatale n'est pas aussi certaine qu'une bonne issue, car les mouvements de la nature sont ordonnés, suivant une seule voie et un seul ordre. Mais les mouvements de la maladie sont très désordonnés, donc le terme de la mort n'est pas aussi certain que celui de la vie».[5] Il ressort de cette constatation que, pour un médecin, ne pas reconnaître l'ordre de la nature – c'est-à-dire de la vie – constituait une faute plus grave que de ne pas prévoir une issue fatale, qui de toute façon relevait d'un désordre à bien des égards imprévisible. Le même Bernard de Gordon usait de l'adjectif *ignominiosum* pour qualifier le cas où un médecin avait été trompé dans son diagnostic d'une maladie qu'il croyait être une phtisie incurable, et qui s'était avérée être une autre pathologie suivie d'une guérison. Un peu plus d'un siècle plus tard à Padoue, Michel Savonarole reprenait les mêmes propos – sans signaler cet emprunt – dans les mêmes termes.[6] Si cette faute était porteuse de honte – bien qu'elle n'ait pas abouti à un échec thérapeutique – elle n'enfreignait pas pour autant la morale ni les pratiques chrétiennes: de ce point de vue, l'erreur inverse aurait été plus préjudiciable, car serait ainsi allé à la mort un patient sans le secours de la religion. L'emploi de l'adjectif *ignominiosum* en ce contexte d'une mort annoncée qui ne survient pas montre clairement que Bernard de Gordon, suivi par Michel Savonarole, ne se plaçait pas sur le plan de la morale chrétienne. La préoccupation principale restait la préservation de la réputation du médecin, de sa *fama*, qui, une fois entachée, non seulement laissait craindre une perte de clientèle, mais aussi enfreignait une règle thérapeutique essentielle: pré-

5 «Et cum hoc intelligendum est quod terminacio ad malum non est ita certa sicut terminacio ad bonum, quia motus nature sunt ordinati adherentes vie uni et ordini uni. Motus autem morbi sunt inordinatissimi, et ideo non est ita certus terminus mortis sicut vite» (A. Alonso Guardo (éd.), *Los pronosticos médicos en la medicina medieval. El «Tractatus de crisi et de diebus creticis» de Bernardo de Gordonio*, Valladolid 2003, pp. 368–370, particula IV, cap. 13, quod docet pronosticare diem et horam mortis). Monographie de référence sur Bernard de Gordon: L. E. Demaitre, *Doctor Bernard de Gordon. Professor and Practitioner*, Toronto 1980.

6 Bernard de Gordon, *Lilium medicine*, IV.7, Lyon 1551, p. 374: «Intelligendum etiam quod sanies in concavitate pectoris existens frequenter deludit medicum, quoniam ut plurimum iudicantur phthisici et incurabiles, et inde sanie mundificata evadunt, quod est medico ignominiosum». Michel Savonarole, *Practica maior*, VI.10.15, Venise 1559: «Item nota quod semper sanies apparens in fundo non significat semper empima. Et similiter etiam neque est sufficiens signum significans super ptisim ut in sequenti rubrica. Unde ex hoc deluduntur quandoque medici iudicantes empicum esse ptisicum, unde iudicant egritudinem incurabilem, et mundificata sanie curantur quidem postea, est eis ignominiosum». Sur Michel Savonarole, le grand-père de Jérôme, voir: C. Crisciani – G. Zuccolin (éds.), *Michele Savonarola. Medicina e cultura di corte* (Micrologus' Library; 37), Florence 2011.

server autant que possible l'espoir et la confiance du patient.[7] Au-delà des déclarations générales et des prescriptions déontologiques, le discours sur les pratiques fait ainsi transparaître des ambiguïtés, des options délicates qui portèrent les médecins à restreindre les questions d'éthique aux limites strictes de leur art et des justifications que pouvaient apporter les fondements théoriques de celui-ci.[8] Le sujet de la morale ordinaire, des bonnes mœurs, ne pouvait toutefois être complètement éludé, qu'il s'agisse des bonnes mœurs du praticien ou de celles des patients.

LE BON MEDECIN DOIT-IL AVOIR DE BONNES MŒURS?

Depuis les temps hippocratiques les qualités morales que doit avoir le médecin ont donné lieu à l'énoncé de préceptes en une répétition souvent stéréotypée.[9] Dans son *Conciliator*, commencé à Paris et terminé à Padoue en 1310, Pietro d'Abano passe en revue l'ensemble de la tradition livresque consacré à ce sujet, tout en tenant des propos déconcertants.[10] La *differentia* 7 pose la question, souvent soulevée dans la médecine médiévale, s'il est souhaitable de recourir à plusieurs médecins. Après une argumentation faisant notamment appel à la *Politique* d'Aristote et une comparaison avec le gouvernement de la cité, Pietro d'Abano déclare qu'il peut être approprié d'avoir plusieurs médecins au chevet d'un patient, tant dans la cure que dans la préservation de la santé, à condition qu'ils soient placés sous l'autorité de l'un d'entre eux, d'un *principalior*. Ce «plus principal» doit être *prudentior*, la vertu de «prudence» étant en effet la qualité requise pour un artisan, qui met en pratique un savoir théorique et a affaire au contingent et au particulier,[11] il doit être aussi *sollertior* («le plus habile»), *magis sollicitus*

7 Une phrase du *De anima* (IV.4) d'Avicenne est en ce contexte souvent citée: «Attende dispositionem infirmi cum credit se convalescere, aut sani cum credit se aegrotare: multotiens enim contingit ex hoc ut cum corroboratur forma in anima eius, patiatur ex ea ipsius materia et proveniat ex hoc sanitas aut infirmitas, et est haec actio efficacior quam id quod agit medicus instrumentis suis et mediis» (*Avicenna Latinus. Liber de anima sive Sextus de naturalibus*, éd. S. van Riet, Louvain / Leyde 1968, p. 64). La dernière partie de cette phrase forma une sorte d'adage.

8 C. Crisciani, «Éthique des consilia et de la consultation. À propos de la cohésion morale de la profession médicale (XIIIe–XIVe siècle)», in: *Éthique et pratiques médicales*, pp. 23–43.

9 Outre les échos de traités déontologiques inclus dans la Collection hippocratique qui circulent en latin dès le haut Moyen Âge, avant la traduction du *De lege* (voir l'article de Michael McVaugh dans le présent volume), cette tradition fut aussi intégrée dans des traductions d'œuvres arabes. Par exemple, dès la fin du XIe siècle, le Pantegni de Constantin l'Africain intègre le traité *Quel doit être le disciple en médecine*, qui forme un chapitre de son original arabe. Sur ce traité hippocratique voir J. Jouanna, «Hippocrate et la Collection hippocratique dans l'Ars medicinae», *Revue d'Histoire des Textes* 23 (1993), pp. 95–111.

10 Monographie de référence sur Pietro d'Abano: E. Paschetto, *Pietro d'Abano medico e filosofo*, Florence 1984. Pour le *Conciliator*, je me référerai à la reproduction (Padoue 1985) de l'édition de Venise 1565.

11 P. Aubenque, *La prudence chez Aristote*, Paris 1963.

(«le plus soucieux», le plus impliqué en quelque sorte) et *ab egroto amplius affectatus* («le plus aimé du patient»). À travers cette dernière indication se retrouve l'idée selon laquelle la confiance portée au praticien contribue grandement à la santé. Après avoir indiqué que les autres médecins réunis autour de ce *principalior* doivent être, en tant que scrupuleux ministres de la nature, savants, compétents et dévoués, Pietro d'Abano insère une remarque qui lui permet de revenir à l'astrologie, son sujet favori. Mais auparavant il avait glissé une perfidie contre les médecins de basse extraction au comportement de parvenus, qui, si elle ne vise pas quelques confrères peu estimés, renvoie peut-être à la Rome antique, où la profession médicale était souvent l'apanage d'esclaves ou d'affranchis, plutôt qu'à une réalité sociologique du temps de Pietro d'Abano.[12]

> Mais il faut savoir que pour la plupart les médecins ont pour des raisons avérées de mauvaises mœurs. Soit parce que d'extraction vile et misérable ils se gonflent et deviennent injurieux lorsqu'ils se sont de quelque manière engraissés. Soit parce que la science médicale dans sa partie absolument curative est surtout assignée au Scorpion et à Mars, dont les propriétés tendant vers le mal ont déjà été évoquées;[13] quant à la partie conservatrice de la médecine elle est plus assignée au Taureau et à Vénus, qui poussent ceux [qui sont sous leur influence] à toute triple luxure. Cependant ceux qui sont astrologiquement de mauvaises mœurs du fait de l'influence du Scorpion et de Mars dominant en eux, en vertu de l'assignation [astrale] se trouvent être des médecins parfaits. D'où il ressort que le bon médecin doit être naturellement de mauvaises mœurs, d'une part parce que cette science ne traite ni des vertus ni des mœurs acquises, comme le font beaucoup d'autres [sciences], mais seulement des naturelles, comme il est dit dans le Tegni, d'autre part en raison d'une mauvaise configuration astrale opposée à la moralité.[14]

On ne saurait être plus clair: la médecine n'a que peu à voir avec la morale, qui n'est pas son objet. Elle ne traite que des dispositions naturelles, innées, non des vertus acquises, ainsi que le dit l'*Ars medica* de Galien dans sa partie dévolue aux tempéraments du cœur: «tout ce qui a été écrit des caractères ou bien à l'instant, ou bien dans quelque autre traité, pour établir un diagnostic du tempérament, a visé non pas les caractères bons ou mauvais résultant d'une attitude philosophique, mais ceux innés en chacun».[15] Relativement à la personne du médecin,

12 J. André, *Être médecin à Rome*, Paris 1987; H. W. Pleket, «The Social Status of Physicians in the Graeco-Roman World», in: P. J. van der Eijk – H. F. Horstlanshoff – P. H. Schrijvers (éds.), *Ancient Medicine in its Socio-Cultural Context*, Amsterdam 1995, pp. 27–34.

13 À la *differentia* 2, voir ci-dessous.

14 Pietro d'Abano, *differentia* 7, propter tertium, Venise 1565, fol. 10v: «Est autem sciendum quod medici merito utplurimum malorum extant morum. Tum quia ex vili stirpe et sterili origine contraxerunt, intumescentes demum et contumeliosi facti cum fuerint aliqualiter incrassati, tum quia medicinae scientia et simpliciter curativa maxime Scorpioni attributa est et Marti, quorum proprietates in malum tendentes iam sunt tactae, conservativa vero magis Tauro et Veneri, hos in omnem trinam incitantibus luxuriam, istos tamen qui stellariter pravorum morum existunt propter virtutem Scorpionis et Martis in eis dominantem ob attributionis virtutem perfectos reperio medicos. Unde naturaliter probus medicus malorum debet esse morum, tum etiam quia scientia haec non de virtutibus, sed de naturalibus tantum, in Techni, tumque propter astralitatem quamque pravam moralitati oppositam».

15 Galien, *Art médical*, XI.7 (Collection des universités de France: Série grecque; 402), trad. V. Boudon, Paris 2000, p. 309.

s'ajoutent à cet argument, qui place l'art médical hors du champ moral, des considérations astrologiques: plus l'horoscope du médecin favorise ses compétences, plus il l'induit à avoir de mauvaises mœurs. Faut-il en déduire qu'un praticien puisse afficher ostensiblement des mœurs dépravées? La tradition hippocratique relayée par de nombreux auteurs brosse au contraire un portrait moral des plus flatteurs du bon médecin. Pietro d'Abano avait repris en une longue énumération toutes les qualités requises, telles que décrites dans cette tradition, à la *differentia* 2 qui posait une question *a priori* étrangère à ce sujet: la connaissance de la logique est-elle utile au médecin? Au cours de l'argumentation il était demandé quelles étaient les dispositions et les habitudes «plus extérieures au médecin», c'est-à-dire ne faisant pas partie intrinsèquement de son art, mais touchant à son comportement dans ses relations avec les malades ou ses confrères et à l'image qu'il devait donner dans la société. Une distinction était opérée entre les dispositions relevant de son apparence corporelle et celles relevant de l'âme, ces dernières menant inévitablement à la question de la moralité. Un renvoi était déjà fait à ce qui allait être dit dans la *differentia* 7: «bien que le médecin expert (*peritus medicus*) soit naturellement de mœurs rustres (*agrestium morum*), cependant par l'habitude et par l'art il doit s'efforcer d'acquérir des mœurs louables». Son mérite en sera d'autant plus grand que son horoscope y sera contraire.[16] Outre que décrire le médecin compétent sous les traits d'un rustre débauché n'était guère conforme à la tradition hippocratique, Pietro d'Abano, à cette occasion comme à d'autres, se trouvait confronté à la redoutable question du déterminisme psychologique. L'exemple de la disposition astrale du bon médecin fournissait donc l'occasion de proclamer, à l'intention d'éventuels censeurs ecclésiastiques, la préservation du libre-arbitre. Le long excursus de la *differentia* 2 énumérait ainsi les qualités morales que devaient acquérir le médecin, en dépit de ses dispositions naturelles défavorables. Etaient alors indiqués les caractères à endosser (*habitus*) et les caractères à retrancher (*privatio*). Parmi les premiers figuraient l'amour et la crainte de Dieu, l'assiduité à l'étude, la chasteté, la miséricorde, le zèle auprès des patients, le bon comportement auprès des disciples etc. Parmi les traits de caractère à gommer étaient citées l'envie, la cupidité, l'ivrognerie, la luxure et, en un rappel du serment hippocratique, la prescription de poisons et d'abortifs. Au sein des qualités relevant du corps, qui décrivaient le bon médecin comme ni trop grand, ni trop petit, ni trop beau, ni trop laid, propre et de bonne odeur, était abordé le sujet de la rémunération qui par un détour dont Pietro d'Abano avait le secret ramenait aux prédispositions astrales. Si le médecin ne doit pas pressurer les pauvres, il lui faut veiller à sa rémunération, qui renforce sa réputation et par voie de conséquence la confiance que lui portent les patients. Sa vigilance sur ce point

16 Pietro d'Abano, *Conciliator*, *differentia* 2, propter tertium, fol. 4v: «Licet enim peritus medicus naturaliter agrestium sit morum *differentia* 7, consuetudine tamen et arte conari debet laudabiles acquirere, qui et magis sic erit appreciatus quando contra eius tali freno rationis operabitur nativitatis signatores».

doit être d'autant plus grande que Mars qui préside au traitement curatif est aussi la planète de la non-récompense, des reproches et de l'iniquité.[17]

La question du pronostic et de la prudence qu'il requiert retient longuement Pietro d'Abano, qui cite à ce propos de multiples autorités. Son conseil général est d'user d'astuce et de sagacité et d'éviter de se prononcer de manière absolue sur une issue fatale en se référant au plus probable, à ce qui arrive le plus souvent (*ad plurimum contingens*).[18] Il est bon d'user d'une formule du type: «Cela se passe ainsi dans de tels cas, cependant pas de manière nécessaire, nous voyons en effet des hommes avoir six doigts ou l'un d'entre eux plus court; en effet, la monstruosité arrive dans les maladies, comme dans les natures». Les jugements du médecin doivent être, comme ceux de l'astrologue, liés continuellement à des conditions, «comme d'interprétation multiple (*quasi multiplici intellectu*)». Pietro d'Abano rejoint ici son contemporain Bernard de Gordon, mais plus dans la proposition de modèles de formules à l'intention des malades: il ne s'agit pas tant de préserver le praticien d'une erreur de pronostic que de ménager le patient. La feinte, la dissimulation sont jugées préférables à une annonce certaine de la mort, en arguant des «monstruosités», des anomalies dans le déroulement des maladies qui peuvent mener à une guérison imprévue. Un autre argument, d'ordre religieux, peut être avancé pour faire comprendre au patient que son cas est sérieux, sans pour autant lui ôter tout espoir et sans paraître porter atteinte aux prérogatives du Créateur: un miracle divin est toujours possible.[19] Annoncer la mort avec certitude relève d'une vaine gloire que souhaite acquérir le praticien en montrant sa perspicacité et sa compétence: en filigrane, se lit à nouveau chez Pietro d'Abano une prudente mise à distance d'un déterminisme absolu, surtout si les astres s'en mêlent. Mais surtout l'annonce certaine d'une issue fatale, de toute façon hors de la portée du médecin, risque d'ôter tout espoir au malade et de précipiter sa mort, en le privant de la confiance nécessaire à sa guérison et en incitant son entourage à relâcher son zèle. La prudence est également conseillée pour annoncer une issue favorable et, à ce propos, on retrouve la tradition du commentaire au premier aphorisme d'Hippocrate: pour arriver à la bonne fin espérée, il faut que le malade soit obéissant, l'entourage adapté, et que les contingences extérieures ne viennent pas ap-

17 Ibid., fol. 5r: «Non tamen velis pauperes opprimere neque egenos saltem intuitu pietati disserere, cum inde laudabilis consurgat fama. Quod enim abundanter accepisti, his velis gratis primae amore bonitatis impartiri. Numquam autem sis oblati obnegator, nisi fortassis prius intulerit tanti, et maxime cum minor aut mediocris fueris medicorum, quoniam medicina et maxime curativa Marti est scripta, qui omnibus fere planetis iudicatur odiosior, hic etiam irremunerationis, obiurgii et omnis iniquitatis extat planeta».

18 Ibid.: «Amplius oportet etiam denuo medicum esse astutum ac sagacem in futurorum maxime pronuntiatione, nunquam enim quid absolute pronuntiandum, sed sub conditione dicendum id ad plurimum contingere contrahere».

19 Ibid.: «Ideo medici oportet iudicia, sicut etiam astrologi, fore conditionibus alligata continue quasi multiplici intellectu [...] ut dicatur exempli gratia: 'Ita solet in talibus casibus contingere, non tamen necessario, videmus enim quandoque senos digitos in homine et collobium habentem et huiusmodi. Nam et monstruositas interdum occurrit in egritudinibus velut in naturis' [...] tunc enim dicendum est salutem ipsius quasi ex miraculo divino posse ac non aliter contingere».

porter quelque obstacle.[20] En ce condensé de prescriptions déontologiques que fait Pietro d'Abano, en une sorte d'antidote anticipé aux propos provocateurs sur les prédispositions astrologiques du bon médecin qu'il va tenir dans la *differentia* 7, se discernent les réquisits en ce début du XIVe siècle: préserver la respectabilité du praticien dans la société, en s'appuyant sur la conviction, sincère ou non, que la confiance a des effets physiques;[21] laisser à Dieu ce qui lui revient, en particulier dans la délimitation du nécessaire et du contingent.

LE MEDECIN ET LES MŒURS DU PATIENT

La part laissée obligatoirement au divin fixe au Moyen Âge les limites entre les domaines de la morale, du ressort de l'âme, et de la médecine qui doit se restreindre au corps, avec toute la difficulté, essentielle, de déterminer où se situe précisément la frontière. Qu'ils aient frôlé la transgression, comme Pietro d'Abano, ou observé la plus stricte orthodoxie, les médecins n'eurent pas moins à situer leur propres conseils selon leur évaluation de ce qui revenait respectivement au physiologique et à l'exercice de la raison et de la volonté de leurs patients. Le substrat galénique de leur théorie, avec ses hésitations quant à la nature de l'âme, ne leur facilitait pas la tâche, non plus que les prises de position fermes d'un Avicenne, qui, malgré quelques contradictions dans le détail de son discours médical, considérait en tant que philosophe le niveau rationnel comme totalement détaché des puissances sensitives et donc de toute influence corporelle.[22] Commentant le *Canon* d'Avicenne dans la première moitié du XVe siècle, alors qu'il s'était retiré de la Faculté de médecine de Paris pour vivre durant de longues années à Tournai et à Cambrai, où il était chanoine, Jacques Despars n'élude pas la question de ces frontières, sans pour autant opérer de transgression. Observateur critique de ses contemporains, il déplore autant la dépravation des mœurs de certains que les excès de religiosité d'autres qui aboutissent au même résultat d'une dégradation de la santé.[23] Dès le début de son commentaire, il aborde le sujet de la morale, alors

20 Ibid.: «Evasuros etiam cum conditione et necessitate pronuntiabis predictae simili, iudicando ipsum rationabiliter salvaturum, si medicum diligentem habuerit, sitque infirmus obediens et ministri idonei, ac necessaria preparata extrinseca neque aliquid supervenerit inostensum».

21 Pietro d'Abano consacre un long développement à ce sujet: *differentia* 135.

22 L. G. Ballester, *Alma y enfermedad en la obra de Galeno*, Valence 1972; R. J. Hankinson, «Body and Soul in Galen», in: R. A. King (éd.), *Common to Body and Soul*, Berlin 2006, pp. 231–257; P. Manuli – M. Vegetti (éds.), *Le opere psicologiche di Galeno*, Naples 1988; J. Barnes – J. Jouanna (éds.), *Galien et la philosophie* (Entretiens sur l'Antiquité classique; 49), Vandœuvres / Genève 2003. M. Sebti, *Avicenne. L'âme humaine*, Paris 2000; D. Jacquart, «Avicenne et la nosologie galénique. L'exemple des maladies du cerveau», in: A. Hasnawi – A. Elamrani-Jamal – M. Aouad (éds.), *Perspectives arabes et médiévales sur la tradition scientifique et philosophique grecque*, Louvain / Paris 1997, pp. 217–226; D. N. Hasse, *Avicenna's «De anima» in the Latin West. The formation of a peripatetic philosophy of the soul 1160–1300* (Warburg Institute Studies and Texts; 1), Londres / Turin 2000.

23 D. Jacquart, «Le regard d'un médecin sur son temps. Jacques Despars (1380?–1458)», *Bibliothèque de l'Ecole des chartes* 138 (1980), pp. 35–86 [reproduit dans D. Jacquart, *La sci-*

que le texte du *Canon* n'y incitait pas. Avicenne rappelait la subdivision de la médecine en théorique et pratique, précisant que par «pratique» il ne fallait pas entendre l'opération effective ni l'intervention manuelle sur les corps, mais la science du mode d'opérer. Parmi les *dubia* soulevés par ce passage fameux, Jacques Despars pose la question classique de savoir si la médecine est un art libéral ou un art mécanique. Après une série d'arguments plaidant en faveur de son statut d'art libéral, est évoquée la manière dont elle peut être considérée aussi comme un art mécanique.

> Un art est dit libéral car il tend au bien de l'âme et en traite, et un art est dit mécanique car il œuvre pour le bien du corps. Ainsi l'art de la médecine n'est libéral que par voie de conséquence, en tant qu'il tempère la complexion humaine, une tempérance que suivent la répression des mauvaises inclinations et le penchant aux bonnes mœurs, mais l'art de la médecine est d'une certaine manière mécanique et assujetti à la philosophie morale.[24]

Si la discussion du statut de la médecine menait traditionnellement à postuler ses liens avec toutes les branches de la philosophie, y compris l'éthique, il est intéressant de noter ici que ce n'est pas par son versant théorique, spéculatif, que Jacques Despars établit un lien avec la morale, mais par son action sur la complexion, qui peut mener *de facto* à l'amendement des mœurs. À l'appui de ce qui vient d'être énoncé est cité un passage du début de la *Méthode thérapeutique* où Galien se référait lui-même au *Phèdre* (270c–d) de Platon et s'adressant à Thessalos déclarait: «Homme de très noble naissance, tu l'as entendu, Platon demande que les efforts pour faire des découvertes dans le domaine de l'âme s'effectuent avec une méthode exactement semblable à celle d'Hippocrate pour le domaine corporel».[25] La version arabo-latine qu'utilise Jacques Despars déforme quelque peu le propos de cette phrase en faisant de l'étude de la médecine un préalable à l'étude plus noble de l'âme humaine, ce qui mène le commentateur à citer une formule devenue de son temps une sorte d'adage: «si l'on veut soigner l'âme il faut d'abord soigner le corps».[26] Sans le reconnaître ouvertement, Jacques Despars, dans son œuvre tout entière, comme la plupart de ses contemporains médecins, délivre une morale en même temps qu'une médecine, une morale de la tempérance.[27] En

ence médicale occidentale entre deux renaissances (XIIes.–XVes.) (Variorum Collected Studies Series; 567), Aldershot 1997, n. 14].

24 Jacques Despars, commentaire au *Canon* d'Avicenne, I.1.1.1, Lyon 1498: «Quarto dicitur liberalis aliqua ars, quoniam ad bonum anime dirigit et de ipso tractat, et mechanica, quia agit de bono corporis, sic ars medicine non est liberalis nisi ex consequenti inquantum scilicet temperat humanam complexionem, ad cuius temperiem sequitur repressio malarum inclinationum et pronitas ad bonos mores, sed quodammodo mechanica est subiectaque morali philosophie».

25 Galien, *Méthode de traitement*, trad. et annot. par J. Boulogne, Paris 2009, p. 54 (*Prolégomènes*).

26 Jacques Despars, comm., I.1.1.1: «Iuxta illud Galieni primo de ingenio sanitatis: si animus alicuius ad artem ceteris digniorem transcendere cupit id est ad tutelam sanitatis anime, necesse est tamen ut primitus in hac, scilicet medicina, que minus est digna studiosius laboret. Nam si quis animam curare voluerit oportet ut ante curet corpus».

27 D. Jacquart, «Médecine et morale. Les cinq sens chez Evrard de Conty (m. 1405)», *Micrologus* 10 (2002), pp. 365–378.

outre, s'il est d'avis, à la suite de Galien et de ce qu'énonce la *Physiognomonie* du pseudo-Aristote, que les états de l'âme suivent les dispositions du corps, tout particulièrement sa complexion, il ne néglige pas de faire appel à la responsabilité des patients, à leur volonté.

La question de savoir s'il est possible de trouver un homme tempéré *ad iustitiam* – selon le vocabulaire technique qui distingue cet état d'équilibre relatif des qualités d'une complexion de l'équilibre parfait (*ad pondus*) jugé inatteignable chez un homme ordinaire[28] – mène au topos de l'affaiblissement de la nature humaine depuis les temps anciens, un topos que les dernières années de la Guerre de Cent ans et les poussées répétées de la peste ne peuvent que renforcer. Les principes de la génération et de la vie sont affaiblis, tant en raison des épidémies, des mutations de l'air dues en partie au ciel et en partie aux corruptions provoquées par les cadavres engendrés par les guerres atroces des hommes que du fait de la débauche, de l'intempérance en matière de boissons et de nourriture: *omnes enim hodie pene filii sunt crapule*. Ivrognerie et gloutonnerie se joignent dans cette *crapula*, qui touche spécialement les princes et les nobles. Si l'on parcourt le monde, conclut Jacques Despars, et que l'on rencontre autant d'hommes que possible, on trouvera plus vite un phénix qu'un homme tempéré *ad iustitiam*.[29] Les distinctions des complexions en fonction des âges de la vie conduisent de même à relier intimement dispositions corporelles et attitudes mentales. L'âge dit de l'*adolescentia*, qui correspond au développement de l'individu et le mène jusque vers trente ans, est le plus difficile à délimiter car d'un homme à un autre des variations sont induites par le régime, l'exercice, les maladies, mais aussi les mœurs.[30] Alors que sur le sujet de l'équilibre de la complexion en fonction de l'âge, Avicenne restait sur le strict plan des qualités corporelles, son commentateur fait intervenir les aptitudes intellectuelles et l'exercice de la volonté. Ainsi le temps de la vieillesse (ou de l'âge mûr, entre environ quarante et soixante ans), qui précède le grand âge, est celui de la sagesse, car les activités qui sont le propre de l'homme atteignent la perfection; les facultés supérieures fleurissent, car la volonté est alors mieux réglée et suit très peu les passions: la raison est en cet âge parée de vertus et l'intellect nourri de savoir. Puisque une complexion tempérée se décèle dans les actions de l'homme qui en est doté, l'âge de la vieillesse, qui permet les opérations les plus parfaites dans les activités humaines les plus élevées,

28 Sur cette distinction, voir: P. G. Ottosson, *Scholastic Medicine and Philosophy. A Study of Commentaries on Galen's «Tegni»*, Naples 1988.

29 Jacques Despars, comm., I.1.3.1: «Dubitatur circa primam et secundam partes utrum sit dare hominem temperatum ad iustitiam. Quod non arguitur primo: principia generationis et vite sunt debilitata ab eo quod olim, tum propter pestes et alias magnas immutationes aeris ex parte celi et corruptiones cadaverales ex atrocibus hominum bellis, tum propter luxus et intemperantias ebrietatum et comestionum. Omnes enim hodie pene filii sunt crapule [...] Incede per orbem et vide homines quot volueris citius fenicem invenies quam hominem talem [temperatum ad iustitiam]».

30 Ibid., I.1.3.3: «maior est diversitas in adolescentia quoad regimen et motus et mores et egritudines occurentes quam in quacunque alia etate».

pourrait bien le mieux répondre à cet état. Toutefois, ce n'est pas à mettre au compte véritablement de l'équilibre de la complexion.

> À propos de l'argument selon lequel la vieillesse a les actions de l'âme rationnelle et les vertus de celle-ci, à savoir l'intellect, la volonté et la raison, les plus achevées. Dis premièrement que cela ne vient pas de l'équilibre de la complexion car celles-ci n'usent ni de la complexion ni d'un organe corporel dans leurs actions [...] Dis deuxièmement que les actions de l'âme rationnelle ne sont pas plus achevées chez les hommes âgés que chez les jeunes en raison de leur âge, mais du fait des études et des expériences rassemblées depuis longtemps, d'où ils ont tiré une manière d'être en sciences et en vertus, et parce que de nature plus froide ils sont moins tyrannisés par les passions.[31]

Sur un sujet hautement médical comme celui de l'équilibre de la complexion, Jacques Despars n'a pu se limiter aux seules caractéristiques physiques et a envisagé l'être humain tout entier, corps et âme. Bien qu'il s'en tienne à l'orthodoxie en réaffirmant que l'âme rationnelle n'use ni de la complexion ni d'un organe corporel, il insinue que le refroidissement naturel propre à l'âge dit de la vieillesse joue quelque rôle dans la plénitude des facultés qui en dépendent en diminuant la tyrannie exercée par les passions.

S'écartant de la ligne indiquée par Avicenne, Jacques Despars considère que le médecin ne peut s'abstenir de s'intéresser à la rationalité et à la volonté humaines. La question du mal est même posée à l'occasion d'un développement sur la mort dite «naturelle», c'est-à-dire celle qui intervient à un terme déterminé pour chaque individu par sa complexion première et sa capacité à préserver son humide radical, lorsque quelque accident ou faute de régime ne vient pas provoquer un abrègement. Selon Avicenne, aussi bien le terme naturel que l'abrègement proviennent d'un ordre divin. Le commentateur éprouve une réticence à considérer que des maux tels que le crime, le suicide ou la débauche qui entraîne un abrègement de la vie puissent avoir une origine divine. En effet, il n'y a pas de déterminisme absolu, pas de *fatum*: l'homme dispose de son libre-arbitre. Tout en laissant aux théologiens le sujet de la prédestination, il rappelle que si Dieu permet les actions mauvaises, il n'est pas la cause de celles-ci.[32]

31 Ibid.: «Ad rationem de senectute quod habet operationes anime rationalis et virtutes eius, id est intellectum, voluntatem et rationem, perfectiores. Dic primo quod illud non est ex parte temperamenti complexionis cum nec complexione nec organo corporeo utantur in suis operationibus [...] Dic secundo quod operationes anime rationalis non sunt perfectiores in senibus quam in iuvenibus ratione etatis, sed propter studia et experientias diu ante frequentatas, unde contraxerunt habitus scientiarum et virtutum et quia refrigerati minus ab animi passionibus tyrannisantur».

32 Ibid.: «Dubitatur tertio utrum termini abbreviati individuorum divino proveniant precepto. Videtur quod sic per principem [Avicennam] hic dicentem: 'Sunt vero et alii termini abbreviati, totum tamen provenit divino precepto' [...] Oppositum arguitur, quia multi termini abbreviantur per proditiones, intoxicationes, desperationes, homicidia, luxus, crapulas. Tales autem difformitates et seva scelera nephas videtur ascribere divino precepto [...] Dic ergo ad quesitum relinquendo materias predestinationis et prescientie divine theologis que sunt de altissimis et difficilioribus apud eos quod termini abbreviati quicumque proveniant divina permissione [...] dic quod deus actus difformes permittit, sed non est causa difformitatis, cum difformitas sit boni privatio et deus sit summa bonitas».

Les chapitres du *Canon* consacrés aux facultés cérébrales fixent la limite de la compétence médicale, à laquelle échappent, selon Avicenne, les facultés dépendant de l'âme rationnelle.[33] Malgré cette mise à l'écart, Jacques Despars dit ne pouvoir se retenir d'en traiter quelque peu, «par amour de la philosophie» et en raison de l'alliance de celle-ci avec la médecine. La faculté humaine rationnelle est ce qui forme le propre de l'homme, et le rend différent de tous les autres animaux. Comprenant la volonté, l'intellect et la raison, elle considère ce qu'est la fin de l'homme et les moyens pour parvenir à cette fin. Tandis qu'à la raison est dévolue la recherche des moyens, c'est la volonté qui entre en jeu si la fin visée est le bien et l'intellect, si c'est le vrai.[34] Le statut de la volonté est l'objet d'attention de la part de Jacques Despars, car c'est par elle que le sujet humain choisit de suivre ou non ses penchants naturels, de se laisser dominer par les prédispositions de sa complexion ou d'obéir à la raison en les contrôlant et en les contrecarrant. Il en est longuement traité à propos de la faculté motrice, et en particulier de celle qui régit le mouvement volontaire. Est-elle unique ou est-elle formée de plusieurs? En effet elle ne peut se résumer à un appétit, car, par exemple, «des hommes religieux et continents ont souvent l'appétit d'actes vénériens ou de somptueux et magnifiques festins et d'abondantes libations, mais ils ne suivent pas leurs désirs, et obéissent à la raison».[35] Le sujet des passions mène encore plus directement à situer la responsabilité morale et, par voie de conséquence, la compétence médicale.

> Observe premièrement que les passions de l'âme ont quatre causes subordonnées les unes aux autres. La première [cause] est l'objet délectable ou attristant. La deuxième est la faculté [sensitive] de l'âme qui saisit cet objet. La troisième est la faculté motrice qui commande suivant l'exigence de la passion suscitée à fuir ou à poursuivre. La quatrième est la faculté motrice commandée qui, située dans le cœur, suivant l'ordre de la dite faculté meut le sang et l'esprit [vital] vers l'intérieur ou vers l'extérieur. Observe deuxièmement que relativement au genre il y a deux passions de l'âme auxquelles toutes se réduisent, à savoir le plaisir et la douleur, renvoyant de manière générale à une appréhension d'un bien et d'un mal tant par les sens externes que par les facultés internes de saisie [les sens internes]. En effet au plaisir sont reconduits l'amour, la joie, l'espoir, l'audace. A la douleur, la haine, la tristesse, la peur et le désespoir. Observe troisièmement que les médecins ne considèrent pas les accidents de l'âme

33 Avicenne, *Canon*, I.1.6.5, trad. Gérard de Crémone, Venise 1507 (reprod. Hildesheim 1964), fol. 25r: «Virtus vero comprehensiva que est una de virtutibus anime comprehensivis est humana rationalis. Et quia medici virtutem existimativam non consideraverunt propter causam quam diximus, ideo hanc virtutem non consideraverunt».

34 Jacques Despars, comm., I.1.6.5: «Et licet minus attineat medico de virtutibus rationalis anime tractare quam de estimativa, propterea quod separate sunt a corporeo organo, estimativa vero non, continere tamen nequeo quin de ipsis aliquid dicam amore philosophie et federationis eius cum medicina [...] Attende primo quod virtus humana rationalis est que proprie convenit homini secundum quod homo est et qua differt a ceteris animalibus [...] triplex est virtus humana rationalis, scilicet voluntas et intellectus et ratio. Omnis virtus humana rationalis vel directe respicit finem hominis vel media ad finem. Si media sic est ratio. Si finem vel sub ratione boni et est voluntas, vel sub ratione veri et est intellectus».

35 Ibid., I.1.6.6: «Virtus motiva non est appetitus tantum. Probatur quia viri religiosi et continentes sepe appetunt venereos actus et epulari laute et splendide et abunde bibere, non tamen sequuntur desideria sua, sed parent rationi».

> dans leur relation aux vertus de concupiscible et d'irascible dont ils sont les passions, ni selon le comportement en bien et en mal à l'égard de ceux-ci qui rend une âme vicieuse, mais en tant qu'ils altèrent le corps humain de diverses manières, à savoir en échauffant ou en refroidissant, en desséchant ou en humidifiant, en relâchant ou en affaiblissant.[36]

Dans cet excursus philosophico-médical, il est intéressant de noter le changement de vocabulaire: des «passions de l'âme» on est passé à l'expression devenue technique dans le discours médical d' «accidents de l'âme». Ce passage d'un registre lexical à un autre marque la frontière entre le moral et le médical. Mais un médecin peut-il se borner à traiter les effets physiques des passions? Les interrogations de Jacques Despars tendent à suggérer fortement que le statut particulier de l'homme, qui le rend apte par l'exercice de la raison et de la volonté à réfréner ses passions et à redresser les penchants induits par sa complexion naturelle, impose au médecin de le traiter dans sa globalité et de prendre en compte la part irréductible à son corps seul. Multiples sont les sujets sur lesquels médecine et morale se rejoignent. C'est le cas de l'ivresse. Avicenne indique que, selon certains – sous lesquels on peut notamment reconnaître Râzî –, un enivrement périodique, une à deux fois par mois, est conseillé.[37] Dans son *Lilium medicine* Bernard de Gordon remarquait que le but de cette pratique étant de purifier le corps par le vomissement, la sudation ou la diarrhée consécutifs à l'enivrement, il valait mieux recourir à d'autres modes de purgation. Il considérait cette ivresse périodique comme un moyen *ignominiosum* et non dépourvu de danger, car une apoplexie pouvait intervenir avant le vomissement escompté. En conclusion, il rejetait ce recours hors du domaine de la spéculation médicale. Il se gardait de reprendre l'effet cal-

36 Ibid., I.2.2.1.14: «Attende primo quod passionum anime sunt quattuor cause subinvicem subordinate. Prima est obiectum delectabile vel contristabile. Secunda est virtus anime apprehensiva illius obiecti. Tertia est virtus motiva imperans secundum exigentiam passionis illate fugere aut prosequi. Quarta est virtus motiva imperata cordi insita que secundum imperium nunc dicte virtutis movet sanguinem et spiritus intus aut extra. Attende secundo quod due sunt anime passiones secundum genus ad quas omnes reducuntur, scilicet delectatio et dolor, secundum quod communes sunt apprehensionibus boni et mali tam per sensus exteriores quam per vires apprehensivas interiores. Ad delectationem quidem reducuntur amor, gaudium, spes, audacia. Ad dolorem autem odium, tristitia, timor et desperatio. Attende tertio quod medici non considerant anime accidentia secundum relationem ad virtutes concupuscibilem et irascibilem quarum sunt passiones, neque secundum quod ex bene vel male se habere circa ea redditur anima viciosa, sed secundum quod alterant humanum corpus diversimodo, calefaciendo scilicet aut infrigidando, siccando vel humectando vel laxando vel debilitando». Sur l'arrière-plan philosophique et médical du sujet des passions (ou émotions) au Moyen Âge, voir: S. Knuuttila, *Emotions in Ancient and Medieval Philosophy*, Oxford 2004; P. Gil-Sotres, «Modelo teorico y observacion clinica. Las pasiones del alma en la psicologia medical medieval», in: M. Terrasse (éd.), *Comprendre et maîtriser la nature au Moyen Âge. Mélanges d'histoire des sciences offerts à Guy Beaujouan*, Genève 1994, pp. 181–204.

37 Avicenne, *Canon*, I.3.2.8, éd. cit. fol. 61r: «Quibusdam vero visum est quod semel in mense aut bis inebriari confert propterea quod virtutes alleviant animales et requiescere facit et urinam provocat et sudorem et superfluitatem resolvit». Cf. Abû Bakr Mohammad b. Zakarriyya ar-Râzî, *Guide du médecin nomade*, Aphorismes, prés. et trad. par El-Arbi Moubachir, 2e éd., Arles 1996, p. 91.

mant sur les vertus psychiques indiqué par Avicenne.[38] Jacques Despars envisage la question sous divers angles, en appliquant des distinctions suivant l'intensité de l'ivresse. Un argument d'autorité semblait plaider en faveur d'une ivresse forte. Selon l'un des *Problèmes* aristotéliciens une ivresse profonde, qui interdisait tout jugement, était moins dangereuse qu'une légère ébriété qui portait à juger faussement.[39] Malgré l'autorité d'Aristote et le conseil de Râzî relayé par Avicenne, Jacques Despars, tout comme Bernard de Gordon avant lui, n'est pas disposé à préconiser de forts enivrements périodiques. S'il admet qu'une légère ébriété une fois par mois est tolérable et peut même apporter un bienfait au corps, surtout si elle porte à la joie et non à la violence,[40] l'ivresse forte et véhémente est *periculosa, detestabilis, inutilis et multum damnosa*. Elle est dangereuse de divers points de vue: elle peut mener au spasme et à la mort; un accident peut arriver, parfois mortel, si l'homme ivre se met «à trébucher, à tomber sur des pierres, dans une cave, dans un puits, dans une fosse ou une rivière ou à se précipiter d'une hauteur»; elle est aussi dangereuse pour les autres, du fait de la perte du discernement et de l'usage de la raison qui peut entraîner bagarres, blessures, voire homicides ou incendies. Elle est détestable car l'homme perd la dignité que Dieu lui a conférée en le plaçant juste au-dessous des anges et elle le rend inférieur même aux bêtes, lorsque «sous l'excitation du vin il perd l'usage de la raison sachant moins se dominer et se conduire que les animaux sauvages». Elle est inutile car elle n'apporte ni repos ni allègement des facultés psychiques. Elle est enfin nuisible, car elle emplit le cerveau et les nerfs de superfluités et ne fait pas d'autre bien que de provoquer finalement un vomissement.[41]

38 Bernard de Gordon, *Lilium medicine*, II.21, Lyon 1551, p. 215: «Quarto sciendum quod secundm intentionem Avicenne bonum est inebriari semel in mense, non propter ebrietatem, sed quia ad ebrietatem sequitur vomitus, sudor et secessus, que corpus habent mundificare et talis passio per relaxationem ad finem non est morbus. Et cum multi alii sint modi purgationis et hoc est ignominiosum, et etiam non est omnino tutum, quia ante vomitum bene posset incurrere apoplexiam, ideo ab aula nostre speculationis totaliter sit remotum». Sur le sujet des effets du vin dans les textes médicaux médiévaux, voir: A. Jaboulet-Vercherre, *Wine, the Physician and the Drinker. Late Medieval Medical Views on Wine's Uses, Pleasures and Problems*, PhD dissertation, Yale University, 2011.

39 Aristote, *Problèmes*, III.2 (Collection des universités de France), trad. du texte grec par P. Louis, Paris 1991, p. 58: «Pourquoi n'est-ce pas ceux qui sont complètement ivres qui ont le vin mauvais, mais plutôt ceux qui ne sont qu'éméchés?».

40 Jacques Despars, comm., I.3.2.8: «Attende tertio quod duplex est ebrietas. Quedam levis que non tollit usum rationis sed linguam in sermone vacillare facit et in gressu pedes cancellare et mores immutat vel ad letitiam vel ad iram secundum dispositionem subiecti et iudicium pervertit et somnolentum reddit [...] Attende quarto quod ebrietas levis semel in mense tolerabilis est et conferens corpori propter causas dictas precipue in illis qui non rixantur quando sunt ebrii, sed potius querunt ludere et iocari, vinum simie non canis gerentes ut ait vulgus».

41 Ibid.: «Attende quinto quod ebrietas fortis et vehemens est homini periculosa, detestabilis, inutilis et multum damnosa. Periculosa quidem quia quandoque infert spasmum et mortem. Iuxta illud Hypocratis amphorismorum quinta [V.5]: 'Si inebriatus aliquis repente sine voce fiat spasmo innato moritur'. Periculosa iterum quia ebrius se regere nesciens quandoque cespitat, quandoque cadit vel supra lapides vel in celarium vel in puteum vel in foveam vel fluvium vel se ab alto precipitat, unde contunditur, mutilatur et occiditur. Et iterum periculosa

Ces arguments clairement ordonnés et hiérarchisés, portant à condamner l'enivrement périodique violent, rendent un fidèle écho du rôle qu'entend jouer un médecin à la fin du Moyen Âge, entre préservation physique, morale et sociale. Les dommages portés au bon fonctionnement du corps sont indiqués, mais la morale individuelle est prise aussi en compte par la condamnation de ce qui fait perdre à l'homme sa dignité. Enfin, le souci de «l'utilité commune», revendiqué par des médecins universitaires de plus en plus impliqués dans la vie de la cité[42], porte à dénoncer les dangers de l'ivresse pour l'ordre public. Il est clair que le soin des corps implique une attention à ce qui les met en mouvement, c'est-à-dire leur âme, et à les situer dans leur environnement, non seulement naturel mais social.

quia ebrius discretione carens et usu rationis quandoque rixatur, quandoque pugnat his quibus obviat, quandoque vulnerat, quandoque occidit sicut canis rabidus, quandoque domui impellit ignem. Detestabilis autem quia cum rex regum et dominus dominantium minuerit hominem paulominus ab angelis, gloria et honore coronaverit eum et constituerit eum super opera manuum suarum omnia, subiiciens sub pedibus eius infamis abiectis, detestabilis est inferior bestiis dum lacessitate vini perdit usum rationis minus se regere et conducere sciens animalibus brutis. Inutilis vero quia hec ebrietas nec quiescere facit nec alleviat animales virtutes teste Aristotele tertia particula Porblematum [III. 25 bis] querente propter quid ebriis non fit somnus. Damnosa quidem quia superfluitatibus replet cerebrum et nervos neque aliud bonum facit nisi quod interdum vomitum provocat».

42 M. R. McVaugh, *Medicine Before the Plague. Practitioners and their Patients in the Crown of Aragon, 1285–1345*, Cambridge 1993, pp. 190–235; D. Jacquart, *La médecine médiévale dans le cadre parisien, XIVe–XVe siècle*, Paris 1998, pp. 229–323; Nicoud, *Les régimes de santé*, pp. 638–649.

PETRARCA, ARISTOTELES UND DIE KRITIK AN DER SCHOLASTISCHEN MEDIZIN

Klaus Bergdolt

Francesco Petrarca (1304–1374), der „früheste Humanist", der „das Denken seiner Zeit maßgeblich beeinflusste" (Paul Oskar Kristeller[1]), war nicht nur der hochgerühmte Autor des *Canzoniere*, einer viel bewunderten Gedichtsammlung, die unzähligen späteren Autoren als Vorbild diente,[2] sondern dank seiner politischen, philosophischen und gesellschaftskritischen Schriften einer der einflussreichsten europäischen Intellektuellen seiner Zeit.[3] Vor allem gegen die Ärzte, die er, was heute merkwürdig klingen mag, als verachtenswerte Repräsentanten eines *mundus iam senescens*[4] betrachtete, einer ‚vergreisten', durch die ‚Scholastiker' künstlich am Leben gehaltenen mittelalterlichen Welt, führte er einen geistigen Kampf, der die Haltung späterer Humanisten zur Medizin bis hin zur Zeit Vesals beeinflusste.[5] Eine neue, nicht nur in zahlreichen Briefen, der berühmten Autobiographie[6] oder psychologisierenden Werken wie dem 1242/43 in Avignon verfassten *Secretum*[7] demonstrierte Subjektivität, die in der Regel eine kritische Selbstbespiegelung intendierte, wies weit in die Zukunft und widersetzte sich, wie bereits zahl-

1 P. O. Kristeller, *Acht Philosophen der italienischen Renaissance*, Weinheim 1986, S. 4.

2 Francesco Petrarca, *Canzoniere, Triumphe, Verstreute Gedichte*, Italienisch und Deutsch, aus dem Ital. von K. Förster, hg. und mit einem Nachw. vers. von H. Grote, Düsseldorf / Zürich 2002; Francesco Petrarca, *Canzoniere. 50 Gedichte mit Kommentar*, Italienisch-Deutsch, Ditzingen 2006; Francesco Petrarca, *Canzoniere*, Italienisch-Deutsch, ausgew., eingel. und mit Anmerkungen vers. von G. Regn, übertr. von K. Förster, Mainz 1987.

3 Vgl. die unterschiedlich akzentuierten Übersichtsarbeiten, etwa H. W. Eppelsheimer, *Petrarca*, Frankfurt am Main 1926; K. Bergdolt, *Arzt, Krankheit und Therapie bei Petrarca. Die Kritik an Medizin und Naturwissenschaft im italienischen Frühhumanismus*, Weinheim 1992; F. Neumann, *Francesco Petrarca*, Reinbek bei Hamburg 1998; K. Stierle, *Francesco Petrarca. Ein Intellektueller im Europa des 14. Jahrhunderts*, München 2003.

4 Francesco Petrarca, *Invective contra medicum*, Lib. II, 353 (Storia e Letteratura: Raccolta di studi e testi; 32), hg. von P. G. Ricci, Rom 1978, S. 49.

5 Vgl. K. Bergdolt, *Zwischen ‚scientia' und ‚studia humanitatis'. Die Versöhnung von Medizin und Humanismus um 1500* (Nordrhein-Westfälische Akademie der Wissenschaften: Vorträge; G 379), Wiesbaden 2001.

6 Vgl. Francesco Petrarca, *Dichtungen, Briefe, Schriften* (Insel-Taschenbuch; 486), hg. von H. W. Eppelsheimer, Frankfurt am Main 1980, S. 27–37.

7 Vgl. Francesco Petrarca, *Über den geheimen Widerstreit meiner Sorgen. Wege zur Selbsterkenntnis* (Insel-Taschenbuch; 3021), Frankfurt am Main 2004, S. 23–195; Francesco Petrarca, *Secretum meum* (Mein Geheimnis), Lateinisch-Deutsch, hg., übers. und mit einem Nachw. von G. Regn und B. Huss, Mainz 2004.

reiche Zeitgenossen erkannten, ungeachtet beachtlicher Kontinuitäten[8] den tradierten Grenzen des mittelalterlichen Literatur- und Wissenschaftsverständnisses.

Welches waren aber die tieferen Gründe des Dichters, die zeitgenössische Ärzteschaft, aber auch Juristen und Theologen zu attackieren, ja – wenn auch nach allen Regeln antiker Rhetorik – verbal zu beleidigen? Seiner Meinung zufolge war diesen Berufsgruppen an den Universitäten bzw. den (rangmäßig zunächst gleichstehenden) *Studia* kirchlicher Orden ein rigides, ‚rückwärtsgewandtes' Denken und eine provokante Autoritätsgläubigkeit vermittelt worden.[9] Obgleich es die meisten Mediziner nicht ahnen konnten, standen sie – zumindest aus Petrarcas Perspektive – für eine obsolete, ja gefährliche Geisteshaltung, die seiner Meinung nach – heute, wo Scholastik eher mit Theologie in Verbindung gebracht wird, mag auch dieser Vorwurf überraschen! – atheistisch orientiert war, islamischen Einflüssen offen stand, vom Einfluss der Sterne auf das menschliche Handeln überzeugt war und alles Glück in irdischen Gütern suchte.[10] Den Ärzten wurde ferner unterstellt, als ‚Handwerker' auf nichts anderes als eine gute Bezahlung aus zu sein.[11] Eine solch diesseitsorientierte Kunst erschien Petrarca – wie auch die Jurisprudenz, zu deren Studium in Montpellier und Bologna der Vater den Zwölfjährigen einst gezwungen hatte[12] – als charakteristisches Produkt der scholastischen Universität, ihrer Didaktik, Sprache und Methodik. Sie entsprach, so sein Vorwurf, dem Zeitgeist. Aus der altrömischen Literatur, aber auch aus dem ihm verhassten *medium aevum* (Petrarca prägte damit den Begriff ‚Mittelalter'![13]) übernahm der Dichter gleichzeitig Argumente, die bereits Cato und Plinius den Ärzten entgegengeschleudert hatten.[14] Er vermischte sie mit Verbalinjurien, die noch im 19. Jahrhundert einige Kulturhistoriker, darunter Georg Voigt, den Verfasser der *Wiederbelebung des classischen Alterthums* (1859)[15] sowie seinen Biographen Gustav Koerting (1878)[16] wunderten, ja schockierten. Tatsächlich finden sich in den 1355 vollendeten *Invectivae contra medicum* Ausdrücke wie „tu mihi oles"[17] oder „tu es faex ipsa"[18] sowie Beleidigungen, die, vergegenwärtigt man sich die *dulcedo* Petrarcascher Lyrik, zunächst kaum ein- und demselben

8 Hierzu Bergdolt, *Arzt*, S. 135–191; umfassend auch E. R. Curtius, *Europäische Literatur und Lateinisches Mittelalter*, Bern / München 1967.

9 Petrarca stellt diese scholastisch-mittelalterliche Welt bewusst tendenziös dar, so in den *Invectivae*, vgl. Bergdolt, *Arzt*, S. 35, ferner ibd., S. 41–47.

10 So die Palette der Vorwürfe in den *Invective*, vgl. ibd., S. 33–54.

11 Vgl. Bergdolt, *Arzt*, S. 45.

12 Vgl. Petrarca, *Dichtungen*, S. 31.

13 Zu diesem Begriff vgl. A. Buck, *Die humanistische Tradition in der Romania*, Bad Homburg u. a. 1968, S. 36.

14 Vgl. Bergdolt, *Arzt*, S. 135–152.

15 Vgl. G. Voigt, *Die Wiederbelebung des classischen Alterthums oder das erste Jahrhundert des Humanismus*, Bd. 1, 3. Aufl., Berlin 1893 (unveränderter Nachdruck Berlin 1960), S. 74.

16 So sprach Gustav Koerting von „höchst bedenklichen sittlichen Schwächen" Petrarcas, vgl. Ders., *Petrarca's Leben und Werke* (Geschichte der Literatur Italiens im Zeitalter der Renaissance; 1), Leipzig 1878, S. 619.

17 Petrarca, *Invective*, Liber IV, 271, S. 89.

18 Petrarca, ibd., Lib. III, 340, S. 68.

Autor zuzutrauen sind. Der Adressat, einer der Leibärzte des mit dem Tode ringenden Papstes Clemens VI., erscheint als „Dummkopf" (*stulte*)[19], als „unverschämter Handwerker" (*infamis artifex*)[20] und „lächerlicher Zensor der Sitten" (*gravissime morum censor*)[21], als notorischer Lügner[22] und „arroganter Alter"[23], als jemand, „der den Urin beurteilt und dabei nur ans Geld denkt"[24].

Die Bilder und Vorwürfe Petrarcas wurden Topoi einer zeitlosen antimedizinischen und -naturwissenschaftlichen Polemik. Konsequent verachtete er die Werke bedeutender scholastischer Gelehrter, die sich, wie etwa Roger Bacon, Witello, John Peckham und Albertus Magnus im 13. oder Dietrich von Freiberg, Johannes Buridan und Thomas Bradwardine im 14. Jahrhundert, auf hohem Niveau – und oft mit theologischen Intentionen! – mit naturwissenschaftlichen Fragen auseinandergesetzt hatten.[25] Allein die Unterstellung, deren *Opuscula* (der Diminuitiv war selbstverständlich despektierlich gemeint) gelesen zu haben, empfand „der erste moderne Mensch" (Ernest Renan[26]) als beleidigend.

Noch heute erntet man mit der (historisch längst abgesicherten!) These Erstaunen, ja Widerspruch, die naturwissenschaftliche und medizinische Forschung sei im Mittelalter nicht unterdrückt worden, wie das eine hartnäckige, im 19. Jahrhundert festgemeißelte, bis heute im kulturhistorischen Diskurs überlebende Legende suggeriert, die im allgemeinen auch noch um die Behauptung erweitert wird, mit dem Anbruch der Renaissance seien Naturwissenschaften im eigentlichen Sinn erst möglich geworden. Petrarca steht für das Gegenteil! Die *scientiae naturales* – im 13. Jahrhundert hatten sie sich hoher Wertschätzung erfreut! – wurden von den frühen Humanisten, so auch von Giovanni Boccaccio, Coluccio Salutati oder Leonardo Bruni wegen ihrer scholastischen Prägung verachtet und bekämpft.[27]

Auch das sonstige scholastische Schrifttum wurde abgelehnt. Für Petrarca gab es „keinen Duns Scotus, St. Anselm, Thomas von Aquin, Abaelard nur in seinen Liebesbriefen"[28]. Der neue humanistische Diskurs der Subjektivität und Individualität mit seiner stark moralisierenden Tendenz schien mit den alten Bildungsinhalten unvereinbar. Obgleich Petrarca an anderer Stelle – in einer Art Negativrhetorik – beteuerte, dass er niemals etwas „gegen die Medizin und die wirklich

19 Petrarca, ibd., Lib. II, 437, S. 51.
20 Petrarca, ibd., Lib. I, 5–7, S. 25.
21 Petrarca, ibd., Lib. II, 174, S. 44.
22 Petrarca, ibd., Lib. I, 398–402, S. 36.
23 Petrarca, ibd., Lib. II, 6–8, S. 39.
24 Petrarca, ibd., Lib. II, 639–641, S. 57.
25 Hierzu Bergdolt, *Arzt*, S. 9–15.
26 E. Renan, *Averroes et l'Averroisme. Essai Historique*, Paris 1852, S. 260.
27 A. Buck, „Die Medizin im Verständnis des Renaissance-Humanismus", in: *Humanismus und Medizin* (Mitteilung der Kommission für Humanismusforschung; 11), hg. von R. Schmitz und G. Keil, Weinheim 1984, S. 181–198; vgl. auch F. Bausi, „Medicina e filosofia nelle Invective contra Medicum", in: M. Berté – V. Fera – T. Pesenti (Hgg.), *Petrarca e la Medicina. Atti del Convegno di Capo d'Orlando 27–28 Giugno 2003* (Biblioteca umanistica; 8), Messina 2006, S. 19–52.
28 Zit. Eppelsheimer, *Petrarca*, S. 57.

guten Ärzte" hatte sagen wollen,[29] war seine Ärztekritik programmatisch, ja Ausdruck einer geistesgeschichtlich bedeutsamen Kampagne.[30] Was die Medizin in ihrer damaligen Erscheinungsform nach Petrarca nicht zu leisten imstande war, war die Pflege der Seele, die Introspektion, die Gewissensbildung, die Pflege des Schönen und Erhabenen, die Beschäftigung mit Dingen also, die Ärzten als Gefangenen alltäglicher Geschäftigkeit schon durch ihr unentwegtes Engagement, das freie Zeit nicht vorsah, verwehrt blieb. Dass sie sich oft mit beachtlichem Zeitaufwand um ihre Patienten kümmerten, rechnete ihnen Petrarca nicht etwa positiv an, weil sie dafür, so sein hartes Urteil, als „Lohnabhängige" (*mercennarii*) bezahlt wurden.[31] „Du bist ein Sklave des Geldes", bekam der Arzt des Papstes zu hören.[32] Selbst seine Gespräche mit dem prominenten Patienten wurden ihm negativ angekreidet, hatte Vergil die „ideale" Medizin einst doch als *ars muta* bezeichnet![33] „Die alten Ärzte pflegten schweigend Kranke zu behandeln", warf Petrarca dem Mediziner vor. „Ihr aber haltet Reden, streitet herum und bringt unter lauter Geschrei [eure Patienten] um!"[34]

In den 1355 vollendeten *Invective contra medicum* eskalierte die antiärztliche Polemik, obgleich Petrarca das Thema auch in anderen Schriften abhandelte.[35] Im Mittelpunkt stand ein Briefwechsel mit dem erwähnten Leibarzt Papst Clemens VI., der im Dezember 1351 schwer erkrankt war. Im März 1352 schickte Petrarca dem Pontifex Genesungswünsche, wobei er mit Schmeicheleien nicht geizte („Alle [...] sind, wenn du krank bist, nur scheinbar gesund!"). Doch kommt er bald auf die Mediziner zu sprechen, denen der Papst sein Vertrauen schenkte. „Ich weiß, daß dein Bett von Ärzten belagert wird, und vor allem dies ist für mich Grund zur Sorge",[36] hält er dem Schwerkranken entgegen, um ihn dann, unter Berufung auf Plinius[37], gleich vor deren Lügen und Ignoranz zu warnen („Sie lernen, wenn wir in Gefahr sind und machen ihre Experimente über Leichen"[38]). Der Tatsache eingedenk, daß das römische Volk, wenn man Plinius glaubt[39] (was Petrarca selbstverständlich tat!), mehr als 600 Jahre ohne Ärzte existiert habe, solle

29 Zit. Petrarca, *Invective*, Lib. I, 277f., S. 33.

30 Hierzu auch P. O. Kristeller, „Petrarca, der Humanismus und die Scholastik", in: A. Buck (Hg.), *Petrarca* (Wege der Forschung; 353), Darmstadt 1976, S. 261–281.

31 Bergdolt, *Arzt*, S. 38–40.

32 Vgl. Petrarca, *Invective*, Lib II, 559–561, S. 55: „tu pecuniae servus es".

33 Aeneis XII, 397.

34 Petrarca, *Invective*, Lib. III, 745f., S. 80: „Solebant medici veteres taciti curare: vos perorantes et altercantes et conclamantes occiditis".

35 Etwa in der 1371 fertiggestellten Schrift *De sui ipsius et multorum ignorantia*, vgl. Francesco Petrarca, *De sui ipsius et multorum ignorantia* (Über seine und vieler anderer Unwissenheit), Lateinisch-Deutsch (Philosophische Bibliothek; 455), übers. von K. Kubisch, hg. und eingel. von A. Buck, Hamburg 1993; ferner Bergdolt, *Arzt*, S. 67–76.

36 G. Fracassetti (Hg.), *Francisci Petrarcae Epistulae de Rebus Familiaribus et Variae*, Bd. I, Florenz 1859, S. 300: „Lectum tuum obessum medicis scio. Hinc prima mihi timendi causa est".

37 Plinius, *Naturalis Historia*, XXIX, 5–7.

38 Fracassetti, *Francisci*.

39 Vgl. Plinius, *Naturalis Historia*, XXIX, 5, 11.

sich der Pontifex „einen von vielen" auswählen, „der wenigstens nicht durch Geschwätzigkeit, sondern durch Sachkenntnis und Vertrauenswürdigkeit" besteche.[40] Dass Gott selbst die Heilkunde geschaffen habe, wie der päpstliche Leibarzt offensichtlich eingeworfen hatte, erhöhe ihren Wert keineswegs, denn, wie schon der *Ecclesiasticus* unterstrichen habe, stamme jedes, auch das einfachste Wissen von Gott.[41] Ebenso wenig überzeuge der Hinweis auf die Nützlichkeit der Heilkunde, denn hier werde sie von anderen Berufen weit übertroffen: „O du Verrücktester glaubst also, dass die Nützlichkeit das Ansehen einer Kunst bewirkt. Das Gegenteil ist der Fall. Ein Esel ist viel notwendiger als ein Löwe, eine Henne mehr als ein Adler. Also sollen diese edler sein?"[42] Auf der Basis diverser Briefe stellte Petrarca, unter Zusammenfassung seiner Argumente, in der Folgezeit die *Invective contra medicum* zusammen, die er im Sommer 1355 an den Dichterkollegen Giovanni Boccaccio schickte.[43]

Auch die Fächer des *Quadrivium*, zu denen auch die Musik zählte, sowie zahlreiche seit dem 12. Jahrhundert im Schlepptau des Aristotelismus in Mode gekommene Forschungsthemen, etwa die Kosmologie, Geologie, Botanik, Zoologie und Balneologie[44], schienen dem Gegner der mittelalterlichen Geisteswelt durch die ideologische Klammer der Scholastik abgewertet, die er verabscheute, ja als Hauptursache des kulturellen Niedergangs seiner Epoche empfand. Sein Kampf gegen die Heilkunde wird nur aus dieser profunden Abneigung gegen alle an den traditionell scholastisch geprägten Universitäten gelehrten Disziplinen verständlich, die sich in der Regel aus den sieben *Artes Liberales* ableiteten.[45] Respekt verdienten aus seiner Sicht nur die trivialen Fächer Grammatik und Rhetorik (sie wurden später in den Kanon der erstmals von Coluccio Salutati definierten *studia humanitatis* übernommen[46]). Vehement, wenn auch etwas systemlos rebellierte Petrarca gegen die unbestreitbare Tatsache, dass das geistige Europa im Trecento, vor allem im universitären und kirchlichen Bereich, noch weitgehend vom aristotelischen Gedankengut geprägt war, wohl ahnend, dass dieses Paradigma noch lange Bestand haben würde (noch zu Beginn des 17. Jahrhunderts sollte z. B. Galilei primär gegen ‚Aristoteliker' wie Cremonini ankämpfen![47]). Tatsächlich hatte der Aristotelismus seit dem 12. Jahrhundert an den europäischen Universitäten eine geradezu singuläre Bedeutung erlangt. Pietro d'Abano (1250–1316), einer der führenden Ärzte und Naturforscher des Spätmittelalters, etablierte nach 1306 an der Universität Padua ein aristotelisch geprägtes Curriculum, welches nicht nur das Studium der Medizin, sondern auch das (vor Beginn des eigent-

40 Vgl. Fracassetti, *Francisci*, S. 300f.
41 Petrarca, *Invective*, Lib. I, 219–225, S. 31.
42 Petrarca, *Invective*, Lib. III, 85 und 95–97, S. 60.
43 Bergdolt, *Arzt*, S. 36f.
44 Vor allem in Padua versuchte um 1300 Pietro d'Abano solche Fächer in den Kanon der Medizinerausbildung zu integrieren, vgl. Bergdolt, *Arzt*, S. 18–20.
45 Bergdolt, *Arzt*, S. 7.
46 Vgl. Buck, *Die humanistische Tradition*, S. 135.
47 Hierzu H. C. Freiesleben, *Galilei Galileo. Physik und Glaube an der Wende zur Neuzeit*, 1564–1642 (Große Naturforscher; 20), 2., durchges. Auflage, Stuttgart 1969, S. 30 und 34.

lichen Fachstudiums vorgeschriebene) Propädeutikum der Freien Künste neu akzentuierte.[48] Petrarca, der als Gast der Carrara häufig in der Stadt weilte[49], muss hier, wenn nicht bereits als Student in Montpellier und Bologna, das Weltbild der Ärzte und Universitätsgelehrten in zahlreichen Streitgesprächen kennen gelernt haben. Die Tatsache, dass die westlichen Mediziner seit Gründung der berühmten Medizinschule von Salerno (11. Jh.) zunehmend auf aus dem Arabischen übersetzte Schriften, aber auch zahlreiche im frühen Mittelalter aus dem Griechischen übertragene Werke antiker Philosophen und Ärzte samt ihrer arabischen Kommentatoren zurückgriffen, setzte sie aus seiner Sicht ferner dem (geradezu dramatisch beschworenen) Verdacht aus, islamischen, d.h. nichtchristlichen Interpretationen nahezustehen, allen voran den Lehren des „Höllenhundes" Averroes (12. Jh.), welcher, wie der Dichter sich ereiferte, „von höllischem Zorn aufgepeitscht, mit gotteslästerlichem Bellen und mit von überall hergeholten Flüchen den heiligen Namen von Christus und den katholischen Glauben lästert und schindet".[50]

Die scholastische Bildung hatte die Ärzte nach Petrarcas Meinung zudem dazu verführt, umstrittene autoritative Texte, ob von Aristoteles oder Hippokrates, kritiklos nachzubeten. So waren sie dazu prädisponiert, auch die Lehren des als ‚freigeistig' geltenden Philosophen aus Cordoba unkontrolliert zu rezipieren, d.h. an die Unvergänglichkeit des Kosmos wie die ihm zugeschriebene These von der doppelten Wahrheit (d.h. einer unüberbrückbaren Divergenz theologischer und säkularer Inhalte[51]) zu glauben.[52] Doch erschien auch ihr Idol Aristoteles selbst verdächtig: Wer immer in Paris, Montpellier, Salerno oder Padua Medizin studiert hatte – es war damit zu rechnen, dass er die Lehre des großen griechischen Philosophen, für Petrarca aber auch, angesichts der moralischen Nutzlosigkeit der Naturwissenschaften, Verführers von geradezu metaphysischer Dimension („istorum deus"[53]) und „gottlosen und blasphemischen Gegners Christi"[54], selbst dort bewunderte, wo sie mit dem christlichen Glauben unvereinbar erschien.

In der antischolastischen Abhandlung *De sui ipsius et multorum ignorantia* (1367) schrieb der Dichter später: „Aristoteles lehrt uns, ich leugne es nicht, was Tugend ist, aber jene überzeugenden und begeisternden Worte, die uns zu deren

48 Pietro d'Abano hatte in Paris studiert, der Hochburg des Aristotelismus im 13. Jahrhundert und dort sein Hauptwerk, den *Conciliator differentiarum philosophorum et praecipue medicorum* verfasst, vgl. Nancy G. Siraisi, *Arts and Sciences at Padua. The Studium at Padua before 1350*, (Pontifical Institute of Medieval Studies: Studies and Texts; 25), Toronto 1973, S. 59.

49 Bergdolt, *Arzt*, S. 22.

50 G. Fracassetti (Hg.), *Lettere Senili di Francesco Petrarca*, Bd. II, Florenz 1892, S. 425: „...quel rabioso cane ch'è Averroe, il quale afitato da infernale furore, con empi latrali, e con bestemmie da ogni parte raccolte, oltraggia e lacera il santo nome di Cristo e la cattolica fede".

51 Die Lehre von der doppelten Wahrheit im westlichen Aristotelismus wird heute allerdings relativiert, vgl. P. O. Kristeller, *Humanismus und Renaissance*, Bd. 2: *Philosophie, Bildung und Kunst*, hg. von Eckhard Kessler, München 1964, S. 127f.

52 Bergdolt, *Arzt*, S. 27f.

53 Petrarca, *De sui ipsius*, S. 32.

54 Petrarca, *Invective*, Lib. II, 479f., S. 53.

Liebe und zum Hass des Lasters bewegen, durch die der Geist entzündet und angefeuert wird, kennt er nicht oder nur selten …“[55] Noch deutlicher drückte er sich an anderer Stelle aus:

> Ich glaube bei Gott, und zweifle nicht daran, dass Aristoteles nicht nur, was Dinge von geringerer Bedeutung angeht, wo ein Irrtum weniger Gewicht hat und keineswegs gefährlich ist, sondern auch bei sehr wichtigen, unsere Existenz betreffenden Fragen, und zwar auf der ganzen Linie, geirrt hat.[56]

Der griechische Philosoph und seine arabischen Kommentatoren waren für ihn auch Ursache dafür, dass bereits die Medizinstudenten, wie er glaubte, programmatisch auf ein materialistisches Weltbild eingeschworen wurden. Moralismus und Polemik geschickt vermischend, beschuldigte Petrarca die Mediziner, Gottlosigkeit und Häresie mit Arroganz, Geldgier und hohler Rhetorik zu verbinden. Für alles schienen sie sich zu interessieren, nur nicht für die eine, entscheidende Frage: „Ad quid nati sumus?“[57] Zusammen mit Juristen, Philosophen und Theologen traf sie der Vorwurf, formalistisch-logischen Spitzfindigkeiten zu erliegen, sich von Jugend an in erstarrten Techniken des Denkens und Folgerns zu üben und die antiken Koryphäen nur in hündischer, unkritischer Rezeption zu verehren. Das propädeutische Studium der *artes liberales*, mit dem ihre Universitätsausbildung begann und wo auch historische und sprachliche Themen abgehandelt wurden, eine potentielle Brücke zu den *studia humanitatis*, verhindere keineswegs, dass sie für den Rest ihres Lebens die Zeit mit nutzlosen Dingen vergeudeten:

> Einige bringen grammatische Regeln zusammen, andere bestaunen mit offenem Mund Redensarten und Redefiguren, andere meditieren logische Schlussfolgerungen, und wieder andere zählen, andere verknüpfen Zahlen und Töne, andere vermessen die Erde, andere erforschen den Himmel und die Sterne […].[58]

Die ideologische Einseitigkeit solcher ‚Gelehrter‘, welche den Kanon der freien Künste offenbar komplett missverstanden, führte nach Petrarca dazu, dass sie, „obwohl sie noch zu leben schienen und – zumindest bisher – auch atmeten, doch schon abstoßende und schreckliche Leichname“ darstellten (*spirantia, sed iam obscoena et horrenda cadavera*).[59]

Nicht irdische Güter, primär auch nicht körperliche Gesundheit, sondern seelisches Wohlbefinden und augustinische Frömmigkeit stellen nach Petrarca den Sinn des Lebens dar. Es ging ihm darum, dem Menschen seine Angst zu nehmen, was vor allem durch eine bedingungslose Annahme des zu erwartenden Todes möglich schien. Er sollte lernen,

> den Tod sich zu vergegenwärtigen, sich gegen ihn zu wappnen, sich zu seiner Verachtung wie geduldigen Hinnahme bereitzuhalten, ihm sogar, wenn es die Situation erfordert, entgegenzu-

55 Petrarca, *De sui ipsius*, S. 104.

56 Petrarca, ibd., S. 50f.

57 Petrarca, *De sui ipsius*, S. 22.

58 Petrarca, *Fam.* X, 5, vgl. Stierle, Francesco Petrarca, S. 99.

59 Zit. nach Francesco Petrarca, *Le Familiari* (Edizione Nazionale delle Opere di Francesco Petrarca XI/XIII), hg. von V. Rossi, Florenz 1934/42, S. 78f.

eilen und für das ewige Leben, für Glück und Ruhm dieses kurze und elende Dasein großmütig zu erdulden.[60]

Petrarcas Philosophie mündet damit in eine bemerkenswerte *meditatio mortis*, die als Teil einer umfassenden *ars vivendi* verstanden wird.[61]

Die an den Universitäten übliche wissenschaftliche Kommunikations- und Prüfungsform der *quaestiones* führte nach Petrarca ferner zu einer hohlen „Altweibergeschwätzigkeit" (*garrulitas*), „deren Stolz das Wiederkäuen ihrer alten, ewigen Streitereien ist"[62]. Statt *sapientia*, die schon Dante im *Convivium* eingefordert hatte[63], stand bei den Scholastikern bloße *scientia* im Vordergrund, die angesichts ihrer fragwürdigen Inhalte von Pseudo-Rhetorik und „plumpen Redefloskeln" (*flosculos inutilium verborum ingeris*[64]) begleitet werden musste. Im Falle der Medizin lasse dies, wie der Dichter belustigt betonte, „Cicero lachen, Demosthenes sich empören, Hippokrates weinen und das Volk zugrunde gehen".[65] In seiner Attacke gegen die Universitätsgelehrten nahm Petrarca Thesen vorweg, die eine Generation später der schon erwähnte Salutati in seiner Schrift *De nobilitate legum et medicinae* aufgriff: Die Erforschung der Natur sei sinnlos, weil der Mensch in seiner naturgegebenen Begrenztheit Gottes Werk niemals durchschauen könne.[66] Auch der Florentiner Humanist und Politiker Poggio Bracciolini (1380–1459) verband die scholastische Medizin mit einer fragwürdigen „curiositas quaedam supervacua"[67], während Enea Silvio Piccolomini (1405–1464) in seinem Traktat *De liberorum educatione* die Schädlichkeit der Naturwissenschaften für die Persönlichkeitsbildung herausstellte.[68] Der italienische Frühhumanismus implizierte um 1400 ein charakteristisches, wenn auch nicht absolutes „Schweigen der Naturwissenschaften und der [scholastischen] Philosophie" (Eugenio Garin[69]).

In anderen Worten: Die Medizin erschien eines gebildeten, gewissenhaften Menschen unwürdig. Allerdings hatte sie auch im Alltag versagt. Die Pestkatastrophe von 1348 – Petrarca überlebte sie, nicht zuletzt dank einiger Reisen, mit viel Glück! – zeigte, daß die Schulmedizin, vom bekannten Rat zur Flucht abge-

60 Petrarca, *Invective*, Lib. II, 505–510, S. 53f.: „Illam [mortem] praemeditari, contra illam armari, ad illius contemptum ac patientiam com-poni, illi si res exigat occurrere, et pro aeterna vita, pro felicitate, pro gloria brevem hanc mise-ramque vitam alto animo pacisci [...]".

61 Zur Ars moriendi des Spätmittelalters vgl. auch K. Bergdolt, „Tod und Sterben in der Bildenden Kunst", in: H. Wittwer – D. Schäfer – A. Frewer (Hgg.), *Sterben und Tod. Geschichte – Theorie – Ethik, ein interdisziplinäres Handbuch*, Stuttgart / Weimar 2010, S. 215–219.

62 Vgl. Petrarca, *Dichtungen*, S. 203.

63 Dante, *Il Convivio* (Testi e saggi di letterature moderne; 2), hg. von M. Simonelli, Bologna 1966, S. 108: „li medici e quasi tutti i filosofiche non per sapere studiano ma per acquistare moneta o dignitade...".

64 Petrarca, *Invective*, Lib. I, 22, S. 25.

65 Ibd., Lib. III, 662f., S. 77.

66 Vgl. A. Buck, *Die Medizin im Verständnis*, S. 183.

67 Vgl. Bergdolt, *Arzt*, S. 195.

68 Vgl. Buck, *Die humanistische Tradition*, S. 161.

69 E. Garin, „Gli umanisti e la scienza", in: *Rivista di Filosofia* 52 (1961), S. 259–278, hier S. 260.

sehen, keine wirklich effektiven Mittel kannte. „Weder ein Arzt noch eine Medizin taugten hier etwas“, schrieb der Florentiner Chronist Marchionne di Coppo Stefani, „denn eine derartige Krankheit war bisher unbekannt, und die Ärzte hatten nichts darüber in Erfahrung bringen können“.[70] Das war für die Hippokratiker kein Ruhmesblatt.

Ungeachtet ihres längst erfolgten Aufstiegs zu einer den freien Künsten zumindest gleichrangigen Gelehrtendisziplin, welche sich nicht nur durch die inhaltliche Verwandtschaft zum naturwissenschaftlich geprägten Quadrivium, sondern auch durch wissenschaftliche Methodik und ein breites Bildungsspektrum auszeichnete, erscheint die Heilkunde in Petrarcas *Invectivae* als plumpes Handwerk. In der erwähnten Schrift *De sui ipsius et multorum ignorantia* wurden die in den *Invective* vorgebrachten Argumente noch einmal präzisiert. Wiederum attackierte Petrarca die Adepten des Aristoteles, welche schon dessen „bloße[r] Name...mit diesen fünf Silben“ in Verzückung geraten lasse.[71] Im Vergleich zu den *Invective* ist der Ton freilich gedämpfter. Fünfzehn Jahre nach der Auseinandersetzung von Avignon argumentiert er eher philosophisch (was allerdings Verbalinjurien und beleidigende Vorwürfe noch nicht ausschließt!) und bietet – zumindest teilweise – die Hand zur Versöhnung. Nicht die Gegner, vier jüngere Vertreter verschiedenster scholastischer Wissenschaften, sondern ihre Irrtümer und Laster werden angeprangert. Die jungen Intellektuellen, darunter der Sohn seines Freundes, des venezianischen Dogen Andrea Dandolo, hatten Petrarca vorgeworfen, zwar „ein guter, ja trefflicher Mensch zu sein“, aber „ohne Bildung“[72]. Damit hatten sie, wie der Dichter zugab, aus ihrer Sicht sogar recht. Allerdings dachte er nicht daran, sich ihre Art von Wissen anzueignen, da es ihm untauglich schien, das Wesen des Menschen zu erklären. Für die meisten Ärzte und Naturforscher stellte die akademische Szene – so sein Urteil, er bleibt dabei – nur ein *instrumentum dementiae* dar.[73] Was nütze es dem Menschen, nach aristotelischem Vorbild Details der Natur zu erforschen, die spirituellen Werte des Lebens aber, wie sie Augustinus nahe legte, zu verkennen? Geradezu karikierend klingt folgende Feststellung:

> Viel weiß er [der Mensch] von den wilden Tieren, von den Vögeln und Fischen; wieviel Haare der Löwe auf dem Kopf, wie viel Federn der Falke am Schwanz hat, mit wieviel Armen der Krake den Schiffbrüchigen umschlingt; dass sich die Elephanten von hinten begatten und ihre Tragzeit zwei Jahre beträgt. Auch weiß er, dass der Elephant ein gelehriges Tier voller Lebenskraft ist, fast so verständig wie der Mensch, und zwei- bis dreihundert Jahre alt werden kann, oder dass der Phoenix in wohlriechendem Feuer verbrennt und aus seiner Asche wiederentsteht; dass der Seeigel ein Schiff, wie schnell es auch fährt, anzuhalten vermag, während er außerhalb der Fluten nichts ausrichten kann ..., dass das Bärenjunge nach seiner Geburt unförmig ist, das Maultier nur selten Junge zur Welt bringt und die Viper nur ein einziges Mal und dabei selber zugrunde geht.[74]

70 Vgl. die Übersetzung von K. Bergdolt in: K. Bergdolt (Hg.), *Die Pest 1348 in Italien. 50 zeitgenössische Quellen*, mit einem Nachw. von G. Keil, Heidelberg 1989, S. 66.

71 Petrarca, *De sui ipsius*, S. 30: „quod his quinque sillabis multos delectat ignaros“.

72 Ibd., S. 16.

73 Ibd., S. 20.

74 Ibd.

Der *literata ignorantia* der Masse (*multorum*), ihrem auf das Innerweltliche beschränkten, die metaphysischen Komponenten des Seins vergessenden Daseins- und Berufsverständnis wird die entscheidende, religiös motivierte, letztlich bildungsunabhängige *virtus illiterata* Petrarcas (*sui ipsius*) gegenübergestellt. Erstere ist vergänglich, oberflächlich und mit religiöser Gleichgültigkeit verbunden. Wirkliche *sapientia* bezieht sich dagegen nicht auf irdisches Wissen (und schon gar nicht auf die Naturwissenschaften), sondern ist nach Augustinus mit *pietas* identisch.[75] Die Gegner lassen sich freilich, so Petrarcas Behauptung, „vom Glanz (des Aristoteles) blenden und in den Graben des Irrtums stürzen". Herablassend lässt er ihnen „ihre ungeheure Überheblichkeit …, ihre Freude und stolze Einbildung, die unbegründet ist und fragwürdig, sowie all die süßen Früchte, welcher sich Ignoranten und solche, die sich mit falschen Lehren brüsten, in eitlem, hohlen Selbstvertrauen pflücken".[76] „Mir aber sei Demut zu eigen, das Wissen um meine Unwissenheit und Hinfälligkeit", fügt er in allzu demonstrativer Bescheidenheit hinzu![77]

Die programmatische Ablehnung der scholastischen Medizin und den Naturwissenschaften wurde von einer beachtlichen Sachkritik begleitet. Vom Fiasko des Schwarzen Todes einmal abgesehen, monierte Petrarca immer wieder, dass die scholastischen Gegner die Behauptungen des Aristoteles und anderer antiker Naturforscher kaum hinterfragten. Es störte ihn (auch da deutet sich ein neuer Umgang mit autoritativen Texten an), dass die antiken und mittelalterlichen ‚Gewährsleute' Einzelheiten aus der Tier- und Pflanzenwelt nicht selbst erforscht, „sondern aufgrund der weiten Entfernung allzu bereitwillig geglaubt oder allzu freizügig erfunden haben".[78] Ausnahmegestalten wie Albertus Magnus, der schon hundert Jahre zuvor die Reproduzierbarkeit eines wissenschaftlichen *experimentum* gefordert hatte und im Übrigen, wie Petrarca, den Averroismus bekämpfte, wurden natürlich nicht zur Kenntnis genommen![79]

Ungeachtet der unbestreitbaren Abhängigkeit seines Menschenbildes und Bildungskonzepts auch von mittelalterlichen Autoren – sowohl für die antischolastische wie antimedizinische Kritik lassen sich viele Beispiele anführen![80] – artikulierte sich der Gegensatz zwischen *sapientia* und *scientia*, zwischen *studia humanitatis* und Naturwissenschaften, zwischen Religion und Skepsis, Platon und Aristoteles, zwischen Augustinus und der kalten Dialektik, zwischen seelischer und körperlicher Gesundheit erstmals in aller Schärfe und radikaler Konsequenz bei dem großen Dichter und Humanisten des 14. Jahrhunderts, von dem Giosuè Carducci später sagte, er habe „als erster sein Gewissen in der Dichtung entblößt,

75 Dieses Thema wird besonders im *Secretum* abgehandelt, einem fiktiven Dialog mit Augustinus, vgl. Bergdolt, *Arzt*, S. 77–82.

76 Petrarca, *De sui ipsius*, S. 30.

77 Vgl. ibd.

78 Ibd., S. 22.

79 Vgl. *Albertus Magnus. Ausstellungskatalog zum 700. Geburtstag*, Historisches Archiv der Stadt Köln, Köln 1980, S. 88 und 144.

80 Hierzu ausführlich Bergdolt, *Arzt*, S. 164–191.

um es zu befragen und zu analysieren".[81] Durch Petrarcas Schrifttum wehte, ungeachtet aller Unterschiede zwischen heutigen Geisteswissenschaften und den spätmittelalterlichen *studia humanitatis*, ein Hauch des von P. C. Snow in seinem Essay *The Two Cultures and the Scientific Revolution* (1959) verdeutlichten, fundamentalen Konflikts um die Vorherrschaft der Disziplinen.[82]

81 G. Carducci, *Prose di Giosue Carducci 1859–1903*, Bologna 1904, S. 721.

82 Vgl. C. P. Snow, *The Two Cultures*, Cambridge u. a. 2002 (reprint); hierzu auch Stierle, *Francesco Petrarca*, S. 468.

MEDICAL VALUES AND BEHAVIOR. A VIEW FROM 1380s MONTPELLIER

Michael McVaugh

It is a commonplace that a medieval manuscript can tell us a great deal about the person who put it together, even if he did not bother to leave us his name. This is certainly the case with MS 1320 among the Palatine manuscripts in the Vatican Library.[1] As far as I can judge from studying it on microfilm, virtually the entire codex was written out in the same cursive fourteenth-century hand. I think it quite likely that the original owner copied it out himself, but even if he merely commissioned its writing by another scribe, the twenty or so texts he caused to be assembled there reveal a number of things about him and his medical interests.

They tell us first, I think, that he was teaching or studying with the medical faculty of Montpellier, for ten of the works included in that first part of the codex are by fourteenth-century masters at that school, perhaps the latest of whom is Jean Jacme, who was chancellor there in 1364. And we can plausibly date our man to the middle of the second half of the fourteenth century. About four-fifths of the way through the codex comes an anonymous *tractatus de epidimia* that was copied, the explicit says, in 1384, which surely implies that the first part of the volume was copied before that date. Yet perhaps not many years before, for the title of a work in that first part states that it was composed in 1358, and since the scribe evidently found nothing incongruous in setting down that date, we can narrow the period of our owner's activity to 1358–1384. We will certainly not be far off if we suppose these texts contained in the first part of our codex to have been copied out for (or by) its owner by 1380 or so.

But we know more about the owner than that he was a Montpellier academic active in the last quarter of the fourteenth century. We know that he was particularly interested in the treatment of fevers, for the manuscript opens with five major works on that subject, three of them recipe collections by recent Montpellier masters – Bernard Alberti, Gerard de Solo, Jean Jacme – based on the account of fevers in Avicenna's *Canon*. We know that he was also interested in understanding the nature of generation, for he had copied here treatises on that subject by two other recent Montpellier masters, as well as the *Liber de coitu* of Constantine the African. Plague, too, was of great interest to him, for four of the final works in the codex discuss *De pestilentia*, again including one by the Montpellier master

1 The manuscript is described in L. Schuba, *Die medizinischen Handschriften der Codices Palatini Latini in der Vatikanischen Bibliothek*, Wiesbaden 1981, pp. 418–423.

Jean Jacme.[2] That he had no trouble finding Montpellier writings on all these subjects suggests that fevers, conception, and plague may have been topics of interest not only to him but to the faculty more generally, and that our codex is giving us something of a mirror of Montpellier's 'hot topics' as they were about 1380.

In that case, a fourth subject of evident concern to our anonymous Montpellier academic may also be a guide to the thoughts of its faculty at that moment. Immediately preceding the *Tractatus de epidimia* dated to 1384, three short works have been copied close together, all dealing not with diseases or therapeutics but with what we might label 'medical values and behavior': that is, the role, status, and responsibilities of learned medicine. The fourteenth century saw the emergence of a kind of professional sensibility among academic physicians, and these three texts in different but complementary ways show us what this new 'professionalism' may have entailed for Montpellier in the last decades of the fourteenth century.

I

The first of the three is the brief Hippocratic treatise *De lege* (the *Law*). Some historians have found echoes of this work in early medieval literature, but there is no evidence of its actual translation into Latin before the beginning of the fourteenth century.[3] Pearl Kibre's catalogue of Latin Hippocratic texts distinguished among three different versions or translations of *De lege*, but it is unclear why it does so: all three begin and end with exactly the same words, and it seems probable that they all contain the same translation. A number of manuscripts of the work attribute it not implausibly to Niccolò da Reggio (active 1308–45), though there is in fact a slim tradition that it was translated by the thirteenth-century Montpellier master Arnau de Vilanova (d. 1311); but the latter is unlikely to be the case, since Arnau is not known to have been able to read Greek, and the Latin *De lege* was evidently translated from that language, as its resort to a transliteration of the evidently unfamiliar υποκριτα (by "ypocrita") shows.[4] What probably

2 In addition to the text dated 1384 already mentioned, it includes John of Burgundy's *De epidimia* of 1370, and Jean Jacme's Montpellier treatise – which, the scribe notes, helped cure 2000 people when the epidemic struck the city in the summer of 1374. Moreover, the University of Paris's recommendations for the 1349 plague are copied earlier in the codex.

3 P. Kibre, *Hippocrates Latinus*, New York 1985, pp. 182–186.

4 Perhaps, when the Latin text has been edited and compared with the Greek, it will be possible to determine whether there are several translations or only one, and if the latter, whether it shows features characteristic of Niccolò's translation technique. The following slightly expands Kibre's list of manuscripts containing the work: Braunschweig 109; Cesena, Plut. XXIII cod. 1; Cesena, Malatest. S.V.4; Copenhagen, Gl Kgl Saml. 3479, 8vo; Gdansk, Mar. F. 238; Krakow, Bib. Jag. 799; Krakow, Bib. Jag. 809; Kues 293; Laon 414; Laon 418; Leipzig, Univ. 1227; Madrid, BN 1978; Milan, Ambros. E 78 inf.; Munich, CLM 31; Munich, CLM 640; Munich, CLM 18444; Naples, BN VIII.D.25; Nurnberg, Stadtbibl. Cent. VI, 4; Oxford, BL Ashm. 1471; Paris, Acad. Med. 51; Paris, BN 6845; Paris, BN 6865; Paris, BN n.a.l. 481; Paris, Sorbonne 128; Rome, Angelica 1338; St. Petersburg, Acad. Sci. O. 216;

gave rise to the ascription of the translation to Arnau (as in the fifteenth-century manuscript Paris, BN n.a.l. 481) was the fact that he quotes its first words ("Medicina artium excellentissima propter indisciplinam utentium") virtually verbatim at the beginning of his *Antidotarium*: "Lamentabatur Ypocras eo quod medicina artium preclarissima propter indisciplinam utentium et indicantium vane in defectu est magis artibus cunctis."

But if Arnau did not translate it himself, how and where could he have encountered the translation? In fact, there is indirect evidence that in his last years Arnau met Niccolò da Reggio on a visit to the court of Robert of Naples and actually saw some of his translations,[5] and this now seems to be reinforced by Arnau's citation of *De lege* in his *Antidotarium*. The colophon to the copy of the work in MS Vienna, ÖNB 2328, dates its writing to 1314, an independent indication that *De lege* must have been translated very early in Niccolò's career, assuming always that he was its translator.[6]

The *Law* seems to have aroused immediate attention, for there exist quite a number of fourteenth-century manuscripts containing the text, which often copy it together with the even shorter *Oath* (though that is not the case in this manuscript); but the two works are very different. The *Oath* is a statement of commitments to be undertaken by an individual, a disciple; in contrast, the *Law* is the manifesto of a learned community. It begins by anticipating the later *topos* that most self-professed physicians are ignorant and incompetent – *sic autem medici nomine quidem multi, opere vero pauci* – and then proceeds to spell out what is needed for anyone who wishes to master *medicinalis scientia*: a natural talent for the subject, good teaching, dedication, a setting suited to study, and time to devote to it. It expands on this list with an extended simile:

> The discipline of medicine is like the practice of agriculture. Our complexion or nature is like the furrow; the masters' learning is like the seed; instruction is when it is sown in the right season into the prepared earth; the school in which instruction is given is like the air which

Vatican City, BAV lat. 2428; Vatican City, BAV lat. 2369; Vatican City, BAV lat. 2417; Vatican City, BAV lat. 2381; Vatican City, BAV lat. 2382; Vatican City, BAV lat. 2418; Vatican City, BAV Palat. lat. 1068; Vatican City, BAV Palat. lat. 1096; Vatican City, BAV Palat. lat. 1098; Vatican City, BAV Palat. lat. 1320; Vatican City, BAV Barb. 179; Venice, San Marco CL VII, cod. XI [2496]; Vienna, ÖNB 2328.

5 M. R. McVaugh, "Two Texts, One Problem. The Authorship of the *Antidotarium* and *De venenis* Attributed to Arnau de Vilanova", *Arxiu de Textos Catalans Antics* 14 (1995), pp. 75–94, at 82–84.

6 Jacques Jouanna has shown that the Greek text of *Law* found in an Ambrosian manuscript contains an important passage missing from the versions in the manuscripts from Venice and the Vatican from which J. L. Heiberg edited the text for the Corpus Medicorum Grecorum: see J. Jouanna, "Un témoin méconnu de la tradition Hippocratique: L'Ambrosianus Gr. 134 (B 113 sup.), fol. 1–2", in: A. Garzya – J. Jouanna (eds.), *Storia e ecdotica dei testi medici Greci. Atti del II Convegno Internazionale, Parigi 24–26 maggio 1994*, Naples 1996, pp. 253–272, esp. 266–68. It is perhaps worth noting here that the medieval Latin translation omits the same passage.

> nourishes the plants. Effort corresponds to cultivation, and time is what consolidates everything and creates the perfect nutriment.[7]

Those who follow this plan, Hippocrates concludes, will be acclaimed as they travel from city to city as physicians "non verbo sed opere".

The *Law* was apparently composed in the fourth century BCE,[8] but it would have had a powerful affinity for university physicians in the very different world of fourteenth-century Europe. The first Latin authors to cite it were writing at the beginning of the fourteenth century, at a moment when European medical schools had been self-conscious centers of systematic directed study for only about fifty years, and even then in a very small way. For several more decades, medical degrees of any sort would be rarities, and academically-trained practitioners would ordinarily be quite isolated individuals. Thus those earliest readers of *De lege*, like Arnau de Vilanova, perceived it merely as a celebration of medicine as an art, not as a discipline requiring formal study. Arnau's contemporary, Pietro d'Abano, epitomized this aspect of the work even more succinctly in his *Conciliator*: "unde Hippocras [...] in de lege: Medicina artium excellentissima vel praeclarissima".[9]

By the time our Vatican manuscript was being assembled, however, university medicine had become more widespread, and within most of Western Europe medical graduates going out in the world could expect to find nearby colleagues with shared training and values wherever they ended up. *De lege* was beautifully fitted to encourage this development. Its language spoke of the mastery of medical *scientia* requiring time and effort in centers specially fitted for medical teaching, and it thus encouraged the emergent new community of academic physicians to make common cause against the ignorant many who claimed to heal but had no preparation for doing so. If *De lege* had been a kind of manifesto for Hippocratic medicine, it was no less so for the later fourteenth century, and its central importance to the profession was rapidly acknowledged. When at century's end master Jacopo da Forlì (d. 1414) delivered a formal *commendatio* at Padua, an oration celebrating the excellence and status of medicine, it was natural that he should choose to make *De lege* the starting point of his celebration of the subject,[10] and by the end of the fifteenth century it was the foundation for Gabriele Zerbi's dis-

7 "Qualis autem est speculatio vegetabilium que est in terra, talis est et medicine disciplina. Nostra enim complexio vel natura qualis est regio; doctrine autem docentium qualia semina; disciplina autem est quod ipsa cadit in terram cultam ad tempus; locus in quo est disciplina est quale nutrimentum quod est ex convenienti aere factum vegetabilibus; labor autem cultura; tempus ut corroboravit omnia et fecit nutrimenti perfecti."; Hippocrates, *De lege*, MS Vatican City, BAV Palat. lat. 1320, fol. 116r, with modifications from the text printed in *Articella*, Venice 1523, fol. 156rb.

8 Vivian Nutton has recently put its date at 410–350 BCE: "Beyond the Hippocratic Oath", in: A. Wear – J. Geyer-Kordesch – R. French (eds.), *Doctors and Ethics. The Earlier Historical Setting of Professional Ethics*, Amsterdam 1993, pp. 10–37, at 28 n. 2.

9 Pietro d'Abano, *Conciliator*, *differentia* 3, Venice 1565, reprint Padua 1985, fol. 6ra. The date of the *Conciliator* is still uncertain, but Pietro died in 1315, so this citation is a further proof of the early date of *De lege*'s translation.

10 J. Agrimi – C. Crisciani, *Edocere medicos. Medicina scolastica nei secoli XIII–XV*, Naples 1988, pp. 263–73, provide an edition of the oration.

cussion of the training proper to a physician.[11] But the compiler of our Vatican manuscript, over a hundred years before Zerbi, had understood intuitively where academic medicine was going.

II

Immediately after the concluding line of this text, "Explicit Ypocratis de lege", a new work begins in the Vatican manuscript, this time with no title or author's name: it simply starts abruptly "Sicut legitur in Genesi", and I will refer to it by the descriptive title that Ludwig Schuba gave it in his catalogue, *De commendatione medicine.*[12] It too is a manifesto, complementing *De lege* by using Christian doctrine and Aristotelian philosophy to defend a high status for medicine. Adam's fall, it explains, entailed the weakness of the human race in both soul and body, but philosophy has helped make up for the former and medicine for the latter – and medicine is the more important of the two, because rationality is only possible if the body is already healthy. Furthermore, all nature is oriented towards man, and he is therefore the noblest object of study. Some disciplines proceed by the *via resolutiva*, like philosophy, others by the *via compositiva*, like geometry, but medicine uses both, which is a further sign of its superiority. Its achievements begin far back in the past, with all civilizations contributing to its advance: with Solomon, Apollo and Aesculapeius, Hippocrates and Galen, Hunain, Rasis and Constantine. Scripture itself insists that medicine is necessary to mankind, and Aristotle – in his *De anima*, above all, but also in his *Physics* and *Metaphysics* – supports its claims.

Yet not all who claim the title of physician are equally good, the text goes on. Its author would have agreed with the assertion of *De lege*, that some are physicians in name alone, but for him these so-called physicians are no longer just the ignorant and unlearned: some of them are now evidently within the learned medical community itself, but without sharing the values of true physicians:

> They sit in their lofty seats and from there intone imposing words to their students, but they know no more of what happens when someone is sick than they do about measuring the depth of the sea. Knowledgeable about imaginary subtleties but ignorant of medicine, seeking to make up for their lack of skill, they depart from the ways of medicine: instead of Hippocrates they take up Aristotle, instead of Galen they quote Priscian, instead of Avicenna they cite Cicero, abandoning their proper paths [...]. Such men do not deserve to enjoy the title of 'learned physician'.

These are the physicians of whom Galen complained that they dispute only about words that have no value in practice. They hold tight to the shell but discard the

11 D. J. Linden, "Gabriele Zerbi's De cautelis medicorum and the Tradition of Medical Prudence", *Bulletin of the History of Medicine* 73 (1999), pp. 19–37.

12 The text is transcribed in an appendix to this paper. I gratefully acknowledge the help of Luke Demaitre in correcting a number of my initial readings. There remain a number of problematic passages, and a few of the author's references to other works have still to be identified.

kernel, trying merely to keep their listeners entertained; they are uselessly pursuing some other art, not medicine. And the author closes the *De commendatione* with a list of authoritative definitions of what medicine should truly be.

I have come across no other copies of this little text, so it might even be the original reflections of the anonymous compiler of our manuscript, but even if he copied it from another source he presumably shared its views.[13] A not unnatural reaction might be to look for a parallel to those views in Petrarch's attack on learned medicine (*Invectiva contra medicum*) written only twenty-five years before and fewer than a hundred kilometers away from the place where our manuscript was assembled. But of course the two critiques are very different, indeed diametrically opposed. Petrarch's bitter unhappiness with medicine stems from its dependence upon Aristotelian-Averroistic scholastic philosophy and its dialectics, an empty pseudo-rhetoric and a sham substitute for what the patient really wants.[14] For Petrarch, medicine is a mechanic rather than a liberal art, certainly not philosophy. The only true philosophy is moral philosophy, and it is Cicero who is the real philosopher. The medicine Petrarch is attacking is in fact the one that the author of *De commendatione* is determined to maintain, while the targets of the latter's criticism are Petrarch's heroes, those who prefer Priscian and Cicero to Galen and Avicenna. Petrarch's was a personal view of learned medicine seen from the outside, and he found it impossible to appreciate or even understand it in its own terms, but our anonymous author identifies with it entirely. His judgments of contemporary medicine are no less personal, but they are driven by an inherent sympathy for its established methods and goals.

Whether composing *De commendatione* or merely copying it approvingly, our compiler of the Vatican manuscript was evidently not just identifying with learned medicine but with one particular community within it. He is contemptuous of those physicians who are absorbed by philosophy and the liberal arts because they know nothing about illnesses or remedies and thus have nothing to offer their patients. This of course does not mean that he rejects learned medicine outright: like Hippocrates in *De lege*, he wants to distinguish true medicine from that which the ignorant and unlearned practice. One of several scribal jottings (still in the same scribal hand) filling the empty space on the leaf where the *De commendatione* ends reads sarcastically: "Three things the vulgar and ignorant doctor must do: dress modestly, lie skilfully, slay boldly," and then goes on more positively: "Three things the rational and prudent physician must observe in medicine: he must anticipate what will be said, understand the art, and achieve his end."[15] If our academic is indeed also the author of the *De commendatione*, he is no radical, no

13 Against the possibility that this is the compiler's own composition is the existence of at least two apparent scribal confusions in the text, the writing of *fluminis* for *fulminis* and of *domum* for *donum* in nn. 11 and 18 respectively to the transcription given below.

14 K. Bergdolt, *Arzt, Krankheit und Therapie bei Petrarcha*, Weinheim 1992, esp. pp. 38–42.

15 "Nota tria sunt que a vulgo et ignaris expetuntur ut honeste vestiri, subtiliter mentiri, audacter interficere; Tria autem a communibus racionabilibus ut magnorum noticia, divicie et affabilitas. Tria autem expetuntur in medicina a viris prudentibus racionabilibus ut sermonis previsio artis cognitio et finis assequcio." Schuba, *Die medizinischen Handschriften*, p. 421.

iconoclast: he believes in the relevance of Aristotle to medical thought, for he quotes often from his works to make his points; he fully identifies with Galen, and thinks he is following his lead; and he admires some aspects of contemporary medical scholarship, for he has copied Gerard of Solo and Jean Jacme into his own manuscript. But we should note that the works he admires in his contemporaries are practical rather than theoretical: recipes for fevers, recipes for pestilence. This orientation is what he believes separates him from his academic colleagues who are so enthusiastic about word-play. A true physician is not merely learned, he must be learned in practice, in *operatio*. But what exactly does that term encompass, and how does he go about learning it? Starting three leaves after the end of the *De commendatione*, following two brief snippets on anatomy and uroscopy, our physician has caused to be copied into the manuscript a little treatise that goes a considerable way towards answering that question: the *Tabula super vita brevis* supposedly written by his famous predecessor at Montpellier, Arnau de Villanova.

III

In 1301, just before setting out for Rome to defend his orthodoxy before the pope, Arnau de Vilanova delivered what would be his last formal commentary to his Montpellier students, a commentary on the first Hippocratic aphorism: "Ars longa, vita brevis." He was pleased enough with the result to circulate a written text, and to refer back to its contents in his *Speculum medicine* of 1308, but in fact the commentary itself was never popular. Arnau had divided it into three *lectiones*, admitting apologetically that the first was unusually abstract, and indeed the scribe of the copy from which the work was printed in the sixteenth century chose to omit most of that *lectio*, pleading time pressures. The second *lectio* was heavily theoretical as well, and it is perhaps understandable that only one manuscript of the complete commentary survives today.

But its third *lectio* was another matter. Here Arnau had taken from the aphorism Hippocrates' list of the four factors involved in a physician's encounter with a patient – the physician, the patient himself, friends or family who may be present, and external circumstances – and around them had constructed a unique concrete, detailed account of the way in which a physician needs to act when called upon, at each successive stage in the case: from the moment when the patients' friends first come to fetch him, through his examination of the patient and his attempt at diagnosis, to the moment when he settles upon a therapy appropriate to the patient's illness. Only a few years later another academic physician, Alberto de Zancariis of Bologna, presented somewhat similar material in his little *De cautelis medicorum*, but in much less detail, and significantly in a very different spirit.[16] Arnau's account of the physician-patient encounter focused on the physi-

16 M. Morris, *Die Schrift des Albertus de Zancariis aus Bologna 'De cautelis medicorum habendis'*, Diss. Leipzig 1914.

cian's continuing responsiveness to the patient and his needs, while Alberto's used it to lay out "devices and strategies that the doctor can employ to enhance his reputation"[17] (and his wealth), themes that Arnau touches on not at all. As adopted by Gabriele Zerbi, whose own *De cautelis* quotes liberally and without acknowledgement from Alberto, Alberto's approach has been described a little cynically as constituting a 'textbook of ethics'.[18] If so, the third *lectio* of Arnau's commentary has to be seen, too, as implicitly embodying an ethical program, but a sharply contrasting one.

Given its ready applicability to the physician's practice, it is not surprising that the third *lectio* was soon extracted from the commentary and copied separately under the title *De circumspectione medicorum* – two copies of this extract survive. A little later on, someone else took *De circumspectione* and recast it as a series of headings enumerating the physician's actions in a kind of tabular summary which still preserved some of the language of Arnau's original commentary but had now been given a number of thoughtful new illustrative examples to make more meaningful the kinds of choices that a physician might have to make. This new schematic outline circulated as the *Tabula super vita brevis Arnaldi de Villanova*, though of course it was only indirectly Arnau's, and it was vastly more popular than the original scholastic commentary that he had composed. At least fifteen manuscript copies of the *Tabula* exist today.[19] Like the original from which it was drawn, but more succinct and with its organizational skeleton more apparent, it was a manual not only of diagnostic and therapeutic technique, but to some extent of professional behavior as well: it touched on the relationships that the physician needed to maintain with his patients, their families, and even his colleagues when they lent a hand in his cases.

The *Tabula* is therefore a wholly understandable companion to our Montpellier owner's other two texts promoting professional identity. It had evidently been prepared in an academic environment by an editor who understood and fully appreciated its analysis of ideal medical behavior, as the wholly relevant examples he added to it indicate. It would not be surprising, indeed, if both *De circumspectione* and the *Tabula* had been produced at Montpellier and were in circulation there, where the memory of Arnau's teaching must still have been reasonably fresh, but we have no way of knowing. The copy in our manuscript from Montpellier is so far the earliest dated text of the work that has turned up (which is itself a fact of some interest), but comparing it with the sixteenth-century editions shows

17 The quotation is applied to Zerbi's work by R. French, "The Medical Ethics of Gabriele de Zerbi", in: Wear – Geyer-Kordesch – French (eds.), *Doctors and Ethics*, pp. 72–97, at 74, but it seems to me equally applicable to Alberto's, and, given the dependence of Zerbi's text on Alberto's, entirely appropriate to extend it to the latter. Zerbi certainly enlarges upon Alberto's presentation, and introduces new topics, but his language is regularly drawn directly from the earlier text.

18 Ibid.

19 The evolution of the text is examined in more detail in Arnau de Vilanova, *Repetitio super aphorismo Hippocratis 'Vita brevis'*, in: *Arnaldi de Villanova Opera Medica Omnia*, XIV, ed. by M. R. McVaugh and F. Salmón, in press.

that it has a number of instances of homoioteleuton and suggests that our version of the text had already had a long scribal history when it was copied in the 1380s.

For our purposes, the most interesting part of the ideal presented by the *Tabula* is its portrayal of the attitudes the physician should adopt towards others. Actually, for the most part it deals with his responsibilities somewhat summarily. To his patients, it says, he owes *diligentia*, which is a label encompassing the series of diagnostic procedures to which the bulk of the *Tabula* is dedicated; in turn, from them he should expect *obedientia*. But there comes a moment in every case when the patient wants to know what is wrong with him, a moment when the physician may or may not know the answer and yet must somehow respond to his client. In either case (but especially the latter), what should the physician say? How candid, how truthful should he be? Should he lie skillfully, as the *vulgi et ignari* do, in order to keep the patient happy and his own reputation intact? The steadily professionalizing tendency of fourteenth-century medicine made it much less easy for a physician to do that now than would have been the case, say, a hundred years before.

On these matters, therefore, the editor of the *Tabula* chose to set out especially detailed and thoughtful answers for his readers. In preparing the work, he had been typically somewhat selective in what he took over from Arnau's original text (that is, as embodied in *De circumspectione*), leaving out entire topics and abbreviating its language drastically, but when he came to Arnau's discussion of physician-client exchanges he evidently found it to be of particular value. Not only was he careful to preserve the details of Arnau's approach to the topic, he actually adopted much of Arnau's own wording. And to make his recommendations still more powerful, he gave them a particular vividness by recasting Arnau's general counsels into specific phrases that the physician was told to use when responding to the typical concerns of his patients and their friends. Thus, if the patient's friends ask about his condition, do not lie or try to mislead them by saying that you are hopeful, for example, when you are not at all hopeful. Say instead cautiously that there are still some things you need to check, or say simply and truthfully that you aren't sure yet. As for the patient himself, even if you do not understand his illness, you should continue to visit him to check on his symptoms, and if he asks you why he is not getting any medicines from you, reply to him in these words: "Ego antequam vobis medicinalia administrare visito et interrogo vos propter quedam dubia que mihi occurrunt. Nam ego volo vos ducere per securiorem atque tutam viam." If he persists in asking for medication, you can give him something that may help but cannot possibly hurt, but whatever medicine you decide to give to a patient, never say that it will make him well, because this in the end may not be true. Say instead: "ego ordino hunc sirupum vel electuarium ad talem vel talem operationem"; that is, restrict your promise to the specific effect you know that drug will have – purging, for example – so that the patient will gain confidence that whatever statements you do make are true, and will always be looking forward to the next stage in his treatment.[20] The text thus emphasizes how carefully you must pick your words whenever you speak with a patient, so as to ensure that whatever you say will be perfectly true and accurate and yet as reassuring as possible – while carefully avoiding any broad promises about the future.

This recommended language is self-protective, of course, yet the author is clearly also concerned that his readers should not put reputation ahead of *honestas*. This had been a favorite term of Arnau in his commentary, and the *Tabula* maintains and extends his use of it. The physician's responsibility of *diligentia*, of always aiming at the restoration of the patient's health (which distinguishes him from his over-theoretical colleagues), means that he must try to keep his patient from alarm and despair, which will inevitably make an illness worse; a positive attitude in the patient is an enormously powerful therapeutic agent. Yet *honestas* requires that he not lie in order to evoke it. This ideal of *honestas*, of truthfulness, is not always easy to reconcile with that responsibility of diligence. Arnau de Vi-

20 The passage in the Vatican manuscript includes important material omitted from the text of the *Tabula* printed in the editions of the *Opera Arnaldi*, though similar language is present in *De circumspectione*, and it therefore seems important to give it in full: "Ordinato regimine egri in hospitio eius, […] <si> ab amicis interrogetur quid sentiat de statu patientis, respondere debet non cum duplicitate maliciosa aut fallacia vel mendacio, quod poterit contingere duobus modis, aut dicendo sperare se quod non sperat aut dicendo se timere quod non timet, sed cum cautela discretionis honeste, ut non exprimat in quibus dubitat, sed de quibusdam articulis de quibus per examen artificiale intendit certificari, aut cum lima veritatis ut dicat quod non est certus de statu patientis. […] Si proprio studio ex eis non posset iudicium elicere qualiter alterius auxilio seu iudicio poterit iudicare, hoc autem poterit facere si ad alium peritiorem medicum eo recurrat cum eo de accidentibus collectis conferendo; aut est sibi ille medicus propinquus, et tunc aut satisfacit sibi et tunc ordinet regimen curationis secundum quod particularia patientem et morbus tolerabunt, aut non satisfacit et tunc recurrat ad distantem. Aut non est sibi propinquus sed distans, et in hoc casu si patiens fuerit dives, debet medicus persuadere parentibus ut ipsum vel ipsos vocent et venire faciant. Si autem mittatur pro medico distante, restat videre quid faciet medicus in toto tempore medio donec alter medicus veniat. Certe dico quod debet visitare suum infirmum, et debet videre si aliquod signum de novo appareat, scilicet per quod possit illuminari, et debet interrogare infirmum de his de quibus non recordatur eum interrogasse, et debet ei temptando dicere: 'Ego antequam vobis medicinalia administrarem visito et interrogo vos propter quedam dubia que mihi occurrunt. Nam ego volo vos ducere per securiorem atque tutam viam.' Si autem medicus cognoscet quod infirmus esset impatiens vel festinus vel modo importunus, aut dimittat eum si cum honestate possit dimittere, aut si non posset eum dimittere ordinet aliqua medicinalia que aliquo modo possint perficere et nullo modo nocere. Dicat ergo patienti: 'protinus ordinabo vobis salubre antidotum,' et per hoc cessat angustia patientis et murmur amicorum. In tali allocutione loquatur medicus circumspecte ne dictis suis sit contrarius, nam circumspectio est virtus precavens lapsum in contrarium vicium ut proinde considerando futura. Cum ergo ignoraverit medicus quantum debeat durare morbus vel inde in futuro quid debeat accidere, nunquam debet dicere de aliqua particulari dispositione quam exercet quod naturalis sit operatio id est quod sit operatio ordinata ad sanationem egritudinis precise, nam si sanitas non sequeretur esset mendax, sed debet dicere 'ego ordino hunc sirupum vel electuarium ad talem vel talen operationem' et ita sub spe ulterioris operationis debet eos tenere." *Tabula super vita brevis*, MS Vatican City, BAV Palat. lat. 1320, fols. 121v, 122r. The italicized words are missing in the *Tabula* as printed in the *Opera Arnaldi*, Lugduni 1504, fol. 346v.

lanova had implicitly exposed the basic tension between these two ethical ideals in his commentary on *Vita brevis*, but the more tightly structured *Tabula* makes his advice rather more explicit in explaining how to cope with it in particular instances.

This impulse to *honestas* had not always been so obvious in fourteenth-century medicine. Alberto de Zancariis had given instructions for a physician's behavior in his *De cautelis medicorum* that were aimed entirely at strengthening the physician's position vis-à-vis his patients; the patients' competing interests were ignored. If the physician believes he can identify the patient's complaint, Alberto says, he should announce it loudly, so that everyone may admire his skill and entrust themselves in turn to his care.[21] In prognosis, he should be *astutus* and not *audax*, predicting a cure as soon as it is safe to do so, but saying only, when he is sure that death is imminent, "Certe mihi videtur quod, si constent quae apparent, et aliud non superveniat quod praesenter non supervenire videtur, sanabitur hic vel morietur alter."[22] There is a world of difference between this deliberate attempt at vagueness, and the *Tabula*'s scrupulous concern to make definite statements that are strictly true. Or Alberto's physician can simply refuse to reply to his client's questions: "Melius est silere quam ut tu erres", Alberto concludes, once again making plain whose interests he is concerned to protect.[23] This is a far cry from the *Tabula Arnaldi*, which never suggests that the physician may properly evade responding to his patients' concerns, indeed indicates that it is his responsibility to address them.

There is also a striking contrast between the two works as regards their attitude towards the physician's reward. Alberto ends his description of the physician-patient encounter by specifying that a fee has to be demanded and fully paid, though he warns his audience that the patient will resist doing so. There was nothing at all improper, of course, about physicians' requesting money for their services, though it was understood (in the words of Humbert of Romans, a hundred years before) that "they should take a moderate fee that will not distress their conscience",[24] but the resistance of their patients to payment in general was a vexa-

21 "Si enim medicus praedictis inhaeserit poterit de passione, causa eius, et loco aliquam sumere notionem, quam dum nuntiaverit patienti, talis illum admirans excellentem in sui arte seu scientia iudicabit et per communes in manibus illius confidentius se committet, queri suo posse sanans confortet, in casu omni ei salutem promittens." Morris, *Die Schrift*, p. 16.

22 Morris, *Die Schrift*, pp. 17–18. Cf. Zerbi, *De cautelis medicorum*, Venice [1495], fol. 9va, in a passage cited by French, Medical Ethics, pp. 87–88. This may be compared with the language of the *Tabula* in a similar situation: "Morbus quem cognoscit medicus aut est periculosus, et tunc debet dicere medicus amicis patientis quod timet de periculo (cave tamen ab indiscretis), aut est salubris, et tunc debet medicus interrogantibus de statu patientis respondere quod si patiens et ministri fuerint obedientes, et alia egro vel aliud accidens non supervenerit, spes poterit haberi sanationis."

23 Morris, *Die Schrift*, p. 18. Cf. Zerbi, *De cautelis medicorum*, fol. 10ra.

24 "Salarium sic temperatum recipiant quod suam conscientiam lesam non relinquent"; Humbert de Romans, *Sermones ad diversos status*, quoted by J. Ziegler, *Medicine and Religion c. 1300. The Case of Arnau de Vilanova*, Oxford 1998, p. 314.

tion that physicians and surgeons regularly had somehow to deal with.[25] So it is quite remarkable that the *Tabula* never makes any allusion to the physician's fee as an element in the medical encounter, certainly not to his probable need to extract it from a reluctant client. Money only makes its appearance once in the work, when the author explains to his readers that when they are at a loss for a diagnosis or treatment, a wealthy patient is more likely to be willing to bring in a practitioner from far away for consultation: wealth thus is simply another factor that *diligentia* needs to keep in mind, for the sake of the patient. For Alberto de Zancariis, on the other hand, it would seem that the patient's ability to pay was of particular importance for the physician's sake: *honestas* and *diligentia* were evidently not the only values that Alberto was concerned to promote.[26]

I began by making the unoriginal observation that the choice of works to copy and bring together in a medieval manuscript often reveals something about the concerns and values of the original owner. It seems to me that the fact of the copying, one after another, of the three works I have been talking about – *De lege*, *De commendatione*, and the *Tabula Arnaldi* – does just that as regards its presumed Montpellier compiler in the 1380s. Assuming that they testify to a subset of his concerns, what do they show us? First, above all, that he was someone deeply thoughtful about what it meant to be a physician trained in an academic setting: he did not take his occupation for granted, unconsidered, but chose to reflect deliberately on what should distinguish the kind of physician he felt he should be, the kind of medicine he should practice: its tradition, its place in Christian society, its aims, its values. He seems to have defined himself against unlearned healers on the one hand, and the impractical theorizers of his own faculty, on the other. *Honestas* and *diligentia* (and of course *scientia operationis*) were the values that he professed to practice by: the former was what he insisted set him apart from the ignorant and untrained, the skillful liars who only pretend to be physicians, the latter was what distinguished him from his hyper-subtle word-spinning academic colleagues.

I use the word "profess" deliberately, because, as I have already said, learned medicine in the later 1300s was becoming what we might recognize as something of a profession.[27] I have suggested elsewhere that a new public enthusiasm for

25 See, e.g., M. R. McVaugh, *Medicine Before the Plague. Practitioners and their Patients in the Crown of Aragon*, 1285–1345, Cambridge 1993, pp. 172–73, 182–83.

26 *Disciplina* never figures in Alberto's little text, *honestas* only in one passage concerned with the physician's behavior towards friends, family, and servants tending to the patient, where it certainly does not carry the meaning it has in the *Tabula*: "Verum cum quandoque dominae seu domicellae in astantia maneant laborantes, debet medicus se circa honestis gestibus exhibere illis non intuens ultra decens, nec illis alloquens inhonesta"; Morris, *Die Schrift*, p. 20. (The parallel passage in Zerbi skips over this part of Alberto's discussion of *astantes*: *De cautelis*, fol. 13r–v.) For Zerbi, *honestas* (or *inhonestas*) has a rather different moral loading too. As far as I can tell, he evokes the concept only in the following passage: concerning women, he says, "diligenter advertat medicus ne infamiam inhonestatis incurrat" (*De cautelis*, fol. 13va).

27 See M. Pelling, "Medical Practice in Early Modern England. Trade or Profession?", in: W. Prest (ed.), *The Professions in Early Modern England*, London 1987, pp. 90–128.

medical learning was forcing a broadened social role on academic physicians in the fourteenth century at the same time that it provided them with more economic opportunities. As a result, the world of learned medicine was beginning to change from a collection of solo practitioners, of independent and competitive entrepreneurs, to a self-conscious community that was building up a coherent identity out of shared traditions and values. In urban areas, it increasingly claimed the right to control medical practice in order to keep up standards, to preserve the public health, and to serve the public good. Taken as a whole, these elements look very much like the first stages of something we might recognize as professionalization.

I do not think it too far-fetched to suggest that these various elements can be seen reflected in our anonymous owner's choice of works for his manuscript: they define his identity as a member of what he sees as a community with common values that rejects those who do not share those values. Naturally the values are historically rooted: we can trace them back to Arnau de Vilanova at Montpellier, as we have seen, and beyond Arnau to Galen and Hippocrates. But they are not just historical curiosities: they are fusing insensibly into a self-conscious code of behavior that is distinctive of learned medicine and potentially justifies its status and authority. *Diligentia et honestas*: perhaps we can say that they comprise this particular physician's rudimentary professional ethics, the moral values that Petrarch had pessimistically believed must be inherently lacking in medicine. It may even be, as I suggested at the beginning of this paper and as I rather suspect, that he reflects views that were circulating still more widely in Montpellier's medical faculty in the 1380s – but that, of course, remains to be seen.[28]

APPENDIX

De commendatione medicine

(transcribed from MS. Vatican City, BAV Palat. lat. 1320, fols. 116r–117r)

Sicut legitur in Genesi, in primo creavit Deus celum et terram et homines ad ymaginem et similitudinem suam et eum in paradyso terrestri reposuit, qui est locus amenissimus sub lunari globo positus a nostro emisperio per longitudinem terre et maris separatus. Et cum homo in tam amenissimo loco pertingeret, denique in eo ratio succubuit et sensus inceperit dominari, nam per suggestionem dyabolice fraudis et appetitum carnis proch dolor in morsu vetito perditionem sui causatur et transgressus, unde in lacum tante miserie est delapsus quod non intellexit, ymmo

28 An interesting subject for investigation would be Jean de Tournemire, with whom Valesco de Taranta studied at Montpellier about 1380, and whose *Clarificatorium* (a commentary on *Almansor* IX) has a number of interesting asides, as in its chapter on *disuria* (cap. 74 in some editions, 75 in others): speaking of a physician who had self-medicated for strangury and died as a result, Tournemire writes "istum errorem tota die incurrunt medici. Deus misereatur nostri! Non sine causa populares dicunt nos homicidas"; P. Pansier, "Jean de Tournemire", *Monspeliensis Hippocrates* 42 (1968), pp. 6–12, at 9.

magis factus est similis brutis animalibus ut imimicis(?). Proinde tota sua successiva generatio usque ad finem seculi condolebit. nam quolibet sue generationis suppositum in originali peccato participans duplici perfectione nascitur imperfectum, anime siquidem et corporis: anime quidem quod arguitur per Aristotelem 3° de anima ubi dicit anima humana in sua prima causatione est sicut tabula rasa in qua nihil depictum est, depingibilis tamen,[29] id est in ea inserta est potentia perfectiones quibus caret acquirendi; corporis enim quia homo nascitur totus nudus, in substantia valde passibilis, cum non sit nisi substantia spermatica de novo coagulata, unde in 2° de complexionibus Galieni: "Creati sumus in fine limositatis et humiditatis"; et Avicenna in primo fen 3ª, capitulo singulari: Nos sumus ex duobus spermatibus fluidis et liquidis que non potuerunt venire ad tantam duriciem sicut lapides et vitrum.[30] Et cum hoc sit digressiva creaturarum perfectione indiguit meliori quatenus defectus istos duplices relevaret.

Ad relevandas autem indigentias ex parte anime invente sunt scientie liberales que sub philosophia continentur, quibus anima nata imperfecta plenius perficitur, per quas suo creatori assimilatur; unde capitulo de erroribus, primi methaphisice, dicit Aristoteles quod Symonides[31] retulit quod Deus in hoc summo bono quod est philosophia nobis invidet solum.[32] Est autem philosophia divinorum assistrix insidium rationis insigne mirandum imperiosum nature (116v) consilium causas illustrans omnium; hec enim est scala virtutum vite beneficium forma sanctitatis iusticie speculum calamus pudicitie via prudencie fidei disciplina. Ad relevandas autem indigentias corporis invente sunt scientie mechanice que ad ea que corpori sunt necessaria ordinantur; mechanice quasi manifeste vel quasi adultere respectu liberalium imaginantur. Si ergo corpus humanum debeat conservari, scientie medicine sunt nobis necessarie, ymo magis liberales que sunt anime perfectiones, qui est actus primus corporis organici potentia vitam habentis, ut dicit philosophus 2° de anima.[33] Sed quia rationabilitas esse nequit in homine sine corporis sanitate, sanitas autem corporis humorum eget temperamentis, humores autem temperamenta medicine expostulant iuvamenta, ideo medicina ceteris est utilior et magis necessaria, quia ipsa est sine qua nulla nobis prodest scientia. Et si philosophus dicat quod est scientia altera dignior et honorabilior[34], aut quia de nobiliori subiecto aut quia nobiliori modo procedit, et propter hoc utraque scientia de anima in primo ordine dignitatis est ponenda, et ideo propter eadem scientia medicine ceteris scientiis magis existit commendanda, tum quia de nobiliori subiecto quia de corpore humano, ut dicit Constantinus in primo pantegni.[35]

Hoc autem finis est omnium, ut dicitur 2° phisicorum; finis autem est ultimum et optimum, ut habetur ibidem.[36] Et propter hoc dicitur quod finis est illud propter

29 *De anima* III.4.
30 Paraphrasing *Canon* (1507) I.3, 52va–b.
31 MS Simonices.
32 Cf. *Metaph.* I.2.
33 *De anima* II.1.
34 Cf. Metaph. I.2.
35 Cf. Constantine, *Pantegni, theorica* I.2, *Opera Ysaac* (1515), 2.1ra.
36 Cf. *Phys.* II.2.

quod omnia fiunt, et quia homo est finis omnium, ut dictum est, ideo in Genesi innuitur quod ad servicium hominis omnia creata sunt.[37] Et Hagazes dicit: homo cognosce teipsum, quod modo cognoscens omnia, quia homo quodammodo est omnia, quia omnia sensibilia per sensum, omnia intelligibilia per intellectum. Et ad hoc advertens philosophus libro phisicorum vocavit hominem unctuosum, id est minorem humidum, et ideo dicitur in de animalibus quod homo est digressivum animalium cum sit finis omnium, ut dictus est supra, quod Averois sic exponit: corpora celestia sunt propter elementa, elementa propter mixtum, mixtum propter vegetabile, vegetabile propter sensibile, sensibile propter hominem, et ibi est status. Item in de celo et mundo: totum posse celi[38] et nature est in homine ex parte complexionis sue esse digressivum sortitur, nam Avicenna in primo[39] canone 2º de complexionibus: Deus donavit homini complexionem temperatiorem que esset possibile in hoc mundo.[40] Unde dicitur merito regula Policleti que et si nexu corporali constitutus sit, recepit cum complexione mirifica complementum.

Ex parte etiam anime tantam nobilitatem dicitur ut pre ceteris creaturis nobilior habeatur ratione perfectionis sue, unde Themistius supra secundum de anima: Quibuscumque naturalium natura dedit intellectum, eis ministravit ceteras potentias in ministerium intelligitur.[41] Ex parte modi procedendi meruit etiam nobilior ceteris appellari, quia cum quedam scientie procedant via resolutiva, ut philosophia naturalis, quedam compositiva, ut geographia et analetica, quedam diffinitiva, ut liber tegni, ista medicina per omnem modum procedit secundum diversas partes, ut patet intuenti. Ex parte suorum inventorum meruit commendari. Inventores fuisse diversi exhibentur(?) secundum diversitatem lingue et nacionum: in lingua hebrea Salomon regis dicitur filius qui librum fecit de naturis rerum, perscribens ab ysopo periens usque ad cedrum extendit libani. Ac refert Maurus(?) in lingua greca primus omnium fuit Apollo, ad cuius honorem statua erecta est, cui successit Esculapius filius eius quo ictu divini fulminis[42] interempto mortales metuerunt ad hanc artem accedere, timentes causam sue mortis, unde latuit hec per quingentos et lx annos usque ad tempora Ariensis regis persarum, in cuius temporibus Ypocras Chous tanquam sydus mirifice lucis efulsit, ut ait Maurus, qui hanc artem ad nichilum redactam in lucem produxit et laude et opere ampliavit. Cui successerunt Tullius et Democritus, magnus Galienus in greco et Unaym in arabico, cui successerunt Rufus Zalon Palomon Locsus Oribasius et alii plures in greco; in arabico, Ysaac et Rasis et Constantinus qui baptismatis gratia[43] consecutus totam artem transtulit in latinum; et alii plures successores, greci arabici ebrei, reges imperatores et sancti, sicut patet per opera nobilis quantitatis que nobis linguam relinquerunt.

37 Cf. *Gen.* 1.26.
38 MS del. est.
39 MS del. can.
40 Paraphrasing *Canon* I.1.iii.2.
41 Themistius *comm. de anima* III.2, ed. Verbeke p. 114.
42 MS fluminis.
43 MS corr. ex gratiam.

Ex parte sui artificis quo a medicina medicus sollicitudini recommendatur(?), nam in Ecclesiastico xxxviii° capitulo legitur "da locum medico, creavit enim eum altissimus, et non recedat a te, quia opera eius sunt necessaria"; et inde "honora medicum propter necessitatem; creavit enim eum altissimus"; et ibidem "disciplina medici exaltavit caput illum et in conspectu magnorum collaudabitur." Et semper intelligi oportet de medico theorico et practico, unde dicit Rasis in sua cyrurgia: nomen plurium medicorum (117r) nomine est multum, operatione vero paucum. Tales enim medici equivoce debent dici, ut sunt illi de quibus loquitur Galienus in tertia particula pronosticorum, quos vocat medicos locutionum.[44] Sedent enim in sedibus altis et loquuntur in illo discipulis locutionem magnam valde et nesciunt plus de hiis que accidunt circa infirmos quam de mensuratione altitudinis maris. Isti enim de medicina non habentes quem proferant in subtilibus et sensum transcendentibus, sue inpericie solacium querentes, a semitis deviant medicine: ymmo loco Ypocratis sumunt philosophum, et loco Galieni narrant Prescianum, loco Avicenne adducunt Tullium, a propria semita deviantes. Sunt autem tales de secta Hierophonis, qui relictis aliis instrumentis iussit sibi littera attollere, aliam impendens. Tales enim sapientis medici nomine non debent congaudere, quoniam secundum philosophum circa principium primi ethicorum:[45] "prudentis est rei certitudinem in terminis inquirere secundum unumquodque genus in quantum natura rei permittit; par enim peccatum est mathematicum probabilia dicentem placere et rethoricum demonstratione experiri. Unusquisque enim iudicat quod novit et eorum est optimus iudex." Contra huiusmodi medicos clamat Galienus, primo de creticis diebus,[46] dicens quod quidam sunt persistentes medicos de nominis significatione disputantes, id est semper de hiis qui nullum auxilium prebent in opere, sed ignorant quod iam recesserunt a semita medicine et ad illud declinant manifeste, de quo grammatici dyalectici et rethores consueverunt perscrutari, quod faciunt multi medicorum hodie. Tales enim duobus modis peccant: uno modo quia ipsi dimittunt inquirere ea de quibus debet esse inquisitio medicorum, secundo conantur et temptant quod est artis alterius preter quam eius noticiam fuerint assecuti verba Galieni libro predicto. Sunt enim nonnulli medici qui cortici adherentes, nucleum pretermittunt seu etiam abiciunt, intentes politicis sermonibus vento persenis mentes auditorum palleare, quod omnino credo inutile; prefectionibus enim rethoricis non eget medicinalis speculatio sed talibus solum sermonibus quibus evidentis comprehenditur intentio proferentis.

Hiis prelibatis, ad commendationem medicine veniamus. Medicina commendatur multipliciter in ecclesiastico capitulo superius allegato: "Altissimus de terra creavit medicinam et vir prudens non abhorrebit illam," et idem "a deo est medela et a rege accipiet donationem." Et Empedocles vocavit eam divine munificencie donum.[47] Constantinus in primo pantegni[48] diffinit theoricam sic: theorica

44 Galen, *Comm. Hipp. Pronost.* III.6, *Articella* (1523), [2].162va.

45 *Eth. Nich.* I.1.

46 Cf. Galen, *De dieb. cret.* I.5, *Opera* (1490), 1.98vb.

47 MS domum. Cf. *Opusculum de plantis*, prol., MS Troyes 951.

48 Constantine, *Pantegni, theorica* I.3, Opera Ysaac, 2.1vb.

est perfecta cognitio rerum solo intellectu capiendarum subiecta memorie rerum operandarum; practicam sic: practica est subiectam theoricam demonstrare in propatulo sensuum et operatione manuum secundum preeuntis theorice intellectum. Quidam Salernitanus eam sic recomendavit: Medicina est quedam scientia excellentissima que suum artificem reddit miraculis tho…tem(?) honestum et amabilem, quem[49] matrona venerat, virgo non abhorret, nupta illecebri ignara consortii sub spe salutis amplectatur. Non illius negatur calamus, non illum repudiat brachium virginalem sed potius se detegit tactui, et si qua sunt securiora illi tanquam sanctorum sanctissimo revelantur. Ab Avicenna sic:[50] Medicina est scientia qua dispositiones corporis humani cognoscuntur etc. A Galieno in tegni:[51] Medicina est scientia sanorum et egrorum et neutrorum. Ab Ysaac in primo febrium:[52] Medicina est scientia regendi complexionem naturalem in eo in quo est et reducendi eam que est extra naturam ad naturalem.

49 MS quam.
50 Avicenna, *Canon* I.1.i.1.
51 Galen, *Tegni* I text 1, *Articella*, [3].86ra.
52 Isaac, *Liber febrium* I.2, *Opera Ysaac*, 1.203vb.

DER KLUGE PATIENT. HUMANISTISCHE ÄRZTEKRITIK IM SPANNUNGSFELD ZWISCHEN ETHIK UND MEDIZIN

Matthias Roick

Ende 1475 ziehen sich dunkle Wolken über dem Königreich Neapel zusammen, und ausnahmsweise sind es nicht die Barone des Königreichs, die für Unruhe sorgen, sondern der König und sein Thronfolger.[1] Am 12. November berichtet Ippolita Sforza ihrem Bruder Galeazzo Maria, dem Herrscher von Mailand, dass ihr Gatte, Herzog Alfonso, schwer erkrankt sei. Bereits den achten Tag sei er bettlägerig, die Ärzte seien damit beschäftigt, ihn wieder auf die Beine zu bringen.[2] Doch noch am selben Tag sieht sie sich gezwungen, eine weitere Depesche zu verfassen. Auch König Ferrante sei erkrankt, schlimmer noch als sein Sohn, der Herzog.[3] Ein Machtvakuum droht, Ippolita berichtet fast jeden Tag nach Mailand.[4]

Die meisten Briefe aus dieser Zeit sind nicht immer von Ippolita selbst verfasst, sondern von einem jungen Mann namens Giovanni Pontano.[5] Als Humanist

1 König Ferrante war seinem Vater Alfonso von Aragon, genannt *il magnanimo*, 1458 auf den Thron gefolgt, konnte seine Herrschaft aber erst 1464 durch einen Sieg gegen aufständische Barone unter der Führung des französischen Thronanwärters Jean d'Anjou festigen. Alfonso selbst hatte das Königreich Neapel erst 1442 durch einen Sieg gegen dessen Vater René d'Anjou erobert. Die Lage blieb auf Dauer gespannt; 1485 sollten die Barone sich erneut gegen Ferrante auflehnen.

2 Ippolita Sforza an Galeazzo Maria Sforza, Neapel, 12. November 1475: «[...] jo al presente ne dono aviso ad V[ostra] Ill[ustrissima] S[ignoria] che oge sonno otto dì che lo dicto S[ignore] mio è malato de febre con fluxo [...] Et però, benché al principio de tal fluxo lì medici fossero multo temerusi questa egritudine portasse periculo, gionti li altri signi che lo [sic] concomitavano, adesso se confortano che con lo aiuto divino questo male haverà presto et ben terminare, vedendo el male minorare.» Zitiert aus Giovanni Pontano, *Lettere inedite di Joviano Pontano in nome de' reali di Napoli*, hg. von F. Gabotto, Bologna 1893, S. 64.

3 Ippolita Sforza an Galeazzo Maria Sforza, Neapel, 12. November 1475: «[...] qui è sopragionta la infermità del S[ignor] Re, el quale se trova a uno loco chiamato Carinole et secundo intendo sta peio de lo Ill[ustrissimo] S[ignor] duca mio, sì che pensa V[ostra] S[ignoria] come sto; chè, se non fusse la gran fede et speranza tegnio ne la S[ignoria] V[ostra] come patre, io sono meza disperata.» Pontano, *Lettere inedite*, S. 67.

4 Ebd., S. 69: «circa lo Statu se fanno dal S[ignor] Duca mio tutte le provisione se iudicano necessarie, imperò con maturità et secundo el casu monstra rechedere. Ho voluto de tutto dare notitia ad la Ill[ustrissima] S[ignoria] V[ostra] secundo el debito mio rechede, et così farrò de giorno in giorno secundo el casu portarà.»

5 Zu Pontano vgl. C. Kidwell, *Pontano. Poet and Prime Minister*, London 1991. Zu verschiedenen Aspekten seines Schaffens und seiner Biographie vgl. L. Monti Sabia – S. Monti, *Studi*

und loyaler Anhänger des Königshauses, ist er prädestiniert für die Aufgabe als Ippolitas Sekretär: Auf der einen Seite erfüllt er die Anforderungen der gebildeten Ippolita; auf der anderen Seite kann er ihr auf die Finger schauen.[6] Eigentlich ist Pontano Dichter, aber in den Briefen, die die Krankheit des Königs und des Herzogs begleiten, sind keine dichterischen Talente gefragt. Hier steht die Sachinformation im Vordergrund. Es geht um Schleimflüsse, Exkremente, Blutungen und Schröpfungen.[7]

Ähnlich wie in anderen Krankenberichten, lässt sich in den präzisen Formulierungen Pontanos der Krankheitsverlauf der Patienten verfolgen: Man hält sich auf dem Laufenden, holt verschiedene Meinungen ein.[8] So heißt es in einem Brief vom 27. November, man habe durch einen Arzt namens Silvestro erfahren, dass die Krankheit des Königs – entgegen den Beteuerungen seiner Kollegen – noch nicht überwunden sei.[9] Nichtsdestotrotz sind König und Herzog Anfang Dezember wieder wohlauf.

su Giovanni Pontano, 2 Bde., Messina 2010. Zu Pontanos humanistischem Denken vgl. M. Roick, *Mercury in Naples. The Moral and Political Thought of Giovanni Pontano*, Leiden, im Erscheinen.

6 Zur Rolle Ippolitas als Mittlerin zwischen Neapel und Mailand sowie ihrem gespannten Verhältnis zu ihrem Mann, dem Herzog von Kalabrien, vgl. E. Welch, „Between Milan and Naples. Ippolita Maria Sforza, Duchess of Calabria“, in: D. Abulafia (Hg.), *The French Descent into Renaissance Italy. Antecedents and Effects*, Aldershot 1995, S. 123–36.

7 Der Brief vom 12. November beschreibt das Fieber des Herzogs von Kalabrien «la quale depende de colèra, perchè con lo fluxo ha emisso assai quantità de materia colerita che ha havuto assai del maligno. Foli data una medicina … et le materie sonno minorate, le orine più retificate» (Pontano, *Lettere inedite*, S. 65). Ein weiterer Brief vom 19. November berichtet von einem Paroxysmus «el quale fo multo grave et affannoso et multo dà da timere ad ciaschun, sì per esser ancho grave et vehemente, et sequì in fine che evacuò uno verme morto con fece ben corrupta in bona quantità» (ebd., S. 72). Am 23. November wird von «due ventose ad sangue et … alcune cose medicinale per la parte inferiore» berichtet (ebd., S. 74). Am 27. November heißt es, «dicta M[aesta] hebbe un grande beneficio naturale, perchè sponte sua li rompì el naso ad sangue» (ebd., S. 80). Ähnlich am 29. November: «Heri … la M[aestà] del S[ignor] Re hebbe [uno al]tro beneficio de natura, che li uscì dal nasu circa tre oncie de sangue» (ebd., S. 83).

8 Zur Beschreibung (*narratio*) des Krankheitsverlaufs hochrangiger Patienten durch Höflinge und Gesandte vgl. C. Crisciani, „Fatti, teorie, narratio e i malati a corte. Note su empirismo in medicina nel trado medioevo“, *Quaderni Storici* 36 (2001), S. 695–717. Zu einer ähnlich gelagerten und zeitlich nahen Situtaion vgl. den Fall von Ippolitas Mutter Bianca Maria Sforza, dargestellt in M. Nicoud, „Expérience de la maladie et échange épistolaire. Les derniers moments de Bianca Maria Visconti (mai–octobre 1468)“, *Mélanges de l'Ecole française de Rome. Moyen Age* 112 (2000), S. 311–458.

9 Ippolita Sforza an Galeazzo Maria Sforza, Neapel, 26. November 1475: «Questa sera per uno mio fidato venuto da Carinola fo advisata ad bocca da parte del medico, mio servitore, cioè messer Silvestro, como luj non è securo de la infirmità del S[ignor] Re et che per tre o quatro altri dì futuri non arderia affirmare che sia fora de periculo, et stane ancho multo sospiso et timido.»

DER PATIENT ALS VERANTWORTLICHER LAIE

Die Geschichte dieser Doppelerkrankung offenbart den politischen Druck, der auf solch hochrangigen Krankheitsfällen lastet. Sie zeigt zudem, wie sehr sich die Behandlung von Kranken nicht nur in der Obhut der Ärzte befand, sondern auch von den Patienten und ihren Angehörigen verfolgt wurde.

In diesem Zusammenhang scheint es sinnvoll, die Frage nach der humanistischen Medizinethik sowohl in Hinsicht auf die behandelnden Ärzte, als auch in Bezug auf die Patientenseite zu stellen, um so der sozialen Dynamik gerecht zu werden, die sich zwischen Arzt und Patient entwickelt. Um dieser Dynamik auf die Spur zu kommen empfiehlt es sich, das Verhältnis von Arzt und Patient analytisch als eine Beziehung zwischen einem Laien und einem Experten zu lesen. Formelhaft ausgedrückt ist der Patient insofern Laie, als er nicht über das medizinische Sonderwissen verfügt, das den Arzt als Experten auszeichnet. Durch diese ungleiche Verteilung von Wissen kommt es in den Worten Frank Rexroths zu einem „dialogischen Widerspruch“: Ist der Laie einerseits auf den Experten angewiesen, da dessen medizinische Kenntnisse seinen eigenen Wissenshorizont übersteigen, bringt er ihm andererseits ein tiefes Misstrauen entgegen, trägt der Experte doch in gewisser Weise zu der Komplexität bei, die dem Laien einen direkten Zugriff auf diese Kenntnisse unmöglich macht.[10]

Genau an diesem Widerspruch setzt die Kritik der italienischen Humanisten an den Expertenkulturen ihrer Zeit ein. Denn das Ziel der humanistischen Bildung ist – ihrem Selbstverständnis nach – nicht der Experte, sondern der verantwortungsvolle Laie, der Mensch als Handelnder.[11] Diese neue Gewichtung des Laien erklärt, warum die Figur des Patienten in der Medizinethik des Humanismus eine strategisch wichtige Rolle spielt: Sie sieht ihn nicht als eine passive Figur, die sich der Autorität der Ärzte fügt, sondern als eine aktive Figur, die selbst eine Autorität entwickelt und das Handeln des Arztes kritisch und verantwortungsvoll verfolgt.

Pontano selbst bringt diese Verantwortlichkeit der Betreuten in einem seiner frühen Dialoge, dem *Charon* zum Ausdruck. Zwischen Spiel und Ernst, Satire und Gesellschaftskritik angelegt, nehmen die Sprecher des Dialogs, die sich im Jenseits befinden, die Missstände im Diesseits aufs Korn. Die Ärzte dürfen in diesem Pandämonium nicht fehlen. Wie der Götterbote Merkur verlauten lässt, leben „die Ärzte freier, weil es ihnen erlaubt ist, ungestraft einen Menschen zu töten.“ „Ist das bei ihnen nicht schwerer Mord?“ fragt Charon, Ruderknecht mit philosophischen Ambitionen, erstaunt zurück. „Gewiß,“ antwortet ihm Merkur, „trotzdem

10 F. Rexroth, *Expertenweisheit. Die Kritik an den Studierten und die Utopie einer geheilten Gesellschaft im späten Mittelalter*, Basel 2008, S. 20.

11 Diese These wird ausführlich behandelt in M. Roick, „Der Fahnenflüchtige lässt sich krönen. Petrarca und die Anfänge der humanistischen Kritik am Experten“, in: F. Rexroth – B. Reich – M. Roick (Hgg.), *Wissen maßgeschneidert. Die Geburt des Experten in der Vormoderne*, München 2012, S. 45–82.

spricht das Gesetz die Ärzte nicht nur frei, sondern legt für sie auch eine Belohnung fest.“[12]

Diese Kritik ist natürlich ein Gemeinplatz der Ärztekritik. So stammt die Zuspitzung, nur der Arzt gehe straflos aus, wenn er einen Menschen zu Tode brächte, aus dem 29. Buch der *Naturkunde* Plinius’ des Älteren, der auch die „Gewinnsucht ohne Maß und Ziel“ der Ärzte geißelt und die *praemia artis* kritisiert, die sie einstreichen. Für Plinius besteht kein Zweifel daran, „dass all diese Ärzte, indem sie durch irgendeine Neuerung von sich reden zu machen suchen, direkt (auf Kosten) unseres Lebens Geschäfte machen“.[13]

Pontanos Kritik hat jedoch nicht nur antike Quellen; ein näher liegender Bezugspunkt ist der Unmut über die *scientiae lucrativae*, der sich mit der Entwicklung der mittelalterlichen Universität einstellt und die Kritik an den Experten speist: „Dat Galienus opes et sanctio Justiniana, / ex aliis paleas, ex istos collige grana“, lautet ein einschlägiger Vers, der sich bereits im 12. Jahrhundert nachweisen lässt. In der Fächerwahl trennt sich die Spreu vom Weizen und beschert den Anhängern Galens und des *Codex Iustinianus*, also den studierten Ärzten und Medizinern, Geld wie Heu, um das Bild leicht abzuwandeln.[14] Entscheidend an Pontanos Argument ist allerdings, dass er einen Schritt weitergeht, als es in der herkömmlichen Kritik an den Ärzten der Fall ist. Als sich der etwas naive Charon über die Ungerechtigkeit beschwert, Ärzte straffrei ausgehen zu lassen und sie für ihre Unfähigkeit zu bezahlen, wendet Merkur listig ein, dass das Gesetz die Ärzte zu Recht freispreche, denn, fährt er fort, „nicht der Arzt tötet, sondern wer den Rat und die Hilfe eines Arztes gebraucht und dabei noch einen hohen Preis bezahlt“.[15] Der gewitzte Merkur kann durchaus beim Wort genommen werden: Die Behandlungsverantwortung liegt auf beiden Seiten. Patient und Arzt sind nicht durch ein einseitiges Verhältnis aneinander gebunden; medizinisches Handeln ist zugleich ein Verhandeln. Die Frage ist, welche Faktoren im Einzelnen dazu beitragen, das der nötige Spielraum für ein solches Verhandeln entsteht. Natürlich spielt gerade die vielgescholtene Bezahlung des Arztes eine strategische Rolle in der Schaffung einer Verhandlungssituation. Dennoch reicht die Tatsache, dass der Arzt auf die

12 Giovanni Pontano, *Dialoge*, übers. von H. Kiefer, München 1984, S. 72: „Mercurius: [...] liberius medici, ut quibus permissum sit hominem impune occidere. – Charon: An non capitale apud ilos est parricidium? – Mercurius: Etiam; medicos tamen lex non modo absolvit, verum mercedem quoque eis statuit.“

13 Plinius d. Ä., *Naturalis historia*, 29.5.11: „nec dubium est omnes istos famam novitate aliqua aucupantes anima statim nostra negotiari.“ Ebd. 29.8.18: „discunt periculis nostris et experimenta per mortes agunt, medicoque tantum hominem occidisse inpunitas summa est.“

14 S. Kuttner, „Dat Galienus opes et sanctio Iustiniana“, in: A. S. Chrysafulli (Hg.), *Literary and Linguistic Studies in Honor of Helmut A. Hatzfeld*, Washington, D.C. 1964, S. 237–46. Vgl. auch die Bemerkungen in J. Miethke, „Karrierechancen eines Theologiestudiums im späteren Mittelalter“, in: Ders., *Studieren an mittelalterlichen Universitäten. Chancen und Risiken*, gesammelte Aufsätze, Leiden / Boston 2004, S. 97–132.

15 Pontano, *Dialoge*, S. 72: „Charon: Quam inique comparatum! – Mercurius: Quinimo ire eos lex absolvit, siquidem medicus non occidit, verum qui medici utitur consilio et opera, quam quidem vel magno conducunt precio.“

Bezahlung durch den Patienten angewiesen ist, nicht aus, um die Autoritätsverteilung zwischen Arzt und Patient neu zu bestimmen.

DER KLUGE PATIENT

Die Aufwertung der Patientenseite verlangt vielmehr nach einer Ethik, die es dem Patienten erlaubt, den Arzt unabhängig von seinen medizinischen Fachkenntnissen zu beurteilen. Schon bei Petrarca zeigt sich deswegen eine große Aufmerksamkeit für den verantwortungsvollen Umgang des Patienten mit seinen Ärzten.[16] Sein berühmter, im März 1352 verfasster Brief an Papst Clemens VI. (*Fam.* 5.19) ist in dieser Hinsicht besonders aufschlussreich: In den *Invective* verteidigt Petrarca diesen Brief mit dem Argument, sein einziges Ziel sei es gewesen, dem sich in Behandlung befindlichen Papst zur Vorsicht (*cautio*) zu raten – ein klassischer Teilbereich der *prudentia*.[17] Ein Großteil der Menschen begehe den Fehler, sich trotz besseren Wissens immer wieder an inkompetente Ärzte zu wenden. Gebildete Menschen dagegen würden dieser Versuchung widerstehen. Dem dummen Rest, heißt es schon bei Petrarca mit ähnlich viel Mitgefühl wie später bei Pontanos Merkur, solle man keine Träne nachweinen.[18]

Mit seinem Brief will Petrarca also erreichen, dass der Papst als Patient und medizinischer Laie Klugheit gegenüber den Ärzten und Medizinexperten walten lässt. Dabei geht es zunächst weniger um Inhalte, als um die Form der Behandlung. Mit Besorgnis habe er vernommen, dass das Bett des Papstes von Doktoren umlagert sei. Der Situation entsprechend warnt Petrarca den Papst davor, den Rat zu vieler Ärzte zu suchen. Anlass zur Sorge gibt ihm die ‚Gruppendynamik', die sich in dieser Situation entwickelt: Befänden sich nämlich mehrere Ärzte bei-

16 Zu Petrarca und seinem vielseitigen Verhältnis zur Medizin vgl. die Beiträge in: M. Berté – V. Fera – T. Pesenti (Hgg.), *Petrarca e la medicina. Atti del convegno di Capo d'Orlando 27–28 giugno 2003*, Messina 2006. Einschlägig für den deutschsprachigen Bereich sind zudem: K. Bergdolt, *Arzt, Krankheit und Therapie bei Petrarca. Die Kritik an Medizin und Naturwissenschaft im italienischen Frühhumanismus*, Weinheim 1992 sowie K. A. Enenkel, „Ein erster Ansatz zur Konstituierung einer humanistischen Streitkultur. Petrarcas ‚Invective contra medicum'", in: M. Laureys – R. Simons (Hgg.), *Die Kunst des Streitens. Inszenierung, Formen und Funktionen öffentlichen Streits in historischer Perspektive*, Bonn 2010, S. 109–126.

17 Francesco Petrarca, „Invectives Against a Physician", in: Ders., *Invectives*, hg. und übers. von D. Marsh, Cambridge (Mass.) / London 2003, S. 2–179, hier S. 20: „Lege, si libet, et nisi ego quoque tibi grecus videor, epystolam illam totam, que cum ad hoc unum scripta esset, ut universali domino cautionem pareret, tibi nescio cui [...] dolorem peperit ac furorem." Zur Beschreibung der *cautio* als Teilbereich der *prudentia* vgl. z. B. Thomas von Aquin, *Summa Theologiae*, IIa–IIae q. 49 a. 8.

18 Petrarca, *Invective*, S. 62–64: „Tanta est spei humane pertinacia, sic in animis miserorum regnat oblivio, qua fretus multos ante diem in Tartarum premisisti qui si redeant illi veram de te potuerint ferre sententiam! Sed inde quidem tutus es: irremeabilis est regio. Nolo tamen speres latere superstites: notus es publice et, puto, doctos frustra tentabis; ceterorum strages minime flenda est."

sammen, widersprächen sie sich mit Fleiß, da keiner dem anderen nachstehen wolle.[19] An dieser Stelle zitiert Petrarca ausführlich aus dem bereits erwähnten 29. Buch der *Naturkunde* des Plinius, der den Konkurrenzkampf der Ärzte als ein Spiel mit der Hoffnung der Patienten interpretiert:

> Deshalb geschieht es in der Tat bei dieser Kunst allein, dass man jedem, der sich für einen Arzt ausgibt, sofort Glauben schenkt, obwohl doch bei keiner Lüge eine größere Gefahr besteht. Dennoch achten wir nicht darauf, so verführerisch ist für jeden von uns der Zauber des Hoffens.[20]

Plinius selbst bezieht diese Kritik nicht nur auf die Ärzte. Allgemeiner Hintergrund ist seine Polemik gegen die griechische Medizin, der als römisches Vorbild Cato entgegengesetzt wird. Cato habe, schreibt Plinius, nicht als Arzt, sondern als Hausvater für die Gesundheit seiner Familie und seines Gesindes gesorgt und sich auf sein eigenes Rezeptbuch verlassen. Anders die Zeitgenossen des Plinius: Sie verließen sich vor allem auf die griechische Medizin, deren Autorität sie so sehr schätzten, dass selbst römische Ärzte sich in der Art der griechischen Ärzte inszenieren müssten: „Man kommt eben nicht anders zu Ansehen, als wenn man (die Kunst) griechisch betreibt, gerade bei Unerfahrenen und der Sprache Unkundigen; und sie glauben den Vorschriften, die ihr Wohl betreffen, dann weniger, wenn sie diese verstehen."[21] Während Plinius sich gegen diese Art von Inszenierung wendet und die Rückkehr zu einer einfachen, ‚römischen' Medizin fordert – seine Aufzeichnungen sollen in der Tat dem Rezeptbuch Catos ähneln – beschäftigt Petrarca ein anderes Problem. Es geht ihm nicht darum, dass der Papst seine Behandlung hausväterlich selbst in die Hand nehmen soll. Er spricht offen aus, dass man sich mittlerweile „ein Leben ohne Ärzte nicht mehr vorzustellen [wagt]" und empfiehlt dem Papst gerade deswegen, er solle sich „einen von den vielen [aussuchen], der sich nicht durch Beredsamkeit (*eloquentia*), sondern durch sein Wissen (*scientia*) und seine Vertrauenswürdigkeit (*fides*) auszeichnet." Diesen Ratschlag verbindet Petrarca mit einer Kritik an der Praxis einiger Ärzte, am Lager des Kranken eher zu disputieren als zu kurieren.[22]

19 Petrarca, *Familiares*, 5.19.3: „Lectum tuum obsessum medicis scio; hinc prima michi timendi causa est. Discordant enim de industria, dum pudet novi nichil afferentem alterius hesisse vestigiis." Ich zitiere die *Familiares* hier und im Folgenden nach Francesco Petrarca, *Le familiari*, 4 Bde., Florenz 1933–1942.

20 Ebd.: „[...] et in hac sola artium evenire, ut cuicunque se medicum profitenti statim credatur, cum sit periculum in nullo mendacio maius; non tamen illud intuemur, adeo blanda est sperandi pro se cuique dulcedo. Nulla preterea lex que puniat inscitiam capitalem, nullum exemplum vindicte; discunt periculis nostris et experimenta per mortes agunt, medicoque tantum hominem occidisse impunitas summa est." Es handelt sich um ein wörtliches Zitat aus Plinius, *Naturkunde*, 29.5.17–18.

21 Ebd. 29.5.17: „[...] immo vero auctoritas aliter quam Graece eam tractantibus etiam apud inperitos expertesque linguae non est, ac minus credunt quae ad salutem suam pertinent, si intellegant."

22 Petrarca, *Le Familiari*, 5.19.5: „Sed quia iam sine medicis vivere non audemus, [...] unum tibi de multis elige, non eloquentia sed scientia et fide conspicuum. Iam enim professionis sue immemores et dumetis propriis exire ausi, poetarum nemus et rethorum campum petunt, et quasi non curaturi sed persuasuri, circa miserorum grabatulos magno boatu disputant [...]."

In einem Brief an den Arzt Guglielmo da Ravenna (*Seniles* 3.8) nimmt Petrarca diese Kritik wieder auf. In Erinnerung an eine Krankheit während seiner Zeit in Mailand hebt er zwei der Ärzte, die ihn damals behandelten, besonders hervor, die sich nicht so sehr durch ihre Kunstfertigkeit als durch ihr Verhalten (*non tam arte quam moribus*) am Krankenbett unterschieden hätten. Der eine habe sich still zu ihm ans Ruhebett gestellt und seinen Puls gemessen, um sich anschließend mit seinen Kollegen zu beraten und ihm dann Mut zuzusprechen. Der andere habe dagegen Wurzeln an seinem Krankenbett geschlagen und ihm das müde Haupt wirr geredet.[23] Der erste Arzt gewinnt das Vertrauen (*fides*) Petrarcas, den zweiten würde er am liebsten ausschließen. „Kein Kranker möchte einen Arzt, der disputiert (*contionantem*), sondern einen Arzt, der heilt (*curantem*)", stichelt er.[24] Die Medizin ist nach Petrarca eine „stille Kunst" (*ars muta*), in der es um Kräuter, nicht um Worte gehe (*herbis, non verbis*).[25] Die Rede des Arztes soll demnach „kurz, gewichtig und nüchtern" sein (*brevis, gravis, sobria*). Allein auf diese Weise könne der Arzt Hoffnung im Patienten wecken und sich selbst Autorität verschaffen.[26]

Das Raffinierte an Petrarcas Argument ist die Tatsache, dass er sich der ethischen Regeln *für* den Arzt bedient und sie in einen Forderungskatalog *an* den Arzt verwandelt. Es geht eben, anders als in der Kautelenliteratur, nicht um den vorsichtigen Arzt, sondern um den vorsichtigen Patienten. So stellt das Schweigen des Arztes, dass Petrarca vehement von seinem Gegenüber einfordert, eine grundlegende, häufig nachzulesende Regel dar, die ein fester Bestandteil der mittelalterlichen Ärzteausbildung war. „Der Arzt soll nicht geschwätzig sein, sondern die Stille zum Freund haben", heißt es z.B. in einem anonymen Brief „Über die Kunst der Medizin" (*medicum non oportet esse multiloquum, sed amicum debet habere silentium*).[27] Selbst der Ratschlag an Papst Clemens VI. fällt unter diese Kategorie. Im Nachhinein habe er erfahren, dass der Ratschlag, sich nicht auf eine Vielzahl von Ärzten zu verlassen, von Ärzten stammt, schreibt Petrarca Jahre später an einen befreundeten Arzt.[28] Die Schlagkraft des petrarkischen Arguments hängt also nicht von seiner ‚Neuigkeit', sondern gerade von seiner Anlehnung an traditionelle Vorgaben ab, die allerdings eine neue Wendung erfahren, indem sie von Petrarca *gegen* den Arzt gewendet werden. Dem anonymen Verfasser des eben erwähnten Briefes kommt es in der Tat nicht auf ein patientenfreundliches Verhal-

23 Petrarca, *Seniles* 3.8.7–13. Ich zitiere nach der kritischen Ausgabe der medizinischen Briefe Petrarcas in: M. Berté – S. Rizzo, „Le Senili mediche", in: Berté – Fera – Pesenti (Hgg.), *Petrarca e la medicina*, S. 247–375.

24 Ebd. 3.8.14, S. 298.

25 Ebd. 3.8.17–21, S. 299.

26 Ebd. 3.8.24–28, S. 300.

27 Anonymus, „Epistula de disciplina artis medicinae", in: L. Firpo (Hg.), *Medicina Medievale*, Turin 1971, S. 36.

28 Petrarca, *Seniles* 16.3.44, S. 372. Berté und Rizzo (S. 286, Anm. 2) verweisen auf Pietro d'Abano, *Conciliator*, *differentia* 7, in der die Frage behandelt wird, ob der Patient seine Heilung einem oder mehreren Ärzten anvertrauen soll.

ten an, sondern darauf, dass der Arzt seine Berufsgeheimnisse für sich behalten solle.[29]

Ähnlich verhält es sich mit der Kleidung der Ärzte. Ein Regelwerk aus dem Umkreis der ‚Scuola Salernitana' empfiehlt, eine ehrenvolle Bescheidenheit an den Tag zu legen (*modestus cum omni honestate*) und deswegen „glänzende (weiße) Kleider" (*splendida vestimenta*) zu tragen.[30] Petrarca befindet sich eigentlich in Übereinstimmung mit dieser Vorschrift, wenn er die rote oder goldene Kleidung der Ärzte kritisiert. In einem Brief an Giovanni Boccaccio (*Sen.* 5.3) beschwert er sich über den in Mode gekommenen Prunk der Ärztekleidung, ihre feurig roten Roben, die sie besticken lassen, ihre leuchtenden Ringe und goldenen Sporen (*indigni habitus usurpata iactantia, vestes murice ardentes, sub suto vario distintae, annuli radiantes, aurata calcaria*).[31] Aus der Sicht Petrarcas drückt diese Kleidung die Anmaßung (*audacia*) und Lügenhaftigkeit der Ärzte aus. Die Herrscher sollten ein solches Verhalten nicht dulden, schreibt er seinem Freund, und der Dreistigkeit dieser Handwerker ein rechtes Maß auferlegen (*tantae mechanicorum licentiae modum ponat*).[32] Tatsächlich lässt sich Petrarcas Unmut auch institutionell deuten: Wenn zeitgenössische Miniaturen und Tafelgemälde Ärzte häufig in roter Kleidung zeigen, handelt es sich eigentlich um eine Überschreitung des Standesgemäßen – die statuarische Überlieferung bezieht sich nur auf rote Birette.[33]

EIN NEUES LAIENTUM

Dieses letzte Beispiel zeigt, wie eng die moralische Beurteilung von Ärzten – ihre ‚Geschwätzigkeit', ihre angebliche Überheblichkeit und Lügenhaftigkeit – bei Petrarca mit einer institutionellen Polemik verbunden ist. Im Grunde handelt es sich um den Versuch, einen sozialen Raum für sich zu beanspruchen, der immer mehr von Ärzten, aber auch von anderen Expertengruppen wie den Juristen oder den Universitätsphilosophen besetzt worden war. Denn gerade diejenigen Expertengruppen, die seit dem 12. Jahrhundert eine Partikularisierung des Wissens vorantreiben, versuchen im 14. Jahrhundert über ihre Fächer hinaus eine Art ethisch-christliches Wissen zu schaffen, das ihr technisch-wissenschaftliches Wissen ergänzt. Ein berühmter Jurist wie Giovanni d'Andrea (gest. 1348) schreibt nicht nur Glossen und Kommentare zu den Dekretalen, sondern auch ein von Petrarca heftig kritisiertes *Opus Hieronymianum*, das seine Belesenheit und seinen

29 Petrarca, *Seniles* 16.3.44, S. 372: „Non diu debet sermones ambiguos circumire, non secreta curae pandere, aut artis archana publicare, nisi tantum indicia causarum iam sanis exponere. Nam qui vult artis inquisitionem saepius enarrare, tunc incipit in detractionem professionis incurrere."

30 Anonymus, Epistula, S. 40.

31 Petrarca, *Seniles* 5.4, in: Ders., *Opera Omnia*, Bd. 1, Basel 1581, S. 796–801, hier S. 797.

32 Ebd.

33 A. von Hülsen-Esch, *Gelehrte im Bild. Repräsentation, Darstellung und Wahrnehmung einer sozialen Gruppe im Mittelalter*, Göttingen 2006, S. 106f.

Glauben zeigen soll, als wolle er gegen den Spruch des ‚guten Juristen-schlechten Christen' anschreiben.[34] Ganz ähnlich verhält es sich mit den Medizinern. Gerade in Norditalien besteht eine enge Verbindung zwischen der medizinischen Fakultät und den Artisten; viele Ärzte verfassen Schriften über andere als medizinische Themen.[35]

Wenn Petrarca dem Arzt das Recht auf Rhetorik und Disputationen abspricht, steckt hinter dieser Geste mehr als eine persönliche Abneigung gegen zu lange Reden am Krankenbett. Es geht vielmehr darum, die Ärzte in ihrer Kompetenz zu beschneiden und ihre Autorität in den *artes liberales* in Frage zu stellen. Eine herausragende Rolle spielt dabei die Moralphilosophie. In den *Invective* heißt es mit aller Deutlichkeit, die Medizin habe mit der Ethik nichts zu tun (*medicine nichil comune cum ethica*). Damit ist nicht gesagt, die Medizin sei an sich unmoralisch; viel eher geht es darum, den Anspruch der Mediziner auf bestimmte Kompetenzen zurückzuweisen. „Bleib auf deinem Platz", empfiehlt Petrarca seinem Gegenüber, „und überschreite nicht deine Grenzen".[36] Die Herabwürdigung der Ärzte zu bloßen Handwerkern, zu *mechanici*, geschieht vor allem in der Absicht, die Schriften zu delegitimieren, die diese Grenze in Petrarcas Meinung überschreiten.[37] Wie Karl Enenkel pointiert bemerkt, zielt Petrarca in den *Invective* darauf ab, „unliebsame Konkurrenten aus der Gelehrtenrepublik auszugliedern".[38] Zugleich versucht er, sich selbst als Instanz und moralische Autorität zu etablieren. Sabrina Ebbersmeyer spricht in diesem Zusammenhang überzeugend von einer „Übernahme der Kompetenz für Moralphilosophie".[39] Zwar steht die Medizin als *res*, ähnlich wie bei Plinius, nicht in Frage: „Wer würde denn die Medizin hassen außer einem Liebhaber der Krankheiten?" antwortet Petrarca 1372 auf die Frage des Arztes Francesco Casini, ob er denn alle Ärzte hassen würde.[40] Aber anders als Petrarca ständig behauptet, steht die Medizin als *ars*, auch hier in Anlehnung an Plinius, sehr wohl in Frage. Denn die Rede von der falschen Medizin, die Petrarca immer wieder bemüht, lässt sich nicht, wie von ihm behauptet, auf einige Ärzte beschränken, die den moralischen Anforderungen ihrer Disziplin nicht gerecht werden. Vielmehr bezieht sie sich auf die Disziplin selbst, sobald diese sich als Philosophie und Wissenschaft und nicht als Handwerk versteht. „Worte wünsche ich mir von den Rednern und Dichtern", schreibt Petrarca weiter an Casini, „von den Ärzten aber nichts als Genesung (*sanitatem so-*

34 J. Ahern, „Good-bye, Bologna. Johannes Andreae and Familiares IV 15 and 16", in: T. Barolini – W. Storey (Hgg.), *Petrarch and the Textual Origins of Interpretation*, Leiden / Boston 2007, S. 185–204.

35 N. Siraisi, „Die medizinische Fakultät", in: W. Rüegg (Hg.), *Geschichte* der *Universität*, Bd. 1, S. 324–343, bes. S. 332–334.

36 Petrarca, *Invectives*, S. 124, 126.

37 F. Bausi, „Il mechanicus che scrive libri. Per un nuovo commento alle Invective contra medicum di Francesco Petrarca", *Rinascimento* 42 (2002), S. 67–112.

38 Enenkel, *Ein erster Ansatz*, S. 123.

39 S. Ebbersmeyer, *Homo Agens. Studien zur Genese und Struktur frühhumanistischer Moralphilosophie*, Berlin 2010, S. 69.

40 Petrarca, *Seniles* 16.3.49, S. 372.

lam)". Damit ist die Universität als institutioneller Rahmen für medizinische Expertise entwertet: „Kurz gesagt wünsche ich mir keine Professoren der Medizin, sondern der Gesundheit (*non medicine sed salutis professores*)".[41]

DER SCHWIERIGE PATIENT

Mit der Abwertung der Medizinexperten geht eine Aufwertung der medizinischen Laien einher: Aus dem Patienten wird ein schwieriger Patient, der die sozialen und intellektuellen Distinktionsmerkmale der medizinischen Profession kritisch hinterfragt. Dieser Moment kommt vor allem in den *Seniles* an befreundete Ärzte zum Vorschein, die sich weniger polemisch als die *Invective* oder die Briefe an medizinische Laien ausnehmen. Hier sind aus unliebsamen Konkurrenten Freunde geworden, unter der Bedingung, dass sie als Fragesteller, Ratsuchende und Lobredner die kulturelle Autorität Petrarcas anerkennen. Die Briefe, die Petrarca an Guglielmo da Ravenna, Giovanni Dondi oder Tommaso del Garbo richtet, zeugen also nicht von Altersmilde, sondern vom Erfolg seiner sozio-kulturellen Ermächtigungsstrategien. Die „kulturelle und soziale Übermacht der *physici*", wie sie Monica Berté und Silvia Rizzo nennen, scheint zumindest in diesen Briefen gebrochen.[42]

Bemerkenswert ist in dieser Hinsicht vor allem ein auf das Jahr 1370 zurückgehender Briefwechsel mit Giovanni Dondi. In einem ersten Brief gibt Petrarca zwar zu, dass er über keine Kompetenz in der Medizin verfügt, äußert sich aber trotzdem zu den *consilia*, die Giovanni ihm gegeben hat. So schlägt er in seiner *captatio benevolentiae* vor, seinen Brief nicht als eine wissenschaftliche Auseinandersetzung, sondern als ein Spiel oder einen Scherz anzusehen (*non disputatio ergo, sed ludus instituitur*).[43] Wie Chiara Crisciani gezeigt hat, ist der Begriff des *consilium* weitgefächert: In seiner eher ‚technischen' Bedeutung bezeichnet er einen Teilbereich der medizinischen Praxis, einen bestimmten diagnostisch-therapeutischen Ansatz, aber auch das Schriftstück, das im Rahmen dieses Ansatzes verfasst wird. Im weitesten Sinn bezieht sich die Rede vom *consilium* allerdings auf den gesamten Komplex medizinischen Wissens, der nach Crisciani letztendlich den Expertenstatus des Arztes, seine *perizia* ausmacht.[44]

Das Spiel Petrarcas unterläuft aber gerade diesen Expertenstatus. Denn das *consilium* als konkreter Ratschlag hängt vom *standing* des Arztes ab, also von seinem Wissen, seiner Erfahrung und seiner Autorität.[45] Diese Autorität steht trotz aller entgegen lautenden Bekundungen in Frage, wenn Petrarca die Ratschläge Giovannis ablehnt, er solle das Fasten aufgeben, sich nicht mehr vom Fleischver-

41 Petrarca, *Seniles* 16.3.57, S. 373.

42 In den einführenden Bemerkungen zu Petrarca, *Seniles*, S. 279

43 Petrarca, *Seniles* 12.1.4, S. 302.

44 C. Crisciani, „Consilia, responsi, consulti. I pareri del medico tra insegnamento e professione", in: C. Casagrande – C. Crisciani – S. Vecchio, *Consilium. Teorie e pratiche del consigliare nella cultura medievale*, Florenz 2004, S. 260.

45 Ebd.

zehr enthalten, kein Wasser mehr trinken und keine Äpfel mehr essen.[46] Die Gründe für diese Ablehnung können hier nicht im Einzelnen behandelt werden, herausheben lässt sich allerdings ihre wichtigste Voraussetzung: der Zweifel an den *auctoritates*, an den Autoritäten im Gebiet der Medizin:

> Ich bin fest davon überzeugt, dass dir meine Gesundheit ebenso am Herzen liegt wie deine eigene, und nicht weniger bin ich davon überzeugt, dass dir nichts von dem unbekannt ist, was die Größen eures Fachs niedergeschrieben haben, ja dass du selbst mit deinem Geist und deinem Wissen zu diesen Schriften beigetragen hast. [...] Was mich zum Zweifeln bringt, ist die Frage, ob man auf all das, was sie von sich gaben, vertrauen kann, als habe ein göttliches Orakel gesprochen, so dass jede abweichende Meinung einen Frevel darstellt. Hippokrates wird für einen reinen Menschen gehalten, Äskulap aber für einen Gott, nicht nur von seinen Zeitgenossen, sondern, wie ich erfahren musste, auch von uns Heutigen – einen Gott freilich, der von einem mächtigeren Gott mit dem Blitz erschlagen wurde.[47]

Petrarca kommt hier einer Position nahe, die sich auch in dem Wilhelm von Ockham zugeschriebenen *Elementarium logicae* findet. Dort heißt es in Bezug auf den *locus ab auctoritate*:

> Ein weiteres Beweismittel ergibt sich aus der Autorität, und dieses Beweismittel ist wenig wirkungsvoll, wenn die Argumentation nicht von der Autorität einer Person ausgeht, die weder täuschen noch getäuscht werden kann. Also gilt der Schluss ‚Aristoteles sagt X, also ist X wahr' nicht, weil Aristoteles sich täuschen konnte. Genausowenig gilt der Schluss ‚Ein Astrologe sagt X, also ist X wahr', weil ein Astrologe täuschen und getäuscht werden kann. Deswegen muss man nicht mit Notwendigkeit einem jeden Glauben schenken, der in seinem Fach oder in seiner Wissenschaft als erfahren gilt, da in vielen Künsten und Wissenschaften niemand Vollendung erreichen kann, aber ein jeder irren kann.[48]

In seiner Antwort auf Petrarca kommt es Dondi darauf an, diese autoritätskritische Einstellung wieder in traditionelle Bahnen zu lenken:

> Für mich besteht kein Zweifel daran, dass man diejenigen als geeignete Zeugen, Berater und Richter in jeder Angelegenheit ansehen sollte, die im Ruf stehen, über mehr Erfahrung (als andere) in dem Fach zu verfügen, das sich mit dem in Frage stehenden Gegenstand beschäftigt. Welche Wirkungskraft hätte sonst das Autoritätsargument, welche Geltung die nicht nur

46 Petrarca, *Seniles* 12.1.62–63, S. 307.

47 Petrarca, *Seniles* 12.1.20–22, S. 304: „Iam primum illud certum habeo, non aliter tibi salutem meam quam tuam propriam cordi esse; neque illud minus michi persuadeo, eorum que a maioribus vestris scripta sunt nil tibi prorsus incognitum, quin et aliqua forsan ingenio te illis ac studio adiecisse. [...] Illud in dubium venit, an cunta que illis exciderint, quasi divino ore prolata sic fidem mereantur ut contra sentire nefas sit. Et Ypocratem quidem purum hominem, Esculapium vero deum habitum, non apud suos tantum, sed apud nostros etiam novi, a maiori tame fulminatum deum."

48 E. M. Buytaert, „Guillelmi Ockham Elementarium Logicae", *Franciscan Studies* 125 (1965), S. 170–276, hier S. 275: „Alius locus ponitur ab auctoritate; et ille locus debilis est, nisi arguatur ab auctoritate illius qui fallere et falli non potest. Et ideo non sequitur: ‚Aristoteles dicit hoc, ergo hoc est verum,' quia ipse decipi potuit; nec sequitur: ‚Astrologus dicit hoc, ergo ita est,' quia quilibet astrologus decipere et decipi potest. Propter quod non est necesse credere cuilibet, qui putatur expertus in arte vel scientia sua, quia in multis artibus et scientiis nulus potest esse perfectus, sed quilibet errare potest." Vgl. zu dieser Stelle auch J. Miethke, „Die mittelalterlichen Universitäten und das gesprochene Wort", in: Ders., *Studieren an mittelalterlichen Universitäten*, S. 453–492, hier S. 482f.

> unter Gelehrten, sondern auch Ungelehrten allgemein bekannte Maxime: „Ein jeder, der Erfahrung mit sich bringt, ist in den Belangen seiner Kunst oder Wissenschaft glaubwürdig" (cuilibet experto in sua arte vel scientia credendum est)?[49]

In diesem Zusammenhang weisen Berté und Rizzo – nach einem Hinweis Sebastiano Gentiles – auf die Texte eines Anonymus des 14. Jahrhunderts und auf Raimundus Lullus hin.[50] Nahe liegender scheint es allerdings, auf die *Summulae logicales* des Petrus Hispanus zu verweisen.[51] In jedem Fall verschieben sich in den Briefen Petrarcas und Dondis die Koordinaten des Expertentums. Petrarca plädiert für eine Art kritisches Laientum, das sich nicht von medizinischer Fachliteratur abhängig machen will und sich nicht leicht von dem Fachwissen der Ärzte beeindrucken lässt. Das macht ihn zu einem schwierigen Patienten, mit dem nicht leicht umzugehen ist. Dessen ist sich auch Petrarca bewusst: „Du handelst nämlich mit aller Vorsicht", schreibt er Dondi, „wohl wissend, dass du es mit einem zänkischen Menschen zu tun hast".[52] Dondi sieht dagegen das hierarchische Verhältnis zwischen Arzt und Patient gefährdet und versucht, das Autoritätsgefälle zwischen beiden Seiten wieder herzustellen, indem er den Arzt erneut zum Experten kürt, der sich nicht nur durch die Autoritäten, sondern vor allem auch durch seine Erfahrung auszeichnet. Bei allzu hartnäckiger Therapieresistenz weiß er die rhetorische Notbremse zu ziehen. Nochmals Petrarca: „Ich weiß schon, du wirst mir sagen, was du mir immer sagst: ‚Mach was du willst', wird es heißen, ‚aber das eine musst du wissen: Wenn du den Ärzten nicht glaubst, lebst du kürzer'."[53]

DIE ELIXIRE DES ANTONIO

Dieser letzte – und resignative – Satz, der Petrarca öfters zu Ohren gekommen sein muss, zeigt, wie viel eine medizinische Behandlung mit Überzeugungsarbeit zu tun hat. Vielleicht braucht es, wie Petrarca meint, keine Disputationskunst am Krankenbett, ein wenig rhetorisches Geschick braucht es aber auf jeden Fall, will

49 Giovanni Dondi, „Responsiva" 20–21, in: Petrarca, *Seniles*, S. 323–337, hier S. 326: „Nil michi profecto ambiguitatis est quod illos pre aliis ideoneos testes, consultores et iudices in re qualibet crediturus es qui peritiores in ea disciplina habiti sint cuius de re proposita nosse et inquirere proprium sit. Alioquin argumentum ab auctoritate quid vigoris haberet et illa publica non modo literatis sed vulgaribus maxima: ‚Cuilibet experto in sua arte vel scientia credendum est'?"

50 Ebd. in den Anmerkungen.

51 In Petrus Hispanus, *Summulae logicales* 1.36 heißt es zum *locus ab auctoritate*: „Auctoritas, ut hic sumitur, est iudicium sapientis in sua scientia. Unde a rei iudicio solet denominari locus iste. Locus ab auctoritate est habitudo auctoritatis ad id quod per eam probatur, ut ‚astronomus dicit celum esse volubile; ergo celum est volubile'. Unde locus? Ab auctoritate." Zusammengefasst wird dieser *locus* in der Sentenz: „unicuique experto in sua scientia credendum est".

52 Petrarca, *Seniles* 12.1.102, S. 311: „[…] tu enim, sciens, credo, cum litigioso homine tibi rem esse, cautius agis […]."

53 Petrarca, *Seniles* 12.1.192–193, S. 318: „Nec ignoro quid dicturus sis; nempe quod solitus es: ‚Fac ut libet;' inquies ‚scito tamen quod medicis non credendo minus vives'."

man nicht, wie der Bruder des Gorgias, jedes Mal einen Rhetoriker zu Rate ziehen wenn der Patient sich als widerspenstig erweist.

> Nämlich gar oft bin ich mit meinem Bruder oder andern Ärzten zu einem Kranken hingegangen, der entweder keine Arznei nehmen, oder den Arzt nicht wollte schneiden und brennen lassen, und da dieser ihn nicht überreden konnte, habe ich ihn doch überredet durch keine andere Kunst als die Redekunst,

erzählt Gorgias in dem nach ihm benannten platonischen Dialog.[54]

Weder Arzt noch Patient ist also mit Fachwissen allein geholfen. Wer als Arzt Erfolg haben will muss sich, anders als Petrarca das sehen will, nicht nur um die Gesundung seines Patienten kümmern ohne viel Aufhebens darum zu machen. Er muss sich, unter anderem durch seine Kleidung und Haltung, vor dem Patienten ins rechte Licht rücken, seine Autorität in Szene setzen und Strategien des Umgangs entwickeln. Er kommt um „das Prahlen mit der Kunst und das abenteuerliche Angeben mit der Wissenschaft" (*ostentatio artis et portentosa scientiae venditatio*), die bereits Plinius bemängelt,[55] gar nicht umhin, und damit auch nicht um die moralische Zweideutigkeit, die mit dieser Zurschaustellung verbunden ist.

Ein besonders schönes Beispiel einer solchen *ostentatio* findet sich in einem kurzen Prosatext Ludovico Ariostos (1474–1533), der den Titel *Erbolato* trägt, geschrieben um 1530. Es handelt sich um den kurzen Monolog eines gewissen Antonio Faventino, der in diesem Monolog, ganz der ehrwürdigen Tradition des Quacksalbers entsprechend, einen Wundertrank aus Kräutern anpreist (Plinius bezieht sich in der eben zitierten Stelle auch auf einen Kräutertrank, den Theriak). Auf wen sich Ariostos satirischer Text im Einzelnen bezieht ist ungeklärt. Nach Dennis Looney, der in jüngerer Zeit das Interesse der Forschung auf den *Erbolato* gelenkt hat, lässt sich wohl keine einzelne Person mit Antonio identifizieren.[56] Eher scheint es sich um ein Konglomerat verschiedener Personen zu handeln, mit denen Ariosto am Hof von Ferrara in Kontakt stand. Looney nennt hier unter anderen Nicolò Leoniceno, Giovanni Manardi und Antonio Musa Brasavola, also Protagonisten des von Vivian Nutton beschriebenen *medical humanism* in Ferrara.[57] Für diese These spricht vor allem das starke Interesse dieser Ärzte an Botanik und Pharmakologie, die Leitmotive in Ariostos Satire darstellen.

Aber auch ohne die Frage der Zuschreibung endgültig lösen zu können besitzt der *Erbolato* eine hohe Aussagekraft, was den Umgang von Arzt und Patient angeht. Nicht, dass Antonio den idealtypischen Arzt des 16. Jahrhunderts verkörpern würde, vor allem nicht in Hinsicht auf das höfische Umfeld, in dem sich Ariosto bewegt. Seine Rede ist vielmehr deswegen interessant, weil sie die Inszenierungsstrategien seiner Kollegen auf die Spitze treibt. Schon die Darstellung Antonios als eines fahrenden Heilkünstlers, der seinen Wundertrank auf dem Markt feilbie-

54 Platon, *Gorgias*, 456 b (Übersetzung nach Friedrich Schleiermacher).

55 Plinius d. Ä., *Naturalis historia*, 29.8.25.

56 D. Looney, „Introduction", in: L. Ariosto, *‚My Muse Will Have a Story to Paint.' Selected Prose of Ludovico Ariosto*, übers. von D. Looney, Toronto 2010, S. 1–20, hier S. 9.

57 V. Nutton, „The Rise of Medical Humanism. Ferrara, 1464–1555", *Renaissance Studies* 11 (1997), n. 1, S. 2–19.

tet, kann als satirische Übertreibung des Medizingewerbes gelesen werden, das sich ja tatsächlich auf dem freien Markt der Nachfrage bewegt.[58] Von wegen *silentium* – Antonio ist ein Marktschreier, der seine Ware auf einem öffentlichen Platz an den Mann bringen will, und es steht zu vermuten, dass auch seine Gestik nicht dem würdevollen Verhalten entspricht, das von Ärzten am Krankenbett gefordert wird. Der eigentliche Witz an Ariostos Text liegt aber darin, dass er eine voreilige Unterscheidung von ‚unseriöser' und ‚seriöser' Medizin nicht erlaubt. Antonio entnimmt seine Argumente einer reichen medizinisch-ethischen Tradition, derer sich auch seine ‚Kollegen' gerne bedienen. So hebt Meister Antonios Rede mit einer plinianischen Klage über die schwache Stellung des Menschen in der Natur an. Im Gegensatz zu den Tieren ist der Mensch bei seiner Geburt nackt und vollkommen auf seine Umwelt angewiesen. Und doch – ein Allgemeinplatz bleibt selten allein – ist dem Menschen die größte Gabe von allen verliehen: die Vernunft. Mit Hilfe der Vernunft, argumentiert Antonio in klassischer Weise, kann der Mensch seine Schwächen ausgleichen; was zunächst als Nachteil erscheint, stellt sich als Vorteil heraus.[59] Ist der Mensch am Anfang seines Lebens nicht mit bestimmten Fähigkeiten ausgestattet, liegt das nur daran, dass ihm im weiteren Verlauf alle Möglichkeiten offenstehen. Dazu muss er allein seine Erfindungsgabe anstrengen: „Dann kam ihm der Gedanke, dass er allein deswegen an so vielen Krankheiten litt, um seinen Geist, die hauptsächliche und eigentliche Tätigkeit seiner Seele nicht im müßigen Nichtstun verkommen zu lassen".[60] Die Betonung verschiebt sich hier von der *ragione* zum *ingegno*, dem traditionell das Finden und Erfinden zugeschrieben wird. Wie sich im weiteren Verlauf herausstellt, bezieht Antonio das im Schlagwort des *ingegno* enthaltene Suchen bereits auf eine bestimmte Klasse von nutzbringenden Dingen, die speziell der Gesundheit des Menschen dienen:

> [...] so viele Arten von Bäumen, so viele verschiedene Kräuter, so viele Sorten Gummi, so viele unterschiedliche Tränke und so viele andere Dinge sind vom höchsten Schöpfer nicht umsonst hergestellt worden, und wer sie kennt und weiß, wie man richtig mit ihnen umzugehen hat, wird der Krankheit entkommen und sein Leben verlängern und im besten Zustand halten.[61]

Das *ingegno* gleicht also nicht nur die *infermità* im Sinne der menschlichen Schwächen, sondern auch, wie diese Engführung zeigt, die *infermità* im Sinne von Krankheit aus. An dieser Stelle wird zudem, fast noch unmerklich für den Leser

58 Einige Anmerkungen zu fahrenden Heilkünstlern in: K. Bergdolt, *Das Gewissen der Medizin. Ärztliche Moral von der Antike bis heute*, München 2004, S. 151ff.

59 L. Ariosto, *L'Erbolato*, in: Ders., *Opere Minori*, Bd. 2, Firenze 1857, S. 511–526, hier S. 515–516.

60 Ebd. S. 517: «Ebbe considerazione appresso che a tante infirmità non era sottoposto se non perché l'ingegno, il quale era la prencipale e propria operazione dell'anima, non si lasciasse marcire nell'ozio [...].»

61 Ebd.: «[...] tante specie d'alberi, tante varietà di erbe, tante sorte di gummi, tante differenze di liquori e tante e tant'altre cose non erano dal sommo Creatore prodotte indarno, le quali conoscendo, et opportunamente adoperandole, potria fuggire l'infirmità e mantenere in lungo e ottimo stato la sua vita.»

oder Hörer, auf ein Sonderwissen angespielt, das (anders als die allen Menschen zur Verfügung stehenden Fähigkeiten der *ragione* und des *ingegno*) nur wenigen zugänglich ist, da es eines „langen Studiums (*lungo studio*) und einer großen Sorgfalt (*diligenza grande*)" bedarf.[62] Hier klingt bereits ein Topos der medizinethischen Diskussion auf, auf den noch einmal zurückzukommen sein wird: der des Fleißes und der Sorgfalt. Eigentlich gilt diese Bemerkung allen Künsten, doch einer im Besonderen: „Aber mehr als alle anderen schien dem Menschen die Kunstfertigkeit schön, nützlich und eines langen Studiums und größter Sorgfalt wert zu sein, die zeigt, wie man sich gesund hält und von einem schlechten Zustand wieder zu einem guten gelangt, und diese Kunst heißt Medizin."[63] Die Medizin wird als die edelste aller Künste dargestellt: Das Leben, erklärt Antonio, sei das Wertvollste, was wir besitzen; deswegen sei die Medizin, die sich mit der Erhaltung und Verlängerung des Lebens beschäftige, die edelste und zugleich notwendigste Kunst (*la più nobile et necessaria*).[64]

Auch ein Arzt wie Antonio Musa Brasavola wird diesen Topos in der Vorrede zu seinem Galen-Index einbauen, wenn er von der Gesundheit als dem höchsten Gut des Menschen spricht. Für die Widererlangung dieses höchsten Gutes wären die Menschen bereit, keine Kosten und Mühen zu scheuen, heißt es dort: In Aussicht auf Gesundung nähmen sie bittere Tränke zu sich und würden ihr Gold und Silber opfern.[65] Dessen ist sich auch Antonio bewusst, der die Rede von der wertvollen Gesundheit durchaus wörtlich nimmt: „Ich habe mir gedacht, ich überlasse euch einen Edelstein, einen Schatz, einen Reichtum", lässt er sein Publikum wissen und preist seinen Trank als geradezu unbezahlbar an:

> Er sollte euch mehr am Herzen liegen, als machte ich jedem von euch ein Geschenk von zehntausend Gold-Scudi, gleich heute, bar auf die Hand. Was nützen dem Kranken schon Gold und Silber? [...] Ständige Gesundheit und ein langes Leben: das nenne ich wahren und unvergleichlichen Reichtum, und das ist es in der Tat.[66]

Der Trank stellt sozusagen eine Weltneuheit dar. Es handelt sich um das sagenhafte *elettuario Vitae*, von dem Hippokrates, Galen und viele andere berühmte Ärzte geträumt hätten, ohne es je verwirklicht zu haben. Ähnlich wie in Holbeins *Triumph des Arztes*, auf dem der Tod gefesselt zu Füßen des Arztes sitzt, dessen Triumphwagen Krankheiten wie Fieber, Wassersucht und Pest überrollt, besiegt

62 Ariosto, *L'Erbolato*, S. 517.
63 Ebd.: «Ma più di tutte l'altre gli parve bella et utile e di lunghissimo studio e grandissima diligenza degna quell'arte che mostra di tenere l'uomo sano e dalla mala disposizione ritirarlo alla buona, la quale si chiama medicina [...].»
64 Ebd.
65 A. M. Brasavolus, *In omnes Galeni libros refertissimus index*, Venedig 1565, f. *iir–v.
66 Ebd. S. 522: «Ho pensato di lasciarvi una gemma, un tesoro, una ricchezza. vi debbe essere più cara che s'io donassi oggi a ciascuno di voi diecimila scudi d'oro contanti. Che giovano l'oro e l'argento ad uno infermo? [...] la perpetua sanità e la vita lunga si può chiamare, et è in effetto, vera et incomparabile richezza.»

Antonios Trank alle Übel.[67] Auf die richtige Weise eingenommen, schütze er ein ganzes Jahr lang vor Schmerz und Krankheit. Kurz und gut: „Dieses kleine Gefäß enthält in sich ständige Gesundheit und die ein langes Leben, länger als das Leben, das uns die mangelhafte Natur zugestehen kann."[68] Seine Mühen und Wohltaten führt Antonio dem Publikum nicht nur in Worten, sondern auch in Bildern vor. Offensichtlich hat er ein Plakat (*una bandiera*) vorbereiten lassen, das seine Werke darstellt.[69] Sein Publikum soll mit eigenen Augen sehen, was er geleistet hat. Denn während Antonio sich in seinem Streben nach Wissen aufopfert – solche wie ihn gäbe es nur selten – reiche es den meisten aus, sich mit einem Minimalwissen zu schmücken. Auf diese Art greift er noch einmal den Topos der Mühe und Sorgfalt auf:

> Nur wenige wollen die Mühen eines Studiums auf sich nehmen, und schätzen jede andere Art von Verdienst höher ein außer dem, der es mit der Gesundheit und dem Leben zu tun hat; und viele bilden sich ein, dass es ausreicht, gerade soviel zu wissen, dass man ihnen vertraut und sie als Ärzte anerkennt.[70]

Doch Antonios Mühen wollen belohnt sein. Aller Großherzigkeit zum Trotz, umsonst ist nur der Tod. Allerdings bemüht sich Antonio, so wie jeder gute Arzt, die Nerven seiner potentiellen Patienten/Kunden nicht zu sehr zu strapazieren und sie schonend auf die Zahlung vorzubereiten: „Wie ich sagte, ich will euch (meinen Trank) schenken, und ich will ihn euch wirklich schenken: Denn wenn einer euch etwas von größtem Wert für einen verschwindend geringen Preis gibt, dann ist das nichts anderes als geschenkt." Diesem dialektischen Meisterstück fügt er einen pragmatischen Grund hinzu: Die Kosten für seine exotischen (und damit besonders wirksamen) Zutaten würden ihn sonst in den Ruin treiben.[71] Antonio treibt sein Spiel sogar noch weiter:

> Also, wer wird so geizig, so ärmlich sein, dass es ihm aufstößt, einen so geringen Preis für seine Gesundheit und sein Wohlbefinden zu geben? Wer wird so arm sein, dass er nicht seinen Mantel verpfänden oder verkaufen kann?[72]

An diesem Punkt kehren wir zu Pontano und der Kritik Merkurs an den Patienten zurück, die ihr Geld für eine unwirksame Behandlung geben, denn hier versucht Antonio das Publikum wirklich dazu zu bringen, ihm sein Gold und Silber zu op-

67 Vgl. die Abbildung in W. P. Eckert – C. von Imhoff, *Willibald Pirckheimer, Dürers Freund im Spiegel seines Lebens, seiner Werke und seiner Umwelt*, 2., erw. Auflage, Köln 1982, S. 193.

68 Ariosto, *L'Erbolato*, S. 525–526: «Questo picciol vasetto ha in sé rinchiuso la continua sanità e lunghezza della vita umana, e maggiore che non può concedere la difettiva natura.»

69 Ebd. 521.

70 Ebd. S. 518: «Sono pochi che vogliano la fatica dello studio, e fanno più stima di ogn'altro guadagno che di quello della sanità e della vita; et a molti pare abastanza di sapere tanto che loro dia credito e reputazione di medico.»

71 Ebd. S. 526: «Ho detto di donarlovi e ve lo voglio donare veramente: perché dandovi cosa di valuta grandissima per un picciolo e minimo prezzo non si può dire che non si doni [...].»

72 Ebd.: «Ora chi sarà quello sì avaro, quello sì misero, a cui incresca di spendere per salute e per conservazion de la sua vita sì minimo prezzo? Chi sarà quello sì povero che non impegni o venda il mantello?»

fern. Sein Crescendo an Argumenten überspannt den Bogen, seine Sprache und rhetorische Strategie entlarven ihn als moralisch fragwürdig und daher als Quacksalber. Am Ende seiner Rede rutscht er denn auch von seinen hehren Zielen ganz in die Sprache des Krämers ab: „He da! Lasst euch dieses Schnäppchen nicht entgehen" (*non lasciate fuggire l'occasione*), ruft er seinen Zuhörern zu.[73] Gerade in diesem letzten Teil erscheint auch das zweigeteilte Publikum, mit dem Ariosto spielt. Zum einen gibt es das ‚einfache' Volk, das sich das Geld für den vermeintlichen Zaubertrank mühsam zusammensparen muss und an das sich Antonio richtet. Es handelt sich sozusagen um den dummen Rest, von dem Petrarca spricht. Zum anderen gibt es aber das gebildete Publikum am Hof, an das sich Ariosto mit seiner Satire richtet. Dieses Publikum scheint in der Lage zu sein, Antonio zu entlarven, nicht in Bezug auf den Inhalt oder die Wirksamkeit des Tranks, sondern in Hinsicht auf seine rhetorischen Strategien. Sein wildes Durcheinanderwürfeln von Gemeinplätzen und Philosophemen sowie seine ‚niedere' Denkweise, die er am Ende seiner Rede nicht mehr verbergen kann, erweisen ihn als moralisch fragwürdige Person, der auch auf einer medizinischen Ebene nicht zu trauen ist.

In Ariostos Satire treten dem gebildeten Leser damit in verdrehter und übertriebener Weise bestimmte Merkmale der Selbstinszenierung von ärztlicher Autorität entgegen, wie sie eigentlich in der Literatur für Ärzte vorkommen. Damit kann man den *Erbolato* als einen Text sehen, der seine Leser nicht mit einer Ethik im Sinne von normativem Wissen, sondern eher mit einem feinen Gespür für das Auftreten des Arztes versehen will. Ariosto schreibt nicht vor, sondern zeigt auf. Damit ist er letzten Endes einer Ethik der Klugheit verpflichtet, die bereits Petrarca und Pontano für die Patientenseite zu erschließen beginnen.

73 Ariosto, *L'Erbolato*, S. 526.

PRAISE AND PRACTICE OF MEDICINE IN MARSILIO FICINO

Teodoro Katinis

Marsilio Ficino (1433–1499) is one of the most important figures in the fifteenth-century cultural world to try to create a strong connection between philosophy and medicine. As a philosopher, physician, magician, astrologer, author of Latin and vernacular prose he was the embodiment of the typical humanist; yet more importantly he was a translator of and commentator on Platonism. With his work, Ficino displayed Plato's dialogues and the work of Plotinus, among other neoplatonic authors,to the European public, thereby giving life to the 'rebirth of Platonism'. This paper has two main purposes: firstly to analyze the importance given to medicine in Ficino's *Epistolarium*, paying particular attention to the connection between the rebirth of Platonism and the debate on the relationship between philosophy and medicine; secondly to examine some passages of Ficino's *Consilio contro la pestilentia* as examples of medical practice according to the author's theories.

We have evidence that due to his father's work, Ficino had been in contact with the medical field since his youth. In fact, his father Dietifeci d'Agnolo da Figline was a physician, "chyrurgicus Florentie suo seculo singularis"[1], as Ficino mentions in a letter to Francesco Marescalchi, dated September 6th, 1474. He worked for the De' Medici family in Florence, and thanks to him the young Ficino had his first contact with Cosimo 'Il Vecchio' – the first of his patrons. Dietifeci's activity as physician had an enormous impact on Ficino's intellectual formation. Before his death, in 1478, Dietifeci left to his son his sizeable private library with "libros latinos sive grecos aut ebraycos et omnes alios quibus utitur dictus Marsilius."[2] We also have important information on the medical education Ficino received regarding medicine and natural philosophy from Niccolò Tignosi, an Aristotelian philosopher interested in emerging Platonism, who believed in the importance of the collaboration between 'sciences' and 'humanities' – as we call them today. Reading Ficino's medical works, the *Consilio contro la pestilentia* (1481)[3] and *De vita libri tres* (1489)[4], we find evidence of Ficino's knowledge of

1 Marsilio Ficino, *Lettere, I: Epistolarium familiarium liber I*, ed by. S. Gentile, Florence 1990, n. 80: p. 141.

2 *Marsilio Ficino e il ritorno di Platone. Mostra di manoscritti, stampe e documenti 17 maggio–16 giugno 1984*, catalogo ed. by S. Gentile, S. Niccoli and P. Viti, Florence 1984, n. 132: p. 169.

3 The most recent study and edition of this work is in T. Katinis, *Medicina e filosofia in Marsilio Ficino. Il Consilio contro la pestilentia*, Rome 2007. No English translation of Ficino's *Consilio* is available.

many classical and medieval medical sources that he used in his practice, criticizing them when his experience produced different results, or when reason did not support *auctoritas*. It is particularly remarkable that Ficino learned and practiced medicine while translating and commentating on Platonic works. As we shall see in the following pages, Platonism gives a new philosophical basis to the medical theories.

Ficino's *Epistolarium* provides significant argumentation in defense of medicine, which was previously considered a mere 'mechanical art' without any merit. The letter in the first book of the *Epistolarium* addressed to Tomme Valorio and entitled *Nobilitas, utilitas et usus medicine* echoes the considerable fourteenth and fifteenth century debate about the status of the art of medicine. In that letter Ficino discusses the origin of medicine and its real significance for human life. According to the Holy Bible, he claims that God created medicine for mankind and, according to the pagans, he claims that Iside, Apollo and Aesculapius were the divine sources of this art. In addition, the great ancient physician Hippocrates believed medicine and prophecy to be related since Apollo is father of both.[5] Hence, one more piece of evidence to proving the dignity of medicine is that the greatest men in the history of the world used this art.[6] Furthermore, Ficino considers medicine as a 'queen' among arts, since it allows men to pursue every other human activity. He remarks that physicians have a divine power, the power of regenerating the human being.[7]

4 M. Ficino, *Three Books of Life*, Critical Edition and Transl. with Introd. and Notes by C. V. Kaske – J. R. Clark, Binghamton (N.Y.) 1989. Several recent studies on this work are listed in T. Katinis, "Bibliografia ficiniana. Studi ed edizioni delle opere di Marsilio Ficino dal 1986", *Accademia. Revue de la Société Marsile Ficin*, 2 (2000), pp. 101–136; T. Katinis – S. Toussaint, "Bibliographie ficinienne. Mise à jour", *Accademia. Revue de la Société Marsile Ficin* 3 (2001), pp. 9–21 (and further updates).

5 Ficino, *Lettere*, I, n. 81: p. 142: "Medicina vaticinio propinqua est: harum enim duarum artium unus est parens Apollo, scilicet qui progenitor noster est, hic et futuros morbos predicit et eos qui adversa valitudine affecti sunt curat."

6 Ficino, *Lettere*, I, n. 81: p. 143: "Christus ipse, tanquam generis humani medicus, egros egrotosque, quotcunque offerebantur, curabat discipulisque medendi tradidit potestatem. Hanc igitur artem utpote nobilissimam reges meditari et exercere quondam nequaquam dedignabantur, quales fuerunt Sabor et Girges Medorum reges, Sabid rex Arabum, Mithridates Persarum rex, rex Egyptiorum Hermes, Mesues regis Damasci nepos; volunt nonnulli et Avicennam fuisse Cordube principem. Democritus, Timeus Locrus, Plato, Aristoteles, philosophi illustrissimi, in hac arte scripserunt innumerabilesque alii philosophi non ignobiles. Quanta medicine nobilitas sit, ferme quantum patitur epistola dictum est."

7 Ficino, *Lettere*, I, n. 81: pp. 143–144: "quanta vero utilitas ex eo perspicimus, quod artes que ad bene vivendum diriguntur absque huius auxilio parum prodesse videntur. Non enim bene vivere possumus nisi vivamus, neque brevissimo hoc vite tempore in quavis facultate multum proficere nisi valeamus bene, neque facile multum apud homines Deumve mereri nisi diu sobriique vivamus. Omnem vero huiusmodi facultatem diligentia medicine suppeditat. Uti autem hac arte oportet summa tum erga Deum pietate, tum erga homines charitate [...]. Est enim bonorum omnium auctor Deus, est et legitimus medicus quasi deus aliquis inter homines: eos nanque in vitam a morte restituit et tanquam deus colitur vel a regibus et sapientibus, cum egrotant."

A fundamental letter in the development of our topic is the *Oratio de laudibus medicinae*, in the fourth book of Ficino's *Epistolarium*, dedicated to the orator Marco Aurelio. This short treatise begins with an emphatic prologue:

> Thus today, led by an ancient custom and the command of our fathers, we are going to speak in praise of medicine, which is said to be descended from Apollo. Turning the sharp point of the mind away from the darkness towards the light – let us therefore humbly invoke the rays of the true and supreme Apollo, so that, cleansed by his wholesome warmth, we may set forth the praise of this cleansing and bring it to perfection, either through his own worth, or at least through our own native powers. [...] There are three principles by which philosophers have traditionally judged the perfection of any science: the end [i.e. the aim], the source, the substance.[8]

The first source of that passage is the hermetic Latin text entitled *Asclepius*[9] (chapters 6, 22, 37). This text was known and used during the Middle Ages as the work of the author Hermes Trismegistus, a mythical ancient Egyptian revered as a wise ruler and philosopher. In chapter 6, we find the famous definition of the human being: talking with Asclepius, Hermes says "magnum miraculum homo est." The noun *miraculum* is a declaration of the superiority of Man, who should be admired for his wonderful essence. In chapter 22, Hermes claims the superiority of the human being compared to any other divine being, and in chapter 37 he presents his grandfather as the creator of medicine as a divine art. Ficino thereafter defines this art as exceptional, mostly because it cares for the human being as a whole including body and soul.

> [...] Nor would any physician say that his art centres upon Man's body, alone, since Phoebus, as may be read in the Letters of Hippocrates, considered the care of the soul and of the body to come together in one. Thus, among the Egyptians and the Persians the same men were both priests and doctors.[10]

The last sentence is remarkable since it gives us a precise idea of Ficino's point of view regarding the connection between the medical and spiritual spheres. Ficino wanted to embody the connection between this world and that of the divine by becoming "canonicus" and physician at the same time and by taking care of the body as well as the soul. Another interesting point in the *Oratio de laudibus medicinae* is the presence of Plato as a new important source of knowledge and a new *auctoritas*; in other words, Aristotelism is no longer the only philosophical basis for medical knowledge. Ficino quotes the dialogue entitled *Charmides* to support the idea of a close connection between the body and the soul:

> Plato writes in Charmides that those Magi who were physicians of both soul and body, followers of Zalmoxis and Zoroaster, believed that everything belonging to the body, good or

8 *The Letters of Marsilio Ficino*, I, transl. from Latin by members of the Language Department of the School of Economic Science, London 1975, n. 14: p. 22 (Marsilio Ficino, *Opera*, I, Basileae 1576, reimpr. en facsimilé et préf. par S. Toussaint, Ivry sur Seine 2000, p. 759).

9 See *Hermetica. The Greek 'Corpus Hermeticum' and the Latin Asclepius in a new English translation, with notes and introduction*, ed. by B. P. Copenhaver, Cambridge (UK), New York (NY) 1992.

10 *The Letters of Marsilio Ficino*, I, p. 24 (Ficino, *Opera*, I, p. 760).

> bad, flows from the soul into the body itself, just as the nature of the eyes flows from the brain, and the nature of the brain from the whole body. Just as it is impossible to heal the eyes unless the brain is healed, and to heal the brain without healing the whole body, so the whole body cannot be strong unless the soul is strong. [...] Furthermore, Socrates said it was common knowledge among the Thracians that it was customary for doctors, by administering some such treatment, to preserve a few men from death. So great is the dominion of the soul over the body, so great its power.[11]

Ficino presents the organism as a metaphor – one of his favorites – to describe the relationship between the spiritual and the material dimension within the human being. He stresses the fact that within the body the health of every individual part depends on that of the whole. The same connection governs the relationship between body and soul. Socrates conveys the Thracian tradition, which becomes a reliable source thanks to his authority. The main source inspiring Ficino's passage is Plato's *Charmides* (155e–157b), where Socrates explains to his interlocutor, Charmides, how he can heal his head-ache by using a particular herb while simultaneously pronouncing magical words accompanied by a melody. Socrates is referring to a method reported by a student of the wise ancient physician Zalmoxis and in so doing connects present knowledge to an ancient wisdom. According to this *priscus medicus*, medicine is successful only when considering the human being as a whole: paying particular attention to the soul in order to have a healthy body. Ficino must have considered *Charmides* (155e–157b) as a fundamental passage in Plato's dialogue, since it is also mentioned in other works – such as the *Theologia platonica* (XIII, 1) – and highly considered in his *Argumentum in Charmidem de temperantia*.[12] In Ficino's *Argumentum* temperance is presented as the main virtue of the soul, which can be transmitted to the body because of the body-soul organism. At the end of the passage quoted above, Ficino suggests that the body may achieve immortality, a characteristic usually attributed to the soul alone, by practicing temperance. Mankind lost this immortality when Adam was expelled from Paradise, but was able to regain it with the correct use of the art of medicine.

At the end of his *Oratio*, Ficino emphatically exhorts philosophers, priests and physicians to embrace the art of medicine.

> So, my friends, I strongly urge you all, in no way to stint time, money, or labor, so that you may embrace with all your might this most wholesome art, the preserver of human life. Thus you will each be able to watch over the life and prosperity of yourself, then of your family, and finally of everyone else, and to support the other liberal arts, which cannot be learned and practiced without health.[13]

Speaking about medicine, its identity and role, it is worthwhile to note the distance between Ficino's humanistic perspective and the prevalent Western point-

11 *The Letters of Marsilio Ficino*, I, p. 24 (Ficino, *Opera*, I, p. 760).

12 Ficino, *Opera*, II, pp. 1304–1307; the text is also in M. Vanhaelen, "Marsile Ficin, traducteur et interprète du Charmide de Platon", *Accademia. Revue de la Société Marsile Ficin* 3 (2001), pp. 23–52: 48–52 (in the text temperantia is the translation of the Greek word sophrosyne).

13 *The Letters of Marsilio Ficino*, I, p. 25 (Ficino, *Opera*, I, p. 760).

of-view in the twenty-first century. Apparently what Ficino is proposing in his treatise shares almost nothing with 'our' medicine as it is theorized and practiced today. This is even more surprising when one thinks of Ficino as a physician – and not only as a philosopher – involved in healing several patients and writing one of the first medical *consilia*[14] against the plague in vernacular, in which he combines theory and practice, and reveals his original perspective between tradition and innovation.

Ficino wrote his *Consilio contro la pestilentia*, published in that same city in 1481, between 1478 and 1479, when the plague was again in Florence. This work is directed to both the more and the less learned as a useful instrument for understanding, curing and preventing the disease.

> La carità inverso la patria mia mi muove a scrivere qualche consiglio contro la pestilentia, et accioché ogni persona thoscana la intenda et possi con esso medicare, pretermetterò le disputationi sottili et lunghe et etiamdio scriverrò in lingua thoscana. Basti sapere che qualunque cosa io aproverrò, benché per brevità non narri molto, niente di meno è approvata con molte ragioni et auctorità di tutti e doctori antichi e moderni, et sperientie di molti et spetialmente del nostro padre maestro Ficino medico singolare.[15]

In Ficino's *Consilio*, traditional medical theories and practices are put to the test and, alternatively, confirmed, confuted or modified by the author in light of his own hypotheses and experiences. Ficino demonstrates a deep acquaintance with the Western and Arab medical traditions that had already produced a number of texts on the subject of the plague. It cannot be said that Ficino limits himself in the *Consilio* to simply giving practical instructions, for he takes it upon himself to present a coherent treatment of the contagion's nature, its genesis and its modes of diffusion. Ficino's work is almost a treatise and in fact the Latin translation, by Tommaso Benci, published in Augsburg in 1518, is titled *Tractatus Singularis Doctissimi Viri M. Ficini de Epidemiae Morbo*. Ficino's *Consilio* is significant in several respects but we will focus particularly on those related to our topic. The first pages of the text are dedicated to summarizing what plague is, how it affects the body and how the contagion could be avoided. Further, Ficino writes that plague is spread by the poisoned air which works against the human vital spirit ("spirito vitale"), which is generated in the heart and brings life to the body. Therefore the best way to preserve the health is to defend and strengthen the spirit and the heart however possible. Ficino recommends theriaca as the best remedy for plague because of its "friendship" with the vital spirit ("spirito vitale"). Theriaca is the queen of medicines, a divine medical composite made of many ingredients meticulously listed by the author for the reader.[16] Ficino reminds us that Galen wrote about theriaca in his *Ad Pisonem de theriaca liber* saying that it is

14 For an examination of this type of text and further bibliographical information, see J. Agrimi – C. Crisciani, *Les 'Consilia' medicaux*, Turnhout 1994.

15 M. Ficino, *Consilio contro la pestilentia*, apud Sanctum Iacobum de Ripolis, Florence 1481, 1r (T. Katinis, *Medicina e filosofia in Marsilio Ficino. Il Consilio contro la pestilentia*, p. 159).

16 M. Ficino, *Consilio contro la pestilentia*, cc. 10v, 11r (T. Katinis, *Medicina e filosofia in Marsilio Ficino. Il* 'Consilio contro la pestilentia', p. 169).

against all poisons and is wonderfully efficacious where all other remedies are weak. As Gentile da Foligno (c. 1275–1348) already stated in his *Consilium contra pestilentiam*[17], theriaca has some specific feature or form and by consequence it can be used in small quantities avoiding an excessive warming of the body. Ficino defines the theriaca's specific form as spiritual and celestial ("spirituale", "celestiale") coming from the stars.[18]

Other interesting issues in Ficino's *Consilio* are the use of astrology to foreshadow the direction in which plague spreads and the alchemical procedure, taken from Gentile's work, in which drinkable gold is considered a remedy against the plague. But the most significant topic for our purpose is the use of happiness to heal the body. Ficino repeats and expands what Tommaso Del Garbo (c. 1305–1370) suggested in his *Consiglio contro alla peste*[19]. "Letitia" is strongly recommended because of its beneficial effect on the whole human being. Ficino takes his knowledge from different disciplines and from a large number of sources; Platonism is among them for the first time in the *consilia* tradition.[20]

In the twenty-second chapter of the *Consilio*, Ficino offers several ways of preserving oneself against the disease and advocates, among other things, a particular style of life that renders one immune to the plague.

> Debbesi viver lieto, perché la letitia fortifica lo spirito vitale; vivere continente et sobrio, perché la sobrietà et continentia del vivere è di tanto valore che Socrate philosopho, con questa sola, si conservò in molte pestilentie extreme che furono nella citta d'Athene; però Aristotele et Galieno dicono ch'e corpi puri sono tali che quasi è impossibile sentino peste, et invero, sella sentono, almeno non ne periscono.[21]

Abstinence in living, as well as moderate happiness ("letitia"), is a particularly good remedy against the disease. Evidence of this is that Socrates survived the various epidemics that afflicted Athens, including the terrible plague in around 430 B.C., which Ficino could have learned from Thucydides' account of it in *The Pelopennesian War* (IV, 45–58). In his famous description, Thucydides connected the spread of the plague with the growth of moral and civil disorder. One detects an echo of this idea in Ficino, who recommends abstinence as a way of life that will act as a shield against the disease, and proposes Socrates "the philosopher" as the chief example of such a disposition. Apparently Ficino is using for medical purposes what Plato often proposes in his dialogues: the image of a temperate,

17 On Gentile da Foligno and his work see P. Vian, "Gentile da Foligno", in: *Dizionario biografico degli italiani*, vol. 53, Rome 1999, pp. 162–167.

18 J. Beecher, "Ficino, Theriaca and the Stars", in: M. J. B. Allen – V. R. Rees – M. Davies (eds.), *Marsilio Ficino: His Theology, His Philosophy, His Legacy*, Leiden 2002, pp. 243–256.

19 On Tommaso Del Garbo and his work see A. De Ferrari, "Del Garbo, Tommaso", in: *Dizionario biografico degli Italiani*, vol. 36, Rome 1988, pp. 581–585.

20 On Platonism in Ficino's *Consilio*, see T. Katinis, "A Humanist Confronts the Plague: Ficino's Consilio contro la Pestilentia", *Modern Language Notes* 125 (2010, Italian Issue), pp. 72–83.

21 M. Ficino, *Consilio contro la pestilentia*, c. 48v (T. Katinis, *Medicina e filosofia in Marsilio Ficino. Il* 'Consilio contro la pestilentia', p. 206).

continent and sober Socrates, the philosopher *par excellence*. In other words, Socrates embodies the man who avoids excess in all things in favor of an ideal equilibrium, both psycho-physical and moral. The same theory is presented in Ficino's *De Vita Libri Tres*, although in somewhat different contexts. We find, for example, a precise reference to the epidemic in the *De Vita*, in Book III, chapter 4, where Ficino repeats that in order to defend oneself against the disease, one should avoid excess, have a happy soul and steer clear of unhappy or troublesome things. Such conduct revives and fortifies the spirit, placing it under the beneficial influence of the sun – another element quite prominent in the *Consilio* – and rendering it immune from corruption and thus from infection.[22]

For anybody wishing to pursue the research on Ficino's medicine, two directions seem to be particularly promising. Firstly the study of other letters through which it may be possible to enlarge, clarify or modify our understanding of Ficino's philosophy of medicine. Secondly the study of Ficino's legacy in the early modern and modern Western culture. With regard to legacy, I would not be surprised to discover Ficinian influences in any medical practice that stresses the holistic perspective looking at psycho-physical human life. In this way, perhaps, scholars from a variety of disciplines, however diverse they may be, will intensify their collaboration for a common understanding. I like to imagine that at some point, a historian of Platonism, philologist or expert of forgotten hermetic books will be sitting at the same table with a physician, surgeon or biologist, sharing their knowledge for a larger understanding and improvement of the human condition.

22 See M. Ficino, *Three Books of Life*, pp. 259–260.

THE MEDIEVAL FOUNDATIONS OF RENAISSANCE MEDICAL ETHICS: THE CASE OF GABRIELE ZERBI'S *DE CAUTELIS MEDICORUM*

Joseph Ziegler

Francesco Petrarca, who relegated physicians motivated by greed and insatiable quest for fame to the position of the dregs (*faeces*) of the mechanics, exclaimed in one of his many outbursts against the medical profession: "Medicine has nothing in common with ethics, and is in many ways contrary to it" (*Medicina nichil commune cum ethica, sed multe contraria*).[1] The idea that medicine and ethics teach us how to live well (*recte vivere*) seemed to him ridiculously inappropriate. Neither does so, and physicians who confuse medicine with ethics overstep their bounds (*finis, terminus*) and need medical help.[2] I use this well known anecdote to introduce some doubt about my use of the term 'medical ethics', which appears dangerously anachronistic. Nevertheless, I do not intend to pontificate here on whether we are right to call Gabriele Zerbi's De cautelis medicorum a treatise in medical ethics, the first such treatise, and so forth. I shall use the term medical ethics without quotation marks, as a translation of the pre-modern term cautelae medicorum (physicians' prudence or precaution) as it was understood by writers of all treatises so entitled.

While Zerbi's *De cautelis medicorum* seems to be one of the earliest expressions of a group's self-regulatory rules of the Renaissance period,[3] it is necessary to ask what is really new in his text, apart from the banal fact that it is larger and more detailed than all earlier specific treatises on medical ethics. If a mid-fourteenth-century thinker, physician or philosopher had been asked to review Zerbi's *De cautelis medicorum*, would he have been stunned by its novelty? And more specifically, does Zerbi really deserve to be hailed by historians of medical ethics as a pioneer?[4] I shall first draw attention to Zerbi's debt to a long list of medieval and early Renaissance sources which he often cites verbatim and with-

1 Francesco Petrarca, "Invectives Against a Physician", in: Id., *Invectives*, ed. and trans. by D. Marsh, Cambridge (Mass.) 2003, iii. 128, p. 104.

2 Ibid., iii. 149–150, pp. 124–126.

3 R. French, "The Medical Ethics of Gabriele Zerbi", in: A. Wear – J. Geyer-Kordesch – R. French (eds.), *Doctors and Ethics. The Earlier Historical Setting of Professional Ethics*, Amsterdam 1993, pp. 72–97. All references to Zerbi's *De cautelis medicorum* (henceforward Zerbi) are based on the un-paginated first edition: Gabriele Zerbi, *Opus perutile de cautelis medicorum*, Venice 1495.

4 D. E. J. Linden, "Gabriele Zerbi 'De cautelis medicorum' and the Tradition of Medical Prudence", *Bulletin of the History of Medicine* 73 (1999), n. 1, pp. 19–37.

out acknowledgement. Then I shall highlight some of the more significant inflections which undermine the apparent continuity with the medieval discourse on medical ethics.

Zerbi frequently refers to a certain *Nicolus* as his source. It was Katharine Park who in her first book marked in passing the debt that Zerbi owes to a fellow physician Nicolò di Francesco Falcucci da Borgo San Lorenzo (Nicolaus Falcutius; d. 1411 or 1412), the most celebrated Florentine physician of the fourteenth-century, whose fame emerged not from a university association (which he did not have) but from the production of a monumental *Summa* of particular diseases, their causes, symptoms, and cures, entitled *Sermones medicinales*.[5] The book won huge popularity in fifteenth-century Florence among practitioners and academic physicians alike, and in its manuscript form may have contained some 1200 folio pages. It was first printed in Pavia in 1481–84. Nicolò was apparently Thomasso Del Garbo's physician; he probably studied at Bologna and/or in Florence under Thomasso himself.

A close reading of both texts (Falcucci's and Zerbi's) shows the extent to which Zerbi relied on Falcucci in each chapter of his book, often without the attribution. Large parts of Zerbi's *De cautelis* are taken from Falcucci verbatim or with minor amendments (for example chapters 9–13 in Zerbi's *De cautelis medicorum* are borrowed word for word from Falcucci's first *Sermo*). Zerbi used Falcucci also as a handy source for relevant classical and medieval medical authorities who wrote about deontological themes. Falcucci's work embedded in Zerbi's text does not make the latter useless as an independent historical source. Though part of a long medieval tradition of deontological writing, Zerbi's *De cautelis medicorum* still gives a fair picture of medical practice in the urban centres of fifteenth-century Italy, according to Park, who used the fourth and the fifth chapters (how doctors should behave towards the patient and others present at the sickbed of a private client) to reconstruct medical practice in fifteenth-century Florence. Here however I would like to stress the first part of the equation: more than giving a fair picture of medical deontology around 1500 in an urban setting, Zerbi reproduces a much earlier picture from around 1400 with some additions. A quick scan of his sources brings to light an intriguing fact: they are mostly medieval. John of Damascus, Haly Abbas, Pietro d'Abano, and Albertus de Zancariis (never mentioned in name) are the most widely used texts after Falcucci.[6] I even found an intimation of his (Falcucci; and then Zerbi) perhaps being familiar with Arnau de Vilanova's Medicationis parabole. In describing the desired rhetorical skills of physicians, Zerbi maintains (after Falcucci) that the physician should be able to speak courteously, richly and beautifully, with a certain gravitas and with parables. He should not be ashamed to be called parabolanus when the Gospel teaches us that the supreme physician Jesus Christ was a parabolanus. And every

5 K. Park, *Doctors and Medicine in Early Renaissance Florence*, Princeton 1985, pp, 110; 111–117; 133–134; 211 n. 75. I have used Nicolò Falcucci, *Sermonum liber scientie medicine* [*Sermones medicinales*], Venice 1515 [henceforth Falcucci].

6 See the appendix for an illustration of Zerbi's method of using the medieval sources.

action of Christ is our model (*instructio*).[7] It is tempting to read here some reworking of Arnau's last aphorism on why this genre of aphorism is suitable for medicine.

Let us examine a few specific examples of Zerbi's reliance on medieval sources: first, knowledge of the Hippocratic Oath and its ideas.[8] When reading surveys about the Hippocratic Oath in the Latin West, one normally encounters the notion that before the translation from the Greek of the Oath and Hippocrates' other works relating to medical ethics (*Law*, *Precepts* and *Decorum*) by Niccolò da Reggio in Naples between 1308 and 1345,[9] the West was only vaguely familiar with Hippocratic medical ethics. Implied in these narratives is the notion that the story of the actual impact of the Hippocratic Oath on Western ideas of doctor-patient relations dates from the Renaissance if not later.[10] The Oath as the prime document from antiquity attesting to systematic thinking about issues of medical ethics is depicted as the product of the Renaissance, the decline of Galenism and the consequent exaltation of a 'historical Hippocrates'. This approach is supported by the fact that the Oath as such is first used in 1508 Wittenberg and then in the revised humanist statutes of the University of Basel from 1570. We all still depend on Pearl Kibre's *Hippocrates Latinus*, which maintains that only fragments embodying precepts found in the Oath have come to light in Latin manuscripts prior to the early fourteenth-century.[11] Indeed, there is evidence that the Oath was known and perhaps even used in the Latin West from the fourth-century onwards. The continuity of knowledge of the Oath is further evinced for north-western Eu-

7 Zerbi, c.5: "Quom tempus loquendi datur medico, sit ille affabilis, ornate et pulchre cum quadam grauitate loquens, etiam in parabolis aliquando dicuntur sapientes. Non pudeat medicum vocari parabolanum, cum euangelica lectio doceat summum medicum Iesum Christum fuisse parabolanum, id est in parabolis loquutum. Omnis autem Christi actio nostra est instructio" (Falcucci, c. xi verbatim); cf. Arnau de Vilanova, *Medicationis parabole*, in: *Arnaldi de Villanova opera medica omnia*, VI.1, ed. by J. A. Paniagua, Barcelona 1990, pp. 127–129: "Eterni doctoris evangelica lectio testatur eundem fuisse parabolanum. Sapiens igitur ad exemplum iliius premissa reducet in parabolas oportunas." See Zerbi, c. 3 for an earlier reference to the physician as a *parabolanus* attributed to Mondino.

8 I am grateful to Monica Green who encouraged me to look into this theme and supplied me with pertinent bibliographical references.

9 T. Rütten, "Receptions of the Hippocratic *Oath* in the Renaissance. The Prohibition of Abortion as a Case Study in Reception", *Bulletin of the History of Medicine* 51 (1996), pp. 456–483 at 460–461; for the earlier Middle Ages see C. R. Galvão-Sobrinho, "Hippocratic Ideals, Medical Ethics, and the Practice of Medicine in the Early Middle Ages. The Legacy of the Hippocratic Oath", *Bulletin of the History of Medicine* 51 (1996), pp. 438–455.

10 H. von Staden, "The Discourses of Practitioners in Ancient Europe", in: R. B. Baker – L. B. McCullough (eds.), *The Cambridge World History of Medical Ethics*, Cambridge 2009, pp. 352–358; V. Nutton, "The Discourses of European Practitioners in the Tradition of the Hippocratic Texts", ibid., pp. 359–362; K. Bergdolt, "The Discourses of Practitioners in Medieval and Renaissance Europe", ibid., pp. 370–378; V. Nutton, "Beyond the Hippocratic Oath", in: Wear – Geyer-Kordesch – French (eds.), *Doctors and Ethics*, pp. 10–37, esp. 22–28.

11 P. Kibre, *Hippocrates Latinus. Repertorium of Hippocratic Writings in the Latin Middle Ages*, New York 1985, pp. 177–182 (on the Oath).

rope in segments of the Oath repeated in a series of manuscripts dating from the close of the eighth- to the twelfth-century. But all this does not amount to a critical mass of evidence which would allow the Middle Ages a significant place in the history of pre-modern medical ethics seen through the history of the Hippocratic Oath.

Now, the question of the manuscripts of the Oath (and indeed of all the ethical treatises in the Hippocratic corpus) from the early fourteenth-century onwards and their dissemination is certainly crucial (and perhaps needs revisiting). However, and this is known yet not sufficiently reiterated, there were other routes, whereby if not the text itself, some of its essential ideas and the consequent practices, became accessible to Latin readership. It was Loren C. MacKinney who ended his 1952 survey of medical ethics in the early Middle Ages with a reference to the first chapter in the *Pantegni*. This chapter appears to be a synthesis of materials long in circulation and originally derived in large measure from Hippocratic sources such as the Oath.[12] MacKinney ignored the history of the *Pantegni* and its significance for learned Latin medicine, more particularly for twelfth-century natural philosophers and thirteenth-century encyclopedists. Yet while reading MacKinney's survey I could not but cast my mind over all modern surveys of medical ethics in the pre-modern period: despite its shortcomings it is the only one that draws attention to the *Pantegni* as a source of Hippocratic medical ethics before the translations of the fourteenth-century. All recent narratives of medieval deontology or ethics neglect this fact, to my knowledge.

Some time in the last quarter of the eleventh-century, the *Pantegni* exposed to Latin readership Haly Abbas al-Maǧūsī's *Kāmil as-sinā'at at-tibbīya* (*The complete art of medicine*). The first chapter in the *Theorica* part of the *Pantegni*, which draws heavily on Hippocrates' Oath and occasionally paraphrases parts thereof, was entitled *Qualis debeat esse discipulus* (How should the student behave?). A second and more literal translation of the Arabic text (known in Latin as the *Liber regalis* or *Regalis dispositio*) by Stephen of Antioch appeared in 1127. It named the chapter (chapter 2 in the new division) *De hypocratis et aliorum mandato sapientum medicorum quo medicum suos disponere mores*: On the precept of Hippocrates and other wise physicians, by which the physician may ordain his manners.[13] This is the version which Zerbi used, and which is the source for some eight specific references to the Oath in his text. I am unaware of the actual use of these chapters by twelfth- to fourteenth-century physicians – a topic which merits systematic study; though it would be plausible to assume that being the first or the second chapters in such a medical encyclopedia it had a substantial readership (at

12 L. C. MacKinney, "Medical Ethics and Etiquette in the Early Middle Ages. The Persistence of Hippocratic Ideals", in: C. R. Burns (ed.), *Legacies in Ethics and Medicine*, New York 1977, pp. 173–203, at 199 (originally published in *Bulletin of the History of Medicine* 26 (1952), pp. 1–31).

13 C. Burnett, "Stephen, the Disciple of Philosophy, and the Exchange of Medical Learning in Antioch", Crusades 5 (2006), pp. 113–129; Haly filius Abbas, *Liber totius medicine necessaria continens* […], Lyon 1523, fol. 7ra, c. ii (De Hypocratis et aliorum mandato sapientum medicorum quo oportet medicum suos disponere mores).

least until it was eclipsed in the 1240s by Avicenna's *Canon*). But a second and more important problem arises in this context: when expounding the impact of the Oath on medical ethics should we direct our gaze at the late fifteenth-century context represented by Zerbi? Or should we not rather direct our attention to the twelfth- and thirteenth-centuries, which were first exposed to Hippocratic medical ethics through the mediation of the *Pantegni*?

The second theme pertinent to any debate of medical ethics, and which in the case of Zerbi's *De cautelis medicorum* shows clear continuity with the medieval tradition and complete reliance on a series of medieval authors, is the doctor's fee. As Europe was becoming aware of the possibilities of more complex forms of commerce, so the question of fees made its way into the discourse of medical ethics. The financial connection between physician and patient was increasingly viewed as commercial transaction: transition may be detected from a doctor's *honorarium* (a gift determined by satisfaction of employer or client with persons such as teachers, scribes, and other learned professionals) to *salarium* (a fixed sum calculated according to the nature, quality, and success of the work, often agreed by contract or terms of the engagement).[14] But anyone who has read Darrel Amundsen's studies of casuistry and professional obligations of physicians,[15] Luis García-Ballester's[16] and Michael McVaugh's[17] studies of doctor-patient relations around 1300, or Pietro d'Abano himself, knows that the fee became an intrinsic part of the relationship much earlier. Even Humbertus de Romanis in his sermon to the students of medicine composed sometime between 1266 and 1277 already spoke of the physician's duty to demand a moderate salary (*salarium sic temperatum recipient, quod suam conscientiam laesam non relinquent*).[18] The question of its propriety and equity in a competitive world of practice became a central topic at least as early as 1300. At that time Henri de Mondeville included salary as an intrinsic element of the doctor-patient relationship, and Pietro d'Abano clearly linked high fees to the efficacy of a treatment, a position adopted verbatim by Zerbi.[19] Zerbi's chapter on the doctor's fee, partially presented in the appendix to

14 A. R. Jonsen, *A Short History of Medical Ethics*, New York 2000, pp. 44–45.

15 D. W. Amundsen, "Casuistry and Professional Obligations. The Regulation of Physicians by the Court of Conscience in the Late Middle Ages", in: id., *Medicine, Society, and Faith in the Ancient and Medieval Worlds*, Baltimore / London 1996, pp. 248–288 at 261–263 (*Transactions and Studies of the College of Physicians of Philadelphia* n. s. 3 (1981), pp. 22–39, 93–112).

16 L. García-Ballester, "Medical Ethics in Transition in the Latin Medicine of the Thirteenth and Fourteenth Centuries. New Perspectives on the Physician-Patient Relationship and the Doctor's Fee", in: Wear – Geyer-Kordesch – French (eds.), *Doctors and Ethics*, pp. 38–71, at 49.

17 M. R. McVaugh, "Bedside Manners in the Middle Ages", *Bulletin of the History of Medicine* 71 (1997), n. 2, pp. 201–223.

18 Humbertus de Romanis, "Ad studentes in medicina", in: id., *De eruditione religiosorum*, II. 66 (Maxima Bibliotheca Veterum Patrum; 25), Lyon 1677, pp. 488–489.

19 "Empta solet care multis medicina iuvare. si data sit gratis nil confert utilitatis." Pietro d'Abano, *Conciliator*, Padua 1985 (reprint of Venice 1565), Diff. 2 (Utrum medicus oporteat logicum esse nec ne), fol. 5rb; cf. appendix for a partial transcription of Zerbi's discussion en-

this paper, clearly shows how closely he follows the medieval tradition in this respect.

But I am not one of those medievalists who abhor the idea of a change brought about at this or that stage of the Renaissance. Accordingly, I would like to highlight four themes in Zerbi's text suggesting a new development which seems to break the continuity that the medieval sources appear to impose. First, there seems to be a much stronger emphasis on the importance, indeed absolute necessity, of particulars, on learning from practical experience and intense exercise, and on searching for new practical discoveries.[20] Nobody should emerge from his studies to practice before having acquired experience. Nobody should study universals and at the same time despise particulars, and vice versa. When protesting the verbose and quarrelsome consequences inherent in contemporary medicine, and in bitterly criticizing the ambition of the medical establishment striving to develop and expand its reputation by dressing its discourse in philosophical garb, Petrarca may have been a precursor of such a sentiment that was critical of the heavy bias in favour of a theoretical approach to medicine. Doctors, he maintained, were transgressing their disciplinary boundaries and spreading their contentious habit to the fields of rhetoric and poetry also – "knitting Hippocratic knots with a Ciceronian warp".[21] Around 1500 he would have sounded less odd than in the 1350s.

Secondly, I am not sure whether one can claim that there was a more frequent and intensive appearance of *misericordia* and *humanitas*, two Roman categories of medical ethics, which had become fashionable again in the ethical discourse of physicians.[22] But one thing is clear, and may surprise those who still believe in the simplistic dichotomy between the medieval 'Age of Faith' and the more secular hence reasonable Renaissance: both Falcucci and Zerbi produced texts of medical ethics, which were more saturated by far with religious themes than any equivalent medieval predecessor. Zerbi opens his treatise with a call to place God in command of everything (*praeponere*) and links this to two references: one to Haly Abbas's opening chapter in *Liber regalis* mentioned before (*oportet esse ad deum*

titled: *De mercede medici accipienda' accompanied by an identification of the medieval sources* (Haly Abbas, Albertus de Zancariis, Pietro d'Abano, and Nicolò Falcucci).

20 Falcucci, c. x: "ille est melior medicus qui minus errat et talis est qui circa particularia plus exercitatus est. Caveant igitur stadium exeuntes absque exercitiis que nondum operati fuerint ne absque provisione multa properent ad medendum." Zerbi, c. iii: "Non aliter et medicus rationalem siue logycum se prebeat, ut duce hypocrate cum aliis canonicis medicis particularia consideret ut sub universalibus comprehensa sunt. Non sic autem methoycus universalia solum considerans despectis particularibus quod in artificiale est. Neque etiam sit empericus ne despectis universalibus, particularibus solum inhereat. Expedit preterea ut apprehendens sit intelligens et peritus."

21 S. Cracolici, "The Art of Invective", in: V. Kirkham – A. Maggi (eds.), *Petrarch. A Critical Guide to the Complete Works*, Chicago 2009, pp. 255–262.

22 Zerbi, c. 4: "Ratio clamat ad iudicium, si misericordiam deseris propter quod inquit quod oportet medicum cum infirmo languescere et sanitatem eius proxime suscipere. Qui enim respicit super infirmum et egenum in die mala, liberabit eum dominus"; cf. Falcucci, c.x which attributes the approach to Chrisostomos.

suspicientem) and one to John of Damascus. The second chapter in Zerbi's *De cautelis medicorum* is dedicated to a full analysis of the desired relation between the physician and God (*De modo se habendi medici erga Deum*). In addition to a repetition of both mentioned references, the chapter includes a long paraphrastic commentary on *Ecclesiasticus* 38, while Nicolò Falcucci is explicitly mentioned this time as the source for a detailed explanation of how to start a medical treatment (in the name of the Lord, thanking him and acknowledging his role as the source of all cures past and future). The physician should never ascribe the acquired health to his teaching or wisdom, but only to God. He should invoke divine help at the beginning of every curing activity he performs.[23] Zerbi imitates Nicolò Falcucci who about a century earlier devoted the eleventh chapter in the first *Sermo medicinalis* to God (*Qualiter se debet habere medicus versus deum et famam suam*); there he linked to the cult of God the physician's duty to give free medical aid to the poor and needy or to visit patients in hospitals.[24]

The acknowledgment of God as the primary and universal agent of health (*primum et universale agens*), as the source of health-bringing hope, as well as the specific insistence on the physician's duty to verify that the patient has confessed his sins or is committed to doing so in the future along the lines of canon 22 of Lateran IV,[25] would have partially satisfied at least two of the three basic ethical demands that Jean Gerson made to Graduates of medicine in Paris at the second decade of the fifteenth-century in his sermon (*pro licentiandis in medicina*). First, always to be grateful to God and to acknowledge at every stage of the medical

23 Zerbi, c. 2 (De modo se habendi medici erga deum): "Dixit haliabas: Oportet medicum esse ad deum suspicientem. Erit ergo medicus dei dilegentissimus et fidelissimus cultor. Memor continuo preceptorum ioannis Mesue dicentis: Deum o medice in cunctis prepone et preponet te. Honora eum et honorabit te. Time eum et securus cuncta experieris. Sanat enim solus langores deus et de terre solio produxit in largitate suam medicinam. A deo enim est omnis medela dixit Iesus Sirach in ecclesiastico. Etenim altissimus creauit de terra medicinam, quod si feceris sacer fies medicus et diuinus, ut res etiam diuine tibi reuelentur. Nam sacre res hominibus solum ostenduntur, prauis autem nequaquam ut ypocra. in libro de lege. Dixit Nicolus [Cf. Falcucci, c. xi]: Erit sermo medici ad egrotantis curam novissime vocati in nomine domini, eidem gratias agendo, quod ad sui curam et non alterius egrotans inciderit, a quo et gratias petens ut suo nomine infirmum ad pristinam sanitatem restituere queat. Non ascribat medicus sanitatem inductam doctrine aut prudentie sue. Sed salutis omnis auctori deo attribuendum. Imploret medicus diuinum auxilium in componendis, vel exhibendis consiliis sine eius nutu ac voluntate nihil rectum, nihil salutare datur quod si fecerit quia bonus erit, deo similes fiat et ita de eo maior erit dei solicitudo propter quod et sibi potiora beneficia impartietur. Antidoti ex inuentione propria vires et uirtutes commendans medicus in fine omnium ad dat hoc verbum: si deus voluerit [...]."

24 Falcucci, c. xi: "Et debet medicus frequentare et cunctis egenis absque pretio exhibere debet remedium salutare."

25 Zerbi, c. 4: "Salutet itaque, ut decet a corporali malo, dicendo liberet te deus, vel saluus sis, vel tale consimile ut dici sollet consisto sibi egrotantem peccata sua non fuisse confessum antequam ipsum tangat aut aliud de signis suis videat, ipsum interrogare debet si aperuit suorum peccatorum conscientiam sacerdoti. Quod si sic, bene est, si vero non promissionem ab eo recipiat sic se facturum, multe ei egritudines propter peccata emergent"; cf. Falcucci, c. xii.

treatment that he is the source of all medical knowledge and medical remedy, and to maintain the belief in God's ability to perform miracles (hence to be a constant source of salubrious hope). Secondly (thirdly in Gerson's sermon), to always be kind (*benignus*) to the patient and to treat him diligently, receiving well God's gift given to him and lavishing it again equally well and even better for the health of the soul.[26]

Thirdly, there seems to be a heavier stress on the duty to search for new theories and particularly new practices (*novae res*), and to discover (*invenire*) new approaches to medicine.[27] In addition to Zerbi we can find at least two other fifteenth-century sources that hint at the same direction. Falcucci in chapter 13 of his discourse forcefully preaches that the intellectually gifted physician (*medicus intelligens et ingeniosus*) should exhibit both the energy and the ability to produce new inventions, for *in omni medicatione oportet novi aliquid invenire*. A moral duty seems to oblige all physicians to innovate. Their ingenuity is a result of their ability to fill or complete (*suppleare*) what the wise people (*sapientes*) failed to convey orally or in writing. One should thus actively strive to overtake the doctrine of the ancients and free oneself from the constraints of the written word. This approach to innovation is striking when juxtaposed to the instinct of an anonymous fifteenth-century cleric who composed the *Decem quaestiones de medicorum statu*, a Decalogue for Christian medical practitioners.[28] The fourth rule discusses the plurality of physicians. The first argument, supporting the view that this is an unsafe practice, links plurality of opinions with quarrel and discord, for where there are many physicians they will attempt to introduce many novelties (*ubi sunt plures medici, plures nouitates conantur inducere*) – an inevitable result

26 Jean Gerson, *Pro licentiandis in medicina*, in: id., *Oeuvres completes*, vol. 5, # 216, introd., texts and notes by P. Glorieux, Paris 1963, pp. 144–151: "Primum: sit medicus gratus Deo a quo medicinalis scientiae verbum suscepit. Formidet ne sibi contingat illud quod de philosophis ingratis tradit Apostolus... [Rom. 1. 21]. Pellatur suo opere pessimus error ille qui non liberrime sed quadam necessitate naturae posuit Deum agere ad extra; nam hoc errore durante quas Deo gratiarum actiones, qualem de eo spem certam potuerit invenire? Tollit quippe error ille omnem miraculorum operationem et ex consequenti religionem cui adversus est." [Followed by a historical example of Johannes, the Jewish physician of Magister Basilius who predicted his death before dawn, yet Basilius managed to survive till the next morning. Consequently, Johannes converts and is baptized by Basilius 'cognoscens operationem Dei supra naturam']. "Secundum documentum: Sit medicus recollectus in seipsum et supra sensibilium considerationem saepe eleuatus [...]. Tertium documentum: sit medicus diligens atque benignus erga proximum ut diligenter sanet, sibi commissum donum Dei susceptum bene dispensando non minus, immo magis ad salutem animarum, occasione habita, quam corporum. Iis modis perveniet medicus ad eum a quo est medicina efficienter, per quem exemplariter, et ad quem finaliter ducitur, praestante Deo."

27 Zerbi, c. 3: "Ita tamen cum sua peritia se habeat medicus ut non solum antiquorum scriptis omnino insistat, immo solerti ingenio eius est satagare ad novarum rerum inuentionem non minus in traditione doctrine quam in auxiliorum salubrium approximatione."; cf. Falcucci, c. xiii.

28 R. Peitz, *Die 'Decem quaestiones de medicorum statu'. Ein spätmittelaterlicher Dekalog zur ärztlichen Standeskunde* (Würzburger medizinhistorische Forschungen; 11), Hannover 1978, pp. 53–54.

of the clash between diverse opinions and opposing interests. Yet the author's view that plurality of physicians is a good thing removes the danger of novelty: plurality introduces unity, not novelty (*plures medici non debent inducere nouitatem sed unitatem*). Comparison (*collatio*) of the different opinions ends in concord, which is so expedient for the successful cure. The place of innovation and novelty in medical practice according to Falcucci and Zerbi represents a significant shift in expectations from practising physicians. The limited way in which changes were acknowledged as progress and ideas of the 'new' were advocated in learned medicine between the thirteenth- and the early fifteenth-century was no longer the only desirable way to follow.[29]

Fourthly, the attitude to a plurality of physicians treating a single case also underwent a change. The slogan *pluralitas in unitatem redacta* can summarize Pietro d'Abano's discussion in *Conciliator*, Diff. 7: *Utrum corpus humanum sit uni uel pluribus medicis committendum.*[30] Galen's view admitting to have treated many patients who had already been treated by other physicians, and a variety of philosophical sources (among others Aristotle in his *Politics* and *Ethics*) which maintained that an opinion becomes stronger (*potentior*) when it is uttered by several people, fortified the view that plurality of opinions creates sounder knowledge. Confronting this view, Pietro d'Abano introduced Aphorisms 80 and 81 by John of Damascus, who maintained that to reduce the margins of error the patient should commit himself to one faithful physician, and he who consults many physicians will be exposed to the error of each of them.[31] Pietro's solution for the apparent discrepancy is to stick to the middle way (*viam observando mediam*): one should entrust the human body to several physicians, but only after having chosen one of them as the principal (*corpus humanum pluribus committendum est medicis, uno tandem principaliori facto*). In this way it is possible to reduce a plurality of opinions to a single unified judgement (*in unum consurgere*). The analogy that justifies such an arrangement in the medical arena is the similarity between the human and the political body. We should imagine the animal as a city (*aestimandum est animal constare quemadmodum civitatem*): in politics one needs many rulers to maintain order, but they are all ordained by one supreme ruler who procures advice and counsel from these inferior rulers. In the case of the human being, whose nature makes him easily perishable if falsely diagnosed (*propter promptitudinem nature humane ad labendum*), and who has infinite kind of necessary needs, it is impossible for a single person to satisfy perfectly all these

29 Most pertinent here is C. Crisciani, "History, Novelty, and Progress in Scholastic Medicine", *Osiris*, second series, 6 (1990), pp. 118–139. At p. 133 she draws attention to Henri de Mondeville's unique approach to novelty in medicine when he confidently asserts in his *Antidotarium* that God has given each one of us, like Galen, his own natural ingenuity that guides us to resort to new things.

30 Pietro d'Abano, *Conciliator*, fol. 10rb–11rb.

31 Jean Mesue, *Le livre des Axiomes médicaux (Aphorismi)*, ed. by D. Jacquart and G. Troupeau, Geneva 1980, p. 181, no. 80: "Eger uni fideli medicorum commitendus est cuius error ad recti distantiam rarus est." No. 81: "Quod si plurimos consulit, in singulorum errorem plerumque cadit."

unexpected needs. Plurality of doctors is necessary at all stages of the medical engagement, but these treatments should converge into one, determined by the most prudent physician, who is so recognized by the patient (*in unum principalem consurgere prudentiorem, solertiorem, ac magis sollicitum existentem et ab egro-to amplius affectatum, in quo et omnem spem posuerit*). The human body should therefore be entrusted to several physicians, yet at the same time to a single principal one (*Corpus igitur humanum pluribus, uno principaliori facto, medicis committendum*).

On the other side we can find Henri de Mondeville and Francesco Petrarca. Mondeville saw plurality of surgeons as a cause of error. Motivated by his campaign to push the *cyrurgicus expertus* or *litteratus a longo tempore expertus* (the opposite of *juvenis inexpertus*) to the forefront of medical care as an independent agent, hence as an individual practitioner, he likened to a dog's pelage (*vellus canis*) the unhealthy situation in Paris, where people of status summoned several practitioners: it is entirely non-useful (no dog with short hair dies of cold), and when too long it becomes burdensome also because it tends to become infested with flees. The more practitioners surround the patient, the smaller the actual responsibility assumed by each for the object of treatment. Under such circumstances one tends to discuss theoretical explanations and universals, and to hide the simple practical solutions. Henri de Mondeville adopts Pietro d'Abano's compromise: it would suffice to order two or three practitioners for a *consilium* (a few *pauci* in a later debate), but one must appoint one of them to actually draw the information from the others and to run the treatment.[32]

Petrarca's antipathy to physicians reflected the common practice that a patient should be entrusted to one trustworthy (*fidelis*) physician, who seldom errs. For "by consulting many physicians he may be exposed to the errors of many".[33] Like Mondeville, Falcucci too opts for a controlled plurality: two or three physicians, a multitude that will not create confusion and that will choose one of its own to govern the group.[34]

32 J. L. Pagel (ed.), *Die Chirurgie des Heinrich von Mondeville nach Berliner, Erfurter und Pariser Codices*, Berlin 1892, pp. 116–117: "Et re vera id quod dicit Damascenus communiter accidit Parisiis aliquibus, qui in curis suis convocant infinitos diversarum sectarum in collationibus faciendis; tunc enim dicimus nos, quod nos sumus, sicut vellus canis, quod quanto longius et majus, tanto est cani pejus, tum quia magis onerosum tum quia plures pulices se occultant, et utilitas longitudinis velleris canis nulla, quia pauci canes frigore moriuntur. Quanto etenim sumus plures, tanto minus se reputant quilibet operatum, et tunc loquimur de solis universalibus; nam si ad propositum sciat aliquid facile et expertum, nunquam ipsum caute multitudini tevelaret, sed si duo aut tres solum ad consilium vocarentur, tunc deberet sufficere, et quod unicus scilicet ipsorum melior deberet curam prosequi totus solus, tunc ipse extraheret ab aliis quidquid posset, et quia pauci essent non est verisimile, quod aliquid aliquod occultaret. Et ulterius ille, qui prosequeretur negotium totus solus, non solum a se ipso et a sociis eliceret utilia, immo inquireret ab aliis quibuscunque." See also pp. 122–123.

33 Petrarca, *Invectives*, i.5, p. 6.

34 Falcucci, c. xiii: "et ex eis fidelior et magis ab egro affectatus eligatur cuius imperio omnibus aliis auditis medicis regimen ordinetur, dicunt non congregetur caterva medicorum sed duo vel tres ad plus ut non accidat in multitudine confusio."

But for Zerbi there is no longer any issue of doubt. It is a given fact – the common course of things – that several physicians normally treat a single case. He thus dedicated a whole chapter (entitled *De modo se habendi medici erga alios medicos in eadem cura sibi delegatos*) to regulating the difficult dynamics that may develop. From Pietro d'Abano he takes all the references in support of recruiting partners (*socios*) for the cure as a desirable source to increase the scope of knowledge and to reduce error. No physician should presume to treat a deadly disease alone (*Non presumes solus curare egritudinem de qua rationabiliter mors cognoscitur, sed socium vel plures petat*), and he should find such colleagues himself or compel the patient's friends or relatives to do so. He gives detailed instructions on choosing worthy partners: for example, how to avoid an unhelpful association of a learned physician (*canonicus medicus*) and an unlearned practitioner (*plebeius*), how to treat a partner who is of inferior status (a junior physician or even a student), how to maintain efficient and safe collaboration, and how to be silent about mal-practice or the errors of others.

So despite perfect loyalty to the standard medieval texts, a fealty which would have made our imaginary medieval reader of Gabriele Zerbi's *De cautelis medicorum* feel very comfortable with such a text, significant change is also part of the story. I have indicated just four general themes which suggest that we should reflect together more deeply about what was really new in medical ethics in the age of Humanism.

APPENDIX

Gabriele Zerbi Opus perutile de cautelis medicorum, Venice 1495.[35]

De mercede medici accipienda

Licet intentio medici non debeat esse in medendo ad pecuniam sed a deo retributionem et meritum expectare, auctore Haliabate[36]: Attamen quia expedit medico quoad fieri potest celerius, ut eger cuius cura salutis sibi commissa est sanitati pristine restituatur, precipiente ypocrate in suo iureiurando: medicum nemini egritudinem dilaturum. Egritudines enim cum prolongantur non relinquunt medicum omnino immunem ab infamia, saltem apud vulgares. Inter ea autem que opitulantur veloci saluti est ut patientem et qui sui sunt pro uiribus alliciat et obliget: ut mandatis suis obediant.

Ideo studium medici sit: et quod non sit postponendum ut a patiente suo decenter satisfiat. Sic enim medicus maioris apud illum efficietur auctoritatis: il-

35 The discussion concludes chapter four entitled: De modo se habendi medici erga patientes et maxime erga egrotantes.

36 Haly Abbas, *Liber totius*, c. ii, fol. 7ra: "… nec sit eius adquirendam in medicinam, in medendo intentio pecuniam, sed a deo retributionem et meritum."

lum excellentiorem iudicat ipsum sibi ad humanam communicat politiam.[37] Illi omnes obtemperare conantur ne amittantur expense: sicque demum citius sanatur. Iuxta illud: Empta solet care multis medicina iuuare. Si data sit gratis nihil confert utilitatis.[38]

Triplex autem est modus se habendi patientis ad medicum. Unus quo patiens dicitur diuinus, respectu medici et hoc quando infirmus uehementi langore cruciatus medicum deprecatur de restituenda corporis sanitate.

Dyabolicus vero, dum sanitate iam adepta medico ut decet non satisfacit: illum negligit medico obvians: illum fugit ueluti diabolicis uestigiis obsignatum. Sed humanus, si patiens dum sanatur et post adeptam sanitatem medico iuxta merita satisfacit illum sibi reputans dominum et amicum.[39] Mercedem igitur condignam sine intermissione recipiat medicus. Neque unquam sit oblati negator: nisi fortasse sibi quid prius intulerit tanti: et maxime cum minor aut mediocris fuerit medicus. Dignus est enim mercenarius mercede sua.

Meminerit medicus artem medicinalem et precipue curatiuam marti ascribi omnibus fere planetis odiosioris irremunerationis obiurgio et omnis iniquitatis datori: propter quod expetit medici negocium ne decipiatur primitus firmare nisi patiens magnificus fuerit et curialis: uel fuerit tibi affinitate coniunctus: aut pauper: ex hoc enim centuplum accipies. Ex alio lex affinitatis suadet. Pauperes vero et egeni non sunt opprimendi neque deserendi intuitu saltem pietatis, cum inde consurgat medici laudabilis fama. Quod enim habundanter medicus accepit pauperculis velit amore bonitatis Saluatoris nostri impartiri.[40] Ab aliis vero accipiat, omni tamen cum modestia quam ut volens velit, et quasi veluti non aduertens animaduertat, et quasi renuens libenti animo manum cum dexteritate porrigendo recipiat, ne de nimia siti et auiditate notetur [...].

37 Albertus de Zancariis, *De cautelis medicorum habendis*, in: M. Morris, *Die Schrift des Albertus de Zancariis aus Bologna 'De cautelis medicorum habendis'*, Leipzig 1914, pp. 18–19: "Restat de solutione medici ab aegro recipienda, quam debet sollicitare medicus, ut sibi ab aegro plenarie satisfiat. Tunc ipsum autorizabilem et excellentem extimat, illi etiam dum satisfecerit plena manu, ipsum sibi ad humanam communicat policiam."

38 Pietro d'Abano, *Conciliator*, Diff. 2, fol. 5rb: "Empta solet care multis medicina iuuare. Si data sit gratis nil confert utilitatis."

39 Zancariis, *De cautelis medicorum*, in: Morris, *Die Schrift*, p. 19: "Recitatur fabulose vel historice ab antiquis, quod medicis respectu patientis triplex vultus ostenditur: divinus, diabolicus et humanus. Divinus quidem dum infirmus vehementi languore vexatur, ipsum humiliter deprecatur de restituenda corporis sospitate. Diabolicus vero, dum sanatus infirmus medico non satisfecerit condecenter, ipsi non obvians, illum fugat velut diabolicis vestigiis consignatum. Sed humanus, dum curatus infirmus sananti satisfecerit, ut oportet, illum sibi reputans velut dominum et amicum."

40 Pietro d'Abano, *Conciliator*, Diff. 2, fol. 5rb: "Non tamen velis pauperes opprimere, neque egenos saltem intuitu pietatis deserere, cum inde laudabilis consurgat fama. Quod enim abundanter accepisti, his velis gratis primae amore bonitatis impartiri. Nunquam autem sis oblati obnegator: nisi fortassis tibi quid prius intulerit tanti: et maxime cum minor, aut mediocris fueris medicorum: quoniam medicina et maxime curatiua marti est scripta: qui omnibus fere planetis iudicatur odiosior: hic etiam irremunerationis, obiurgii, et omnis iniquitatis extat planeta, propter quod expetit negocium tuum ne decipiaris primitus firmare: nisi aegrotus magnificus esset et curialis omniquaque."

Nisi ergo medicus premia recipiat labor eius vertetur in damnum. Sed cum labor est in damno mortalis crescit egestas, et qui emit rem care et eam vult donare disponat se mendicare. Meminerit quoque medicus quod sine bonis exterioribus quorum fortuna est domina non contingit esse hominem felicem neque ab eius memoria excedat preceptum antiquum. Dum dolet infirmus medicus fit pignore firmus. Expers langoris non est memor huius amoris. Et iterum dum morbus fortis est medico promittitur.[41]

Licet autem hec obseruanda sint in mercedem accipiendo in petendo tamen eam caute procedat medicus: ne ut aiunt in fractione panis dignoscatur: plerumque enim medici ita modum excedunt in petendo ut ars nostra vilescat [...].

Quod si surdum se prebeat patiens, hac cautela ad aliam deveniendum est: ut astantem fidum vel apotecarium vel alium in quo confidet medicus moneat veluti ex se vel patientem vel affines aut amicos moneat ut medici memores sint, si festinam salutem patientis exoptent.

41 Falcucci, c. xiii (Qualiter se debet habere medicus circa alios vel alia), fol. 8vb: "Medicus debet ab infirmis suis condignam recipere mercedem quia dignus est mercenarius mercede sua. Nulli ergo nisi parentela astrictus dimittat quod sibi debetur. Qui enim emit rem care et eam vult donare, disponit se mendicare unde ab aliquis dicebatur. Cum dolet infirmus medicus sit pignore firmus. Expers langoris non est memor huius amoris. Et iterum. Cum locus est morbis medico promittitur orbis. Mox fugit a mente medicus morbo recedente. Empta solet care multos medicina iuuare. Si data sit gratis nil confert utilitatis."

MIT DER VERSTOCKTHEIT EINES KETZERS. DAS BILD DES HÄRETISCHEN ARZTES IN GABRIELE ZERBIS *DE CAUTELIS MEDICORUM*

Kay Peter Jankrift

„Hütet euch sorgsam vor falschen Propheten, das heißt vor ketzerischen Lehren. Sie kommen nämlich zu euch in Schafskleidern. Inwendig aber sind sie wie reißende Wölfe“, heißt es gestützt auf die Worte des Matthäus-Evangeliums im Vorwort von Gabriele Zerbis (1445-1505) *De cautelis medicorum.*[1] Religiöse und medizinische Vorstellungen waren für den Professor für Medizin untrennbar miteinander verbunden. Für ihn stand außer Zweifel, dass ein guter Arzt seine Praxis an den Maßgaben der Evangelien ausrichten und diese ebenso beachten sollte wie die Regeln der Heilkunde.[2] In diesem Sinne empfahl er mit Hinweis auf die Ausführungen Galens, nicht jedweder Schrift Glauben zu schenken.[3] Angesichts solch eindringlicher Mahnungen erscheint es umso erstaunlicher, dass Zerbi angehenden Standeskollegen rät, „von der Ketzerei wie einem gleichsam krankhaften Wahrheitsdrang Besitz zu ergreifen, so als seien sie verrückt“ und unablässig die Werke der ruhmreichen medizinischen Autoritäten zu studieren.[4] Zudem zitiert er offen aus dem *Conciliator* des Pietro d´Abano (um 1250-1316), der von der Inquisition postum als Häretiker verurteilt worden war.[5] Damit stellen sich zwin-

1 Mt 7,7. Gabriele Zerbi, *Opus perutile de cautelis Medicorum*, Venedig 1495, fol.13r. Eine kommentierte, kritische Edition dieses Werkes mit deutscher Übersetzung, die im Rahmen eines von der DFG geförderten und von Mariacarla Gadebusch Bondio geleiteten Forschungsvorhabens am Institut für Geschichte und Ethik der Technischen Universität München erarbeitet wurde, befindet sich im Druck. Der vorliegende Beitrag präsentiert Ergebnisse aus diesem Projekt.

2 Zerbi, *De cautelis Medicorum*, fol. 13r.: „Similis enim videtur observatio canonum medicinae observationi legis evangelicae, quae consimiliter perficitur.“

3 Ebd.: „Non enim oportet cuicumque scripture credere, ut Galienus ait primo de simplicis medicina.“

4 Zerbi, *De cautelis Medicorum*, fol. 14v: „…possidere debet hereticam id est venercam insaniam veritatis acsi pro veritate insaniret et neque die neque nocte deficere et attente addiscere quecumcumque a gloriosissimis dicta sunt veteribus.“

5 Beispielsweise Zerbi, *De cautelis Medicorum*, fol. 14r. J.-P. Boudet – F. Collard – N. Weill-Parot (Hgg.), *Médicine, astrologie et magie entre Moyen Âge et Renaissance: autour de Pietro d'Abano*, Florenz 2013; G. Federici Vescovini, „Profilo di Pietro d'Abano, il conciliatore”, in: G. Bentivegna – S. Burgio – G. Magnano (Hgg.), *Filosofia, scienza e cultura. Studi in onore di Corrado Dollo*, Soveria Mannelli 2002, S. 845–862; D.N. Hasse, „Pietro d'Abano's *Conciliator* and the theory of the soul in Paris“, in: J. A. Aertzen – K. Emery – J. Speer (Hgg.), *Nach der Verurteilung von 1277: Philosophie und Theologie an der Universität von*

gend die Fragen nach den Vorstellungen von Ketzerei am Ende des 15. Jahrhunderts wie auch nach den Hintergründen von Gabriele Zerbis Bild des häretischen Arztes.

HÄRESIE, HEXEREI UND SATANSWERK. GABRIELE ZERBI IM UMFELD DER INQUISITION

Es liegt nahe, die Suche nach Antworten mit einem Blick auf den Lebensweg des Gelehrten zu beginnen und die spezifischen Gegebenheiten, unter denen sein Werk *De cautelis medicorum* entstand, eingehender zu betrachten. Als die Abhandlung im Jahre 1495 bei Christophorus de Pensis in Venedig erstmals im Druck erschien, befand sich Gabriele Zerbi auf dem Höhepunkt seines wissenschaftlichen Ruhmes.[6] Nur wenige Monate zuvor war der Veronese an die hochangesehene Universität von Padua zurückgekehrt, wo sein Werdegang im Sommer 1467 begonnen hatte. Den wenigen bekannten Daten seiner bislang nur bruchstückhaft erschlossenen Biographie zufolge, wechselte er 1475 als Professor für Medizin und Philosophie an die Universität Bologna. Im Jahre 1483 trat er als Leibarzt in den Dienst Papst Sixtus‘ IV. (1414-1484).[7] Daneben lehrte Zerbi an der *Sapienza*. Im August 1484 rückte Innozenz VIII. (1432-1492) auf den Stuhl Petri nach. Auch der neue Papst vertraute auf die Fähigkeiten Gabriele Zerbis, der dem Pontifex sein 1489 bei Eucharius Silber in Rom veröffentlichtes Werk *Gerencontomia* widmete.[8] Der Oberhirte würdigte die Tätigkeit seines Leibarztes, indem er die finanziellen Zuwendungen für diesen im März 1490 von jährlich 150 auf nunmehr 250 Florin in römischer Münze beträchtlich anhob.

Zurzeit von Zerbis Aufenthalt in Rom erlebte inquisitorisches Gedankengut am Heiligen Stuhl einen bedeutenden Aufschwung.[9] Mit seiner Bulle *Exigit sincerae* devotionis, ausgestellt am 1. November 1478, hatte Sixtus IV. den Grundstein

Paris im letzten Viertel des 13. Jahrhunderts, Berlin 2001, S.635–653; L. Olivieri, *Pietro d'Abano e il pensiero neolatino. Filosofia, scienza e ricerca dell'Aristotele greco tra i secoli XIII e XIV* (Saggi e testi; 23), Padua 1988; E. Paschetto, *Pietro d'Abano. Medico e filosopho*, Florenz 1984; L. Norpoth, „Zur Bio-Bibliographie und Wissenschaftslehre des Pietro d'Abano, Mediziners, Philosophen und Astronomen in Padua“, *Kyklos* 3 (1930), S. 292–353; S. Ferrari, *I tempi, la vita, le dottrine di Pietro D'Abano: saggio storico-filosofico*, Genova 1900.

6 J. Haig Gaisser, *Piero Valeriano on the ill fortune of learned men. A Renaissance humanist and his world*, Ann Arbor 1999, S.330; L. Münster, *Studi e ricerche su Gabriele Zerbi*, Bologna 1956.

7 L. G. Marini, *Degli archiatri dei ponifici*, Roma 1784, Vol.1. S.310–311.

8 *Gabrielis Zerbi Veronensis ad Innocentium VIII. Pon. Max. Gerentocomia [i.e. Gerontocomia] feliciter incipt*, Eucharius Silber, Roma 1489.

9 Hierzu unter anderem G. Schwerhoff, *Die Inquisition. Ketzerverfolgung in Mittelalter und Neuzeit*, München 2004; J. Oberste, *Ketzerei und Inquisition im Mittelalter*, Darmstadt 2007, S.132–135; B. Comella, *La Inquisición española*, Madrid 2004; S. Peyronel Rimbaldi (Hg.), *I tribunali della fede: continuità e discontinuità dal Medioevo all'età moderna*, Torino 2008; G. Romeo, *L'Inquisizione nell'Italia moderna*, Roma 2002.

zur Einrichtung der Spanischen Inquisition gelegt.[10] Die Katholischen Könige, Ferdinand II. (1452-1516) und Isabella I. (1451-1504), trieben die Umsetzung des päpstlichen Erlasses in Kastilien mit Eifer voran. Nach dem Tod seines Vaters Johann II. (1397/1398-1479) konnte Ferdinand die Verfügung des Heiligen Stuhls auf Aragón ausweiten. Zwar nutzten die Katholischen Königen die Spanische Inquisition vor allem als herrschaftliches Instrument, doch hatte der Papst nicht zuletzt durch die Ernennung der Generalinquisitoren maßgeblichen Anteil an dieser organisierten Ketzerverfolgung.[11] In deren Zielvisier standen zunächst vor allem Juden, die angesichts des wachsenden gesellschaftlichen Drucks oder unter Zwang das Christentum angenommen hatten und die von den Altchristen spöttisch *marranos*, Schweine, genannt wurden. Diese *Conversos* standen ebenso wie späterhin die konvertierten Muslime, die *Moriscos,* unter dem allgemeinen Verdacht, im Geheimen noch immer dem Glauben ihrer Väter anzuhängen und dessen Riten zu befolgen.[12] Weil sie nach ihrer Taufe als Christen galten, kam ein solches Verhalten einem Abfall vom wahren Bekenntnis und mithin der schwerwiegendsten Form der Häresie überhaupt gleich. Die Vorbereitungen zur Einführung der Inquisition zogen sich über drei Jahre hin. Zu ersten Prozessen gegen vermeintliche Häretiker kam es 1481 in Sevilla. Dort führten Frater Morillo und Frater Martín, ein blutiges Regiment. Will man den Ausführungen des zeitgenössischen Chronisten Andrés Bernáldez (um 1450-1513) glauben, so endeten bis 1488 etwa 700 unbußfertige Ketzer auf dem Scheiterhaufen. In mehr als 5.000 Inquisitionsverfahren kam es zur Aussöhnung.[13]

Das rigorose Vorgehen der Inquisitoren, dem sogar Angehörige des Rates zum Opfer fielen, führte dazu, dass Juden und *Conversos* in wachsender Zahl ihre iberische Heimat verließen.[14] Während die meisten in Gebiete unter islamischer Herrschaft abwanderten, insbesondere das Osmanische Reich, wandten sich andere nach Italien.[15] Einige dieser Flüchtlinge trugen dem Papst ihre Beschwerden über die Willkür vor, mit der Morillo und Martín in Sevilla verfuhren. Zwar wurden die beiden Dominikanerbrüder daraufhin durch andere Inquisitoren ersetzt, doch gingen diese kaum umsichtiger zu Werk als ihre Vorgänger. Der Auftakt der Spanischen Inquisition fällt in etwa in die Zeit von Gabriele Zerbis Ankunft in Rom. Es steht wohl außer Frage, dass sich Nachrichten über die Ereignisse in

10 R. Lemm, *Die spanische Inquisition*, Köln 2005, S.64–67.

11 J. Oberste, *Ketzerei und Inquisition im Mittelalter*, Darmstadt 2007, S.134.

12 Hierzu u.a. Y. Yovel, *The other within. The Marranos – split identity and emerging modernity*, Princeton 2009; M. Bodian, *Dying in the law of Moses. Crypto-Jewish martyrdom in the Iberian World*, Bloomington 2007; J. Valdeón Barruque, *Judíos y Conversos en la Castilia medieval*, Valladolid 2004; N. Roth, *Conversos, Inquisition, and the expulsion of the Jews from Spain*, Madison (Wisconsin) 1995; Y. Kaplan, *Jews and conversos. Studies in society and inquisition*, Jerusalem 1985.

13 Zu den Zahlenangaben siehe R. Lemm, *Die spanische Inquisition*, Köln 2005, S.66.

14 E. Benbassa – A. Rodrigue, *Sephardi Jewry. A history of the Judeo-Spanish community, 14th to 20th centuries*, Berkeley 2000, S.6–7.

15 T. Brechenmacher, *Der Vatikan und die Juden. Geschichte einer unheiligen Beziehung*, München 2005, S.17.

Spanien auch jenseits der Pyrenäen verbreiteten. Als Leibarzt des Pontifex dürften Zerbi die Proteste gegen die rüden Methoden der Inquisition eben so wenig verborgen geblieben sein wie die Vorstellungswelt der Inquisitoren. Diese wurde am Ende des 15. Jahrhunderts nicht allein durch die Eindrücke der Verfolgung von *Conversos* auf der Iberischen Halbinsel geprägt. Vielmehr stellte Zerbis päpstlicher Gönner, Innozenz VIII., die normativen Weichen für die große europäische Hexenverfolgung, der Schätzungen zufolge bis zu 60.000 Frauen, Männer und auch Kinder zum Opfer fielen.[16]

Obwohl in der weiteren Folge vor allem weltliche Gerichte nach dem Vorbild der Inquisitionsverfahren gegen vermeintliche Hexen und Zauberer vorgingen und sich dabei auf eigene jurisdiktionelle Grundlagen wie etwa die *Peinliche Halsgerichtsordnung* (1532) Karls V. stützten, beteiligten sich auch kirchliche Tribunale an dieser Bekämpfung der Hexerei. Vor allem aber lieferte die Kirche die geistig-religiöse Legitimation für die Verfolgungen. Die Verknüpfung zwischen Häresie und Hexerei war keineswegs neu.[17] Wer magische Praktiken gebrauchte, stand nach christlicher Auffassung in Diensten des Satans und galt mithin als Ketzer. In seiner Bulle *Summis desiderantes affectibus* vom 5. Dezember 1484, die er auf Betreiben des dominikanischen Inquisitors Heinrich Kramer, genannt *Institoris* (um 1430-um 1505) erließ, hob Innozenz VIII. diesen Gedanken mit Nachdruck hervor.[18] Darin ist unter anderem davon die Rede, dass Männer und Frauen vom wahren Glauben abfielen, den sie mit der Taufe empfangen hätten, um sich mit Teufeln zu vermischen. Durch seinen Erlass bestätigte der Pontifex offiziell die Existenz von Hexern und Hexen, die sich mit dunklen Kräften zum Schaden der Christenheit und ihrer Mitmenschen verschworen hatten. Zugleich ernannte der Papst Institoris sowie den Kölner Theologieprofessor Jakob Sprenger (um 1437-1495) zu Generalinquisitoren gegen Häretiker, Zauberer und Teufelsbuhlen.[19] Damit leistete Innozenz dem weit verbreiteten Hexenwahn weiteren Vorschub. Gut zwei Jahre später, 1487, erschien die erste Auflage von Heinrich Kramers *Malleus Maleficarum,* der sogenannte *Hexenhammer.* Das Buch, dem die päpstliche Bulle vorangestellt war, wurde vielfach nachgedruckt und etablierte sich rasch als Standardwerk der Hexenverfolgung.[20] Während der Jahre von Gabriele Zerbis

16 Die Zahlenangaben bei G. Schwerhoff, „Vom Alltagsverdacht zur Massenverfolgung. Neuere deutsche Forschungen zum frühneuzeitlichen Hexenwesen“, *Geschichte in Wissenschaft und Unterricht* 46 (1995), S.359–380, hier: S.362 u 365; Ferner W. Rummel – R. Voltmer, *Hexenverfolgung in der Frühen Neuzeit*, Darmstadt 2008; J. B. Durrant, *Witchcraft, Gender, and Society in Early Modern Germany*, Leiden 2007; L. Roper, *Hexenwahn. Geschichte einer Verfolgung*, München 2007; B. P. Levack, *Hexenjagd. Die Geschichte der Hexenverfolgungen in Europa*, München 1999².

17 Exemplarisch B.-U. Hergemöller, *Krötenkuss und schwarzer Kater. Ketzerei, Götzendienst und Unzucht in der inquisitorischen Phantasie des 13. Jahrhunderts*, Warendorf 1996.

18 J. Hansen, *Quellen und Untersuchungen zur Geschichte des Hexenwahns und der Hexenverfolgung im Mittelalter*, Bonn 1901, S. 24–27, Nr. 36.

19 F. Merzbacher, „Institoris, Heinrich“, in: *Neue Deutsche Biographie*, Bd.10, Berlin 1974, S.175–176.

20 P. Segl (Hg.), *Der Hexenhammer. Entstehung und Umfeld des ‚Malleus maleficarum‘ von 1487* (Bayreuther Historisches Kolloquium 2), Köln 1988.

Aufenthalt als päpstlicher Leibarzt und Professor an der *Sapienza* in Rom zwischen 1483 und 1492 spielte die Auseinandersetzung mit Ketzern und unterschiedlichen Formen der Häresie in seinem engsten Umfeld demnach eine herausragende Rolle.

Dass der Veronese zweifelsohne das Vertrauen von Innozenz VIII. besaß und näher über Vorgänge an der Kurie informiert war, bezeugen die Umstände seiner Rückkehr an die Universität von Padua. Der Papst führte nicht nur einen verschärften Kampf gegen Ketzer. Seit dem Krieg von Ferrara befand sich der Heilige Stuhl zugleich in einem politischen Dauerkonflikt mit König Ferrante von Neapel (1423-1494).[21] Wenngleich der Friedensschluss von Bagnolo am 7. August 1484 für eine Atempause sorgte, war die Auseinandersetzung damit noch nicht beendet.[22] Ferrante weigerte sich standhaft, einen Lehenszins an den Pontifex zu zahlen. Aufgrund der militärischen Stärke des Königs von Neapel war Innozenz jedoch nicht in der Lage, seinen Anspruch durchzusetzen. Auch der 1486 geschlossene Friede hielt nur kurze Zeit. Erst 1492 gelang es, unter Vermittlung venezianischer Gesandter den Streit endgültig beizulegen. Einer der Vermittler war der humanistische Gelehrte und Diplomat Girolamo Donato (1457-1511), den die Serenissima 1491 nach Rom entsandt hatte.[23] Bei dieser Gelegenheit traf der Botschafter auch mit Gabriele Zerbi zusammen. Donato, der selbst in Padua studiert hatte, versuchte, den päpstlichen Leibarzt zu einer Rückkehr an seine frühere Wirkungsstätte zu bewegen. Sein diplomatisches Bemühen zeigte schließlich ebenso Erfolg wie sein Werben um Zerbi. Der Tod seines Förderers Papst Innozenz am 25. Juli 1492 mag zur Entscheidung des Arztes beigetragen haben, Rom zu verlassen. Nur wenige Monate zuvor hatte der Oberhirte der Christenheit mit großer Freude die Nachricht vom Fall Granadas und dem siegreichen Abschluss der Reconquista erhalten, die in der Ewigen Stadt mit einem prunkvollen Fest gefeiert wurde.[24] Dem christlichen Sieg folgte mit dem Alhambra-Edikt wenig später die Ausweisung aller Juden aus Spanien.[25] Abermals trafen daraufhin jüdische Flüchtlinge in Italien ein, darunter auch Gelehrte. Der päpstliche Leibarzt war zweifelsohne Augenzeuge all dieser Geschehnisse. Wie viele Heilkundige sich unter den Einwanderern aus Spanien befanden und welche Konkurrenz dies für Gabriele Zerbi und seine übrigen Standeskollegen in Rom möglicherweise bedeutete, lässt sich in Ermangelung einschlägiger Untersuchungen nicht beurteilen. Fest steht nur, dass der Veronese Rom zum Zeitpunkt all dieser Veränderun-

21 M. Gattoni, *Sisto IV, Innocenzo VIII e la geopolitica dello Stato Pontificio (1471-1492)*, Roma 2010; E. Pontieri, *Per la storia di Ferrante I d'Aragona re di Napoli*, Napoli 1969².

22 T. Toulny, *Herculean Ferrara. Ercole d'Este, 1474.1505, and the invention of a ducal capital*, Cambridge 1996.

23 P. Rigo, „Dona (Donati, Donato), Girolamo", in: *Dizionario Biografico degli Italiani*, [http://www.treccani.it/enciclopedia/dona_(Dizionario-Biografico)/ (8.11.2013)].

24 T. Niemeyer, *Geschichte der Stadt Rom*, o.O. 1931, S.1186.

25 G. Bossong, *Die Sepharden. Geschichte und Kultur der spanischen Juden*, München 2008, S.53–69; M. Grüttner, „Die Vertreibung der spanischen Juden 1492", *Geschichte in Wissenschaft und Unterricht* 47 (1996), S.166–188.

gen verließ. Im Jahre 1494 nahm er als Professor für Medizin ein weiteres Mal den Lehrstuhl in Padua an.

Im nächsten Schritt gilt es zu betrachten, in welcher Weise die Eindrücke der Spanischen Inquisition und der beginnenden Hexenverfolgung sich auf das Ketzerbild des Heilkundigen niederschlugen und sich bei der Abfassung seines Werkes *De cautelis medicorum* auf seinen persönlichen Umgang mit den Schriften solcher Gelehrter auswirkten, die wegen ihre Lehren von einem Glaubenstribunal der Häresie für schuldig befunden worden waren.

EINSTAND AN DER NEUEN ALMA MATER. *DE CAUTELIS MEDICORUM*

Der genaue Blick auf Gabriele Zerbis *De cautelis medicorum* lässt einige Rückschlüsse auf die Umstände zu, unter denen das Werk entstanden ist. Der *hochberühmte Philosoph und Arzt*, wie sich der Veronese im Prolog selbst nennt, kompilierte seine Schrift entsprechend der zeitgenössischen Gepflogenheiten weitgehend aus medizinischen und philosophischen Abhandlungen antiker und mittelalterlicher Autoritäten.[26] Auffällig ist, dass ihm dabei eine Reihe von Fehlern unterlief. So weist er etwa den bekannten biblischen Vers Matthäus 7,7 „petite et dabitur vobis" und dessen Folge fälschlich dem zehnten Kapitel dieses Evangeliums zu.[27] An anderer Stelle legt er Mondino dei Liuzzi (1275-1326), der am Beginn des 14. Jahrhunderts als angesehener Anatom an der Universität von Bologna wirkte, irrtümlicherweise ein Zitat aus der *Clavis sanationis* des Simon von Genua (um 1290) in den Mund.[28] Neben solchen Fehlern, deren Liste sich fortsetzen ließe, werden einige Verfasser, deren Schriften Zerbi zur Zusammenstellung seines eigenen Werkes nutzte, gar nicht erwähnt. So etwa der Bibelkommentar des französischen Theologen und Exegeten Nikolaus von Lyra (1270-1349), aus dem Zerbi beispielsweise eine Passage wörtlich und sogar unter Übernahme einer markanten Verschreibung in seine Abhandlung einflechtet, ohne auf den Ursprung der

26 Gabriele Zerbi, *Opus perutile de cautelis Medicorum*, Venedig 1495, fol.13r: Opus perutile de cautelis Medicorum editum a clarissimo philosopho ac medico Magistro Gabriele Zerbo Veronense theoricae medicinae ordinariam studii patavini publice legente sub anno domini MCCCCLXXXXV.

27 Ebd.

28 Ebd., fol. 16v. Vgl. hierzu Simon von Genua, *Simon Ianuensis Incipit Clavis sanationis*, Gulielmus de Tridino, Venedig 1486, unpaginiert: „Parabula dicitur grece parvoli et significat ut proverbium, similitudo, forma, figura rei, non erubescant ergo medici a parabola parabolani dici cum ceteris tam medicis quam literatissimis subtilia arduaque medicine nisi in parabolis dare intelligi non possunt"; ferner G. Pasini, *Mondino de' Liuzzi – Anothomia, Bibliografia dei lavori che danno informazione su Mondino, parte V.*, Bologna 1992; Y. Dahhaoui, *L'atelier de Simon de Genes. Vers une edition de la Clavis sanationis*, Lausanne 2001.

Wendung zu verweisen.[29] Besonders großzügig griff der Paduaner Medizinprofessor auf die *Sermones* des Niccolò Falcucci († 1412) zurück, den er allerdings nur gelegentlich als Urheber der entlehnten Texte ausweist.[30] All diese Befunde deuten darauf hin, dass Gabriele Zerbi keine allzu große Sorgfalt bei der Kompilation seines Buches walten ließ. *De cautelis medicorum* scheint innerhalb weniger Monate während der Übersiedlung des Arztes von Rom nach Padua entstanden und sofort zum Druck gegeben worden zu sein. Diese Umstände sprechen dafür, dass dem Rückkehrer daran gelegen war, seinem Ruf gerecht zu werden und der Universität gewissermaßen als Gabe zu seinem Wiedereinstand als Professor der Medizin ein neues wissenschaftliches Werk zu präsentieren. Dass dieses gleichzeitig der Mehrung des eigenen Ruhmes dienen sollte, veranschaulicht nicht zuletzt der bereits angeführte Beginn des Prologs. Dabei sah sich Zerbi zweifelsohne den Traditionen der Alma Mater von Padua verpflichtet. Als einer ihrer bedeutendsten Vertreter galt der Arzt, Philosoph, Mathematiker und Astrologe Pietro d´Abano (1250-1315).[31]

De cautelis medicorum erschien 1495 erstmals im Druck, genau 180 Jahre nach Pietros Tod. Schon 1420 hatte man dem hochverehrten Gelehrten vor dem Palazzo della Ragione ein Denkmal mit der folgenden Inschrift gesetzt:

> PETRUS APONUS PHILOSOPHIE MEDICINEQUE SCIENTISSIMUS; OB IDQUE CONCILIATORIS NOMEN ADEPTUS, ASTROLOGIA VERO ADEO PERITUS, UT IN MAGIE SUSPICIONEM INCIDERIT, FALSOQUE DE HERESI POSTULATUS, ABSOLUTUS FUIT.[32]

Zweifelsohne kannte Gabriele Zerbi das Monument und dessen Widmungstext bereits aus Studientagen. Doch das Bild Pietros, das die Inschrift vermittelte und welches der angehende Arzt ebenso konservierte wie die Gelehrten seiner und folgender Generationen, entsprach keinesfalls den historischen Gegebenheiten. Dies ist nicht der Ort, um ausführlich auf das bewegte Leben sowie das viel-

29 Vgl. Nikolaus von Lyra, *Biblia. Cum postillis Nicolai de Lyra et expositionibus Guilelmi Britonis in omnis prologos S. Hieroymi et additionibus Paul Burgensis replicisque Matthiae Doering*, Nürnberg 1485, S. 40 mit Gabriele Zerbi, *Opus perutile de cautelis Medicorum*, Venedig 1495, fol.13r: „id est doctoribus hereticis…". Zu Nikolaus von Lyra siehe u.a. G. Dahan (Hg.), *Nicolas de Lyre. Franciscain du XIVe siècle, exégéte et théologien* (Collection des Études Augustiniennes. Série Moyen Age et Temps Modernes 48), Paris 2011.

30 z.B. Gabriele Zerbi, *Opus perutile de cautelis Medicorum*, Venedig 1495, fol.13v. mehrfach, 14v mehrfach; Niccolò Falcucci, *Sermones medicinales septem*, Bernardino Stagnino, Venedig 1491, E. Guarneri – M.A. Manelli, „La vita e l'opera di Niccolò Falcucci medico toscano del secolo XIV", in: *Atti del XXI Congresso internazionale di storia della medicina*, vol. 1, Roma 1970, S.1–10.

31 Das genaue Todesdatum ist unklar. Pietro setzte am 23. Mai 1315 sein Testament auf, wurde in den Listen der Universität Padua für dieses Jahr noch als Angehöriger geführt. Fest steht, dass er vor Ende des Inquisitionsverfahrens 1316 starb. Hierzu E. Paschetto, *Pietro d'Abano. Medico e filosofo*, Florenz 1984, S.23.

32 J.-P. Boudet – F. Collard – N. Weill-Parot, „Introduction", in: diess. (Hgg.), *Médicine, astrologie et magie entre Moyen Âge et Renaissance: autour de Pietro d'Abano*, Florenz 2013, S.VIII Anm. 4.

schichtige Oeuvre Pietros eingehen zu können.[33] Beschränken wir uns daher auf die für unsere Betrachtung relevanten Aspekte.

Fest steht, dass sich Pietro d´Abano für einige seiner Vorstellungen, die er unter anderem in seinem bedeutendsten Werk vertrat, dem *Conciliator differentiarum quae inter philosophos et medicos versantur*, gleich mehrfach vor einem Inquisitionstribunal verantworten musste. Während des Prozesses von 1306 wurde der Gelehrte für nicht weniger als 55 Verstöße gegen die kirchlichen Dogmen angeklagt.[34] Der genaue Inhalt der Anklagepunkte ist zum größten Teil unbekannt. In einer späteren Aussage Pietros ist zu erfahren, dass er sich unter anderem für seine Lehre über die Entwicklung der menschlichen Seele verantworten musste. Aller Wahrscheinlichkeit nach wurden ihm aber vor allem die Leugnung der Existenz von Dämonen, der Totenerweckung und Wundern sowie Zauberei und Nekromantie zur Last gelegt.[35] Dazu kam der Vorwurf, dem christlichen Glauben gegenüber indifferent zu sein. Während er in einem ersten und vielleicht auch zweiten Prozess von der Anklage der Ketzerei freigesprochen wurde – möglicherweise, nachdem er die von der Inquisition als häretisch angesehenen Passagen seiner Werke widerrief – wurde er in einem neuerlichen Verfahren schließlich für schuldig befunden. Pietro d´Abano starb noch vor Verkündung des Schuldspruchs. So entging er einem Tod auf dem Scheiterhaufen, der ihm als rückfälligem Ketzer drohte. Will man der legendenumrankten Überlieferung glauben, so konnten die Inquisitoren nicht einmal seines Leichnams habhaft werden und mussten sich statt dessen mit einer symbolischen Verbrennung zufrieden geben, der sogenannten Verbrennung *in effegie*, bei der ein Bildnis oder eine Strohpuppe anstelle des Delinquenten den Flammen übergeben wurde.[36]

Für die Zeitgenossen Pietros bedeutete die postume Verurteilung zugleich, dass das Werk des Gelehrten nicht benutzt geschweige denn zitiert werden konnte, ohne selbst in den Verdacht der Ketzerei zu geraten. Pietros Zeitgenosse, der spanische Arzt Arnald von Villanova (um 1235-1311), aus dessen Werken Gabriele Zerbi ebenfalls schöpfte, kam weit glimpflicher davon.[37] Eine Verkettung glücklicher Umstände bewahrte ihn davor, dass ihm sein *Tractatus de tempore adventu antichristi*, den er 1297 abschloss und für dessen Inhalt er sich wenig später vor einem Tribunal in Paris verantworten musste, gleichfalls zum Verhängnis wurde.[38] Die Prozesse gegen Pietro d´Abano und Arnald von Villanova fielen

33 Hierzu jetzt insbesondere die Beiträge in Boudet – Collard – Weill-Parot (Hgg.), *Médicine, astrologie et magie*.

34 L. Nordpoth, *Zur Bio-, Bibliographie und Wissenschaftslehre des Pietro d'Abano, Mediziners, Philosophen und Astronomen in Padua*, Leipzig 1930, S.298.

35 L. Thorndike, „Peter of Abano and the Inquisition", *Speculum* 11 (1936), S.132–133; E. Paschetto, *Pietro d'Abano. Medico e filosofo*, Florenz 1984, S.242.

36 Nordpoth, *Zur Bio-, Bibliographie und Wissenschaftslehre des Pietro d'Abano*, S.298 Anm. 7; allgemein G. Schwerhoff, *Die Inquisition. Ketzerverfolgung in Mittelalter und Neuzeit*, München 2004, S.68 u. S.90.

37 z.B. Gabriele Zerbi, *Opus perutile de cautelis Medicorum*, Venedig 1495, fol.14r.

38 J. Ziegler, *Medecine and religion c.1300. The case of Arnau de Vilanova*, Oxford 1998, S.26; M. Gerwing, *Vom Ende der Zeit. Der Traktat des Arnald von Villanova über die Ankunft des*

in Jahre nach dem endgültigen Verlust des Heiligen Landes 1291, die im christlichen Abendland als traumatisches Ereignis empfunden wurde und der gesellschaftliche Entwicklung zu einer „persecuting society" entscheidenden Vorschub leistete.[39] Die weit verbreitete Furch vor dem Wirken dunkler Kräfte und geheimnisvoller, ketzerischer Verschwörer gipfelte im spektakulären Prozess gegen den 1312 zerschlagenen Orden der Templer. Die lange Liste der Anklagepunkte, die gegen die Ritterbrüder vorgebracht wurden, wurde zum Muster für alle späteren Verfahren gegen vermeintliche Häretiker.[40] Darin ist die Rede von Götzendienst, Schändung des Kreuzes, Zauberei, Homosexualität und anderen Formen gotteslästerlichen Handelns. Die Inquisitionsverfahren gegen Arnald und vor allem Pietro d`Abano passen fraglos zu diesem Schema.

Im Einklang mit dem Verbot der Schriften verurteilter Häretiker vermieden die Gelehrten Pietros *Conciliator* offen zu zitieren. Erst um die Mitte des 14. Jahrhunderts findet das Werk wieder wachsende Verwendung, wenngleich – wie etwa bei Gentile da Foligno (1280/90-1348) – anfangs vor allem um Pietros Lehren vehement zu widersprechen.[41] Im Laufe der Jahre scheint sich deren Bewertung allmählich verändert zu haben. Ein solcher Wandel ist mit Blick auf die Entwicklung des Ketzerbegriffs, der in zunehmendem Maße – auch politisch – instrumentalisiert wurde, keinesfalls ungewöhnlich.[42] Stellvertretend dafür, welche Lehrmeinung von der obersten Geistlichkeit als konform angesehen und welche als häretisch verurteilt werden konnte, steht das Aristoteles-Verbot mit der posthumen Zensur von Werken des Thomas von Aquin (um 1225-1274) im Jahre 1277.[43] Jedes Ketzerbild war demzufolge das Produkt des jeweiligen Zeitgeists. Als Gabriele Zerbi seine Abhandlung *De cautelis medicorum* zusammenstellte, konnte er sich mithin wieder gefahrlos auf den *Conciliator* stützen und die Schrift offen zitieren. Für ihn war sein großer Vorgänger an der Alma Mater ebensowenig ein Häretiker wie Arnald von Villanova. Dass man wohl vor allem in Padua mit Erfolg daran gearbeitet hatte, den Ruf Pietros wiederherzustellen belegt nicht zuletzt die Inschrift auf seinem Denkmal. Fest steht, dass Pietros Werke seit dem 16. Jahrhundert weder auf dem römischen noch auf dem spanischen Index stan-

Antichrist in der akademischen Auseinandersetzung des 14. Jahrhunderts (Beiträge zur Geschichte der Philosophie und Theologie des Mittelalters. Neue Folge; 4), Münster 1996, S.39; J. Mensa I Vallis, *Arnau de Villanova, espiritual: Guia bibliográfica* (Institut d'estudis catalans. Treballs de la secció de filosofía i ciènces socials;17), Barcelona 1994.

39 R.I. Moore, *The formation of a persecuting society. Authority and deviance in western Europe, 950–1250*, Oxford 2007²; D. Nirenberg, *Communities of violence. Persecution of minorities in the Middle Ages*, Princeton 1996.

40 B.-U. Hergemöller, *Krötenkuss und schwarzer Kater. Ketzerei, Götzendienst und Unzucht in der inquisitorischen Phantasie des 13. Jahrhunderts*, Warendorf 1996; M. Barber, *The trial of the Templars*, Cambridge 2006²; Peter Partner, *Murdered magicians. The Templars and their myths*, Oxford 1982.

41 J. Chandelier, „Pietro d'Abano et les médecins: réception et réputation du *Conciliator* en Italie dans les premières années du XIVe siècle", in: Boudet – Collard – Weill-Parot (Hgg.), *Médicine, astrologie et magie*, S.183–202.

42 J. Oberste, *Ketzerei und Inquisition im Mittelalter*, Darmstadt 2007, S.3–4 u. S.134.

43 Ebenda, S.111.

den.[44] Lediglich auf dem portugiesischen Index wurden die Schriften des Gelehrten 1624 expurgiert. Die Autoren und Werke, die Gabriele Zerbi für seine Kompilation verwendete, stehen mithin nicht in Verbindung zu dem Bild des häretischen, von krankhaftem Wahrheitsdrang ergriffenen Arztes, der sich nicht um einen guten Ruf schert.[45] Woraus aber nährt sich diese Vorstellung dann?

DER KRANKHAFTE WAHRHEITSDRANG UND DER GUTE RUF

In der Analyse des Textes wird deutlich, dass Zerbi sein Werk nicht zuletzt als ein Manifest der Selbstverortung verstand. Der ketzerische Arzt steht in einem scharfen Kontrast zum umsichtigen, kenntnisreich um das Wohl seines Patienten bemühten und in seinem Lebenswandel untadeligen Heilkundigen. Wenngleich der Kompilator keine direkten Bezüge zwischen seiner Person und dem von ihm gezeichneten Idealtypus des gottesfürchtigen, ethisch handelnden Arztes zieht, so erscheint doch unstrittig, dass er selbst diese Rolle bekleidet. Denn ohne diese auszufüllen, könnte er ja kaum eine solche, auf Erfahrung und das Wissen um die Lehren der alten Autoritäten gestützte Empfehlung für angehende Standeskollegen ausgeben.

Der häretische Arzt ist der negative Gegenentwurf zu diesem Ideal. Die bewusste Wahl von Worten wie „neglegere" und „insania" unterstreicht diesen Aspekt. Dabei ist dieser Mediziner nicht allein ein Gebilde der Theorie. Dass es sich um eine reale Gestalt handelt, zeigt der Rat, ebenso besessen nach der Wahrheit zu suchen und gleichsam unablässig zu lernen, wie dieser Ketzer. Zerbi lässt durch seine Sprachwahl keine Zweifel daran aufkommen, dass die unnachgiebige Verstocktheit, die dem Häretiker grundlegend zu eigen ist, von einem angehenden Heilkundigen als positive Eigenschaft für sein Studium genutzt werden kann. Alles Übrige aber, was mit diesem Eifer verbunden ist, muss als krankhaft und ketzerisch abgelehnt werden.

Aus der Sicht der Zeitgenossen galten die Juden als verstockte, an ihren eigenen Wahrheiten festhaltende Häretiker par excellence. Wenngleich letztendlich Beweise dafür fehlen, dass Gabriele Zerbi jüdische Ärzte vor Augen hatten, so legen seine Erfahrungen mit *Conversos* und Juden, die vor der Spanischen Inquisition nach Italien geflohen waren, diese Möglichkeit zumindest nahe. Dass der Professor der Medizin in Rom, aber auch bereits in Bologna und später in Padua auf die eine oder andere Weise mit jüdischen Heilkundigen in Berührung kam, ist mehr als wahrscheinlich. Immerhin hatte die Medizinische Fakultät von Padua ihre Pforten auch schon für jüdische Studenten geöffnet.[46] Der Eifer, mit dem sich

44 Für die wertvollen Auskünfte danke ich der Kollegin Andrea Badea vom Deutschen Historischen Institut in Rom.

45 Gabriele Zerbi, *Opus perutile de cautelis Medicorum*, Venedig 1495, fol.16r: „Etiam pro inverecundo heretico qui negligit bonam famam."

46 S.M. Shasha – S.G. Massry, „The medical school of Padua and its Jewish graduates", *Harefuah* 141 (2002), S.388–394 [Aufsatz in hebräischer Sprache].

gelehrte Juden dem Studium der religiösen Schriften hingaben und deren Auslegung sie oft hitzig diskutierten, dürfte Zerbi nicht entgangen sein. Immerhin lagen die Synagogen oftmals an zentralen Orten der Stadt.[47] Das Leben fand dort keinesfalls hinter verschlossenen Fenstern und Türen statt.

Zerbis Ausführungen über den ketzerischen Arzt, der sich um seinen Ruf nicht schert, sind untrennbar mit dem Hinweis auf das Vertrauen der Patienten in die Fähigkeiten des gewählten Heilkundigen verbunden.[48] Diese Aussage stützt die Annahme, dass sich hinter dem Bild der *medicorum haereticorum* möglicherweise die jüdischen Konkurrenten des Veronesen verbergen. In Zerbis negativer Bewertung bündelt sich das zeitspezifische Konglomerat aus Vorurteil und Missgunst gegenüber heilkundigen Juden, das in zahlreichen Schriften des 15. und 16. Jahrhunderts zu finden ist.[49] Für seine Leserschaft dürfte die unterschwellige Botschaft in jedem Fall deutlich zu verstehen gewesen sein. Welches Verhältnis Gabriele Zerbi zu seinen jüdischen Standeskollegen hatte und inwieweit seine Nähe zu inquisitorischen Vorstellungen im Umfeld des Papstes seine Haltung gegenüber den Juden prägte, lässt sich nur durch weitere Forschungen zu Leben und Wirken des Medizinprofessors aus Padua klären. Einstweilen lässt sich festhalten, dass sich in seiner Schrift *De cautelis medicorum* nicht nur medizinethische Vorstellungen des späten 15. Jahrhunderts, sondern auch Aspekte des zeitspezifischen Ketzerbegriffs widerspiegeln.

47 Hierzu die Beiträge in C. Cluse (Hg.), *Europas Juden im Mittelalter. Beiträge des internationalen Symposiums in Speyer vom 20. – 25. Oktober 2002*, Trier 2004.

48 Gabriele Zerbi, *Opus perutile de cautelis Medicorum*, Venedig 1495, fol.16r.

49 N. Hortzitz, *Der Judenarzt. Historische und sprachliche Untersuchungen zur Diskriminierung eines Berufsstandes in der frühen Neuzeit*, Heidelberg 1994.

MEDICAL AND ETHICAL ASPECTS OF VEGETARIANISM: ON THE RECEPTION OF PORPHYRY'S *DE ABSTINENTIA* IN THE RENAISSANCE

Cecilia Muratori

In his book *The Bloodless Revolution*, Tristram Stuart[1] reminds the reader of the fact that there are relevant differences in being a vegetarian for ethical reasons rather than for medical reasons: he recollects that Descartes's biographer Baillet, for instance, suggests that the French philosopher preferred a vegetable diet because, as a physiologist, he believed it to be the best diet to prolong human life. This of course does not imply that Descartes considered the killing of animals to be ethically wrong: quite the opposite. In a famous letter to his correspondent Henry More he actually wrote that his understanding of animals as being "like machines" finally freed men from the guilt of slaughtering animals with the purpose of eating them.[2] Ethical vegetarianism and – so to speak – medical vegetarianism were therefore for Descartes two completely different matters.

This categorical differentiation between medical and ethical aspects, such as we find in Descartes, has indeed contributed to shape a view of vegetarianism according to which ethical vegetarianism is concerned with considerations regarding the moral status of animals, while the choice of not eating meat for health reasons can be completely detached from statements on the relation between animals and humans, or on animals considered per se.

In this essay I want to suggest that precisely the combination of, rather than the distinction between, medical and ethical aspects of vegetarianism constitutes an essential part of the history of speculation on the usefulness of a vegetarian diet. In other words, I would like to present vegetarianism as an important point, not just of intersection between medicine and ethics, but even of deep connection. Despite the fact that it is the separation between the medical and the ethical side, which has mostly influenced the way we think of vegetarianism today, in my opinion it is important to stress that it is the convergence of these apparently different aspects that shaped the concept of vegetarianism through relevant phases of its evolution as an idea in the history of philosophy – and of medicine.

I will focus on vegetarianism, then, considered simultaneously as an ethical and as a medical practice, arguing that the first aspect cannot be separated in any

1 T. Stuart, *The Bloodless Revolution. A Cultural History of Vegetarianism from 1600 to Modern Times*, New York 2007, pp. 131–133.

2 See R. Descartes, *Tutte le lettere 1619–1650*, ed. by G. Belgioioso, Milan 2005, p. 2624.

way from the second one in the story I want to reconstruct, and that has at its centre one of the classical texts discussing the benefits of a vegetarian diet: Porphyry's *De abstinentia ab esu carnium*. Medical, ethical and strictly religious themes constantly intertwine in Porphyry's four books, contributing to construct a concept of vegetarianism which was highly influential.

In the following I will concentrate only on a specific phase in the reception of Porphyry's work, that is the influence of this text on its Renaissance editors and translators.[3] On the one hand, the Renaissance reception of Porphyry's *De abstinentia* is a very clear example of the role played by the intersection between medicine and philosophy with regard to the aim of vegetarianism. While the idea of the medical benefits of a vegetable diet was discussed throughout the Middle Ages (one thinks primarily of Arnau de Vilanova's *De esu carnium*), the philosophical and in particular ethical aspects of the debate on vegetarianism, for instance regarding the treatment of animals, do not seem to emerge strongly before the fifteenth century.[4] In this sense I argue that it is possible to detect a shift in the way vegetarianism is understood from the middle ages to the reception of Porphyry in the Renaissance, since a cluster of elements had contributed to reshape the debate on the usefulness of the vegetarian diet by the time the first editions of *De abstinentia* appeared around the beginning of the sixteenth century.[5] On the other hand, this essay aims to establish a basis for a reconstruction of the debate on vegetarianism during the Renaissance, a topic which is yet to be explored in its complexity. It is indeed worth noting that the few works published on the history of vegetarianism either focus entirely on later periods (like Tristram Stuart's above-mentioned volume) or dedicate only a few lines to the Renaissance (like for instance Colin Spencer's *A History of Vegetarianism*).[6] The interest in Porphyry's book and the multiple editions of it during the fifteenth and sixteenth

3 I will not consider the reception of other works by Porphyry, notably the *Isagoge*, on which research has already been done, also with reference to the Renaissance (see for instance B. P. Copenhaver on Valla's reception of Porphyry's *Isagoge* in: "Valla Our Contemporary. Philosophy and Philology", *Journal of the History of Ideas* 66 (2005), n. 4, pp. 507–525, in particular p. 512).

4 Cfr. Arnau de Vilanova, *De esu carnium*, in: id., *Opera medica omnia*, vol. 11, ed. by D. M. Bazell, Barcelona 1999. Diane M. Bazell writes for instance in the introduction (p. 149): "[...] his [Arnau's] argument is not against the eating of meat, but against the notion that meat is a medical necessity." While the focus is set on the medical consequences of abstaining from meat eating, ethical concern for the suffering of animals is not present in Arnau's text. See also J. Ziegler, *Medicine and Religion c. 1300: The Case of Arnau de Vilanova*, Oxford 1998, especially pp. 160–161: "[...] Arnau did not advocate vegetarianism for everyone, since there was no medical justification for doing so, and he himself prescribed meat as a remedy for his patients."

5 A. Guerrini has argued in a similar direction in her essay "A Diet for a Sensitive Soul: Vegetarianism in Eighteenth-Century Britain" (*Eighteenth-Century Life* 23 (1999), n. 2, pp. 34–42), in which she focuses on the connection of medical, moral and religious aspects in the eighteenth-century debate on vegetarianism in England.

6 C. Spencer, *The Heretic's Feast: A History of Vegetarianism*, London 1993. R. Preece dedicates a short chapter to Renaissance authors in his *Sins of the Flesh: A History of Ethical Vegetarian Thought*, Vancouver 2008.

centuries suggest that the impact of Porphyry's concept of vegetarianism in the Renaissance is still to be fully investigated.

A survey of the secondary literature leaves the impression that it was only after Descartes that the topic began to be discussed at all.[7] If this is the case, it could be argued that it would be a mistake to project ethical concern for animals onto a period like the Renaissance.[8] In the following remarks I want to suggest that the problem has to be put in a different way: if questions about the ethical treatment of animals were not discussed independently, they were nevertheless included in broader discussions, such as those concerning the usefulness of vegetarianism. Therefore I propose to look at ethical questions regarding animals as part of a complex of factors that can only artificially be separated from one another. In other words, the question about the treatment of animals can be detected in the Renaissance as well, as long as it is considered as one element that should not be taken out of its context. This is indeed the case in the discussion on vegetarianism.

I'll proceed in two steps: first, I will sketch the reception of Porphyry's text in the Renaissance, paying attention to the various aspects of *De abstinentia* which seem to have had the greatest impact on Renaissance readers. I will then investigate the reasons for the interest in Porphyry's text displayed by its Renaissance editors and translators, and in particular by Giovanni Bernardo Feliciano, Piero Vettori and Marsilio Ficino. This reconstruction will concentrate on one key concept that in my opinion allows us to interpret Renaissance readings of Porphyry as a combination of medical, ethical and religious interests: *abstinentia*.

1. A DIET FOR THE BODY AND THE SOUL: PORPHYRY'S FOUR-BOOK *DE ABSTINENTIA*

The correspondence of the humanist Piero Vettori with Ugolino Martelli shows that around 1538 Porphyry's *De abstinentia* was not an easy text to get hold of. Vettori had asked Martelli to inquire in Padua and in Venice about copies of the manuscript. In the month of March 1538 Martelli answered that the book was not even to be found in the big library of San Marco.[9] Finally, Vettori published an

7 Among the many studies concerned with the so-called bête-machine debate, see for instance: L. Cohen Rosenfield, *From Beast-Machine to Man-Machine: The Theme of Animal Soul in French Letters from Descartes to La Mettrie*, New York 1940; M. T. Marcialis, *Filosofia e psicologia animale da Rorario a Leroy*, Cagliari 1982.

8 For a discussion of ethical reflections in the Renaissance, especially in the reception of Aristotle and Plato, see A. Poppi, *L'etica del rinascimento tra Platone e Aristotele*, Napoli 1997.

9 Ugolino Martelli, *Lettere a Piero Vettori (1536–1577)*, ed. by V. Bramanti, Manziana 2009, p. 36 (4 March 1538). Also p. 39 (19 March 1538), and p. 40 (21 April 1538). See also p. 13 of Bramanti's introduction to the letters. For concise information regarding the activity of Vettori as a translator see P. O. Kristeller (ed.), *Catalogus translationum et commentariorum. Medieval and Renaissance Latin Translations and Commentaries*, annotated Lists and Guides, vol. 2, Washington 1971, pp. 34–36.

edition of the Greek text ten years later, in 1548.[10] In the preface to his edition he laments the fact that the manuscripts he could finally work on contained many mistakes, so that he had to compare several of them in order to obtain a better version of the text, while being aware that he could not possibly eliminate every defect.[11] Indeed Porphyry had until then been neglected – Vettori argues – and badly dealt with.[12] A year before, in 1547, the first Latin edition had appeared, translated by Giovanni Bernardo Feliciano under the title *De abstinentia ab esu animalium*. Previously, Marsilio Ficino had actually translated extracts from *De abstinentia*, some of which are included in a letter, while the rest was published in an edition containing several translations of Neoplatonic texts (1497) on which Ficino had worked between 1486 and 1489.[13] Interest in Porphyry's text was thus growing between the end of the fifteenth and the beginning of the sixteenth centuries.

But from which contexts did this interest emerge? In order to answer this question I shall first briefly sketch the contents of Porphyry's text, paying attention to the different topics that intertwine in his defense of vegetarianism. Written in the form of a long speech or a letter addressed to a friend of Porphryry, Firmus Castricius, *Peri apochê empsuchôn* – so the Greek title of the text, probably written soon after Plotinus' death[14] – consists of four books, each of them addressing a specific question regarding the advantages and disadvantages of vegetarianism.

10 Porphyry, *De non necandis ad epulandum animantibus libri IIII*, trans. by P. Vettori, Firenze 1548. Cod. graec. 171 of the Bayerische Staatsbibliothek contains Piero Vettori's copy of *De abstinentia*, used to prepare the 1548 edition of the text.

11 See Vettori's preface (without page numbers) in: Porphyry, *De non necandis ad epulandum animantibus* (1548): "Quod vero ad scripturae integritatem: diligentiamque in lectione purganda adhibitam, pertinet, non inficiabor Porphyrii libros pessime habitos inscitia superiorum temporum: vitioque librariorum valde corruptos fuisse: tantum tamen studii, collatis plurimis exemplaribus, in illis emendandis posuimus, ut multum auxilii ipsis tulisse nobis videamur: quamvis non omnes maculas delere, nec manca imminutaque nonnulla loca restituere, potuerimus: fides certe illis nostra diligentiaque non defuit. quod etiam in scholiis Ephesii, magna cum eorum utilitate, praestitimus."

12 See ibid. the final address to the learned (*studiosis*) at the end of Vettori's edition (without page numbers): "Cum pluribus spectatis codicibus male habito undique ac neglecto Porphyrio non parum consuluissem, multisque partibus ipsum meliorem reddidissem, tentavi si possem alia via ei opem ferre, quam etiam non inutilem expertus sum […]."

13 Marsilio Ficino, *Epistolae*, Venice 1495, p. 149r–150r (letter to Braccio Martelli). For the English translation see *The Letters of Marsilio Ficino*, vol. 7, translated from the Latin by members of the Language Department of the School of Economic Science, London 2003, pp. 33–39. This edition is henceforth abbreviated as *Letters*. Where possible, I quote from this English translation, in order to facilitate the reading. The original Latin version of relevant passages is provided in the footnotes: M. Ficino, *Epistolae*, Venice 1495 (abbreviated as *Epistolae*). For the 1497 edition see the facsimile reproduction by S. Toussaint, and his introduction to the text: Cf. Iamblichus, *De mysteriis Ægyptiorum, Chaldæorum, Assyriorum*, Venetiis 1497 [= Paris 2006].

14 Porphyry, *On Abstinence*, ed. by G. Clark, London 2000, p. 7 (from now on abbreviated as *On Abstinence*). See also Porphyry, *De l'abstinence*, vol. 1, ed. by J. Bouffartigue and M. Patillon, Paris 1977, p. xviii (from now on abbreviated as *De l'abstinence*).

Firmus Castricius had previously followed a vegetarian diet, but had then gone back to meat-eating: for this reason Porphyry's method is to present in each book very detailed arguments for and against the consumption of meat, with the aim of convincing the friend that vegetarianism is the diet appropriate to a philosopher.

As Jean Bouffartigue and Michel Patillon note in their French edition of *De abstinentia*, each of the four books appear to be solidly structured around a main topic (this is particularly true of books two, three and four).[15] For instance book two focuses on a crucial problem in religious practices, that is the role of sacrifice, and whether fruit and cereals should not be immolated to the gods instead of sentient beings. On the other hand, book three deals with doctrines concerning the nature of the human and of the animal souls, introducing the famous theory that animals should not be considered as completely deprived of reason or more generally of wisdom.[16] Book four then invites the reader to take into account yet another element in the discussion on vegetarianism, that is its diffusion among various cultures, with particular insistence on the fact that the vegetarian diet is accompanied by moderation and purity. In mentioning the diffusion of abstinence from eating animals amongst the Greeks, the Egyptians, and also the Jews, Porphyry argues that this practice is also reflected in a general conduct of purification, promoting not just the health of the body but also the self-control and purity of the soul.[17]

Playing the role of an introduction, book one is dedicated to a more general discussion of the benefits of a vegetarian diet, also responding to the main objections to which vegetarianism is exposed (and which Porphyry's friend Firmus Castricius might have embraced). The following question, for instance, is directly asked: will not the refusal to use animals as food (including medicines, such as viper poison) damage the body? Porphyry's answer to this question also provides a starting point to understand the Renaissance reception of his text, a reception which highlights the intimate relation between the philosophical, the medical and the religious point of view in Porphyry's arguments in favour of vegetarianism. First, Porphyry explains who will benefit from his argumentation, that is:

> [...] the person who has thought about who he is and whence he has come and where he should try to go, and who has principles about food, and about other proper behaviour, which are different from those in other ways of life.[18]

The text is therefore directed to the philosopher, who cares about his nature; but such a person will also want to know what would be the best nutrition for his body, and what is the ethical way of life (and this last question is in Porphyry's argument directly linked to the one regarding the 'principles about food'). It is therefore clear that Porphyry's discourse to Firmus Castricius aims at showing precisely the relevance of this link between purely speculative investigation, ethi-

15 *De l'abstinence*, vol. 1, p. xxiv.

16 See for instance *On Abstinence*, p. 86: "Now it is to be demonstrated that there is also a rational [soul] in animals and that they are not deprived of wisdom."

17 See for instance ibid., p. 102; also p. 103 and p. 106.

18 Ibid., p. 40.

cal concerns and medical or hygienic practice: the choice of the right food for the philosopher encompasses all these aspects.[19] The key to understand this cluster of various aspects is for Porphyry the concept of moderation through abstinence, which guides us toward purification of body and soul:

> A person who has accustomed himself to being satisfied with the minimum has got rid not just of one thing, but of thousands: excess of riches, the service of too many slaves, a mass of belongings, a condition of somnolence, intensity and frequency of illness, need for doctors, provocation of sexual desire, thicker exhalations, much residue, heavy chains, robustness which prompts action, an Iliad of evils. An inanimate [that is: without flesh, CM], simple diet, available to all, takes these away from us, offering peace for the reasoning power which provides us with security.[20]

The vegetarian diet is then presented as a moderate diet, which allows the philosopher to think better because the brain is awake, the body is strong, and he doesn't feel the need for unnecessary things. The editors of the French translation already mentioned thus point out that for Porphyry abstinence is therefore a means to achieve health: «Pour Porphyre l'abstinence est un moyen non suffisant mais indispensable pour parvenir au salut».[21] Health – I underline – for the body and for the soul, because the one is deeply linked to the other.

Abstinence, then, constitutes both a medical and a philosophical way to sharpen the mind and promote the health of the body. This is the main denotation of the term *abstinentia* to which I would like to draw attention, and which will provide a provisional answer to the question I asked above, that is: from what contexts did interest in Porphyry's *De abstinentia* emerge in the Renaissance? This double effect of *abstinentia* – at the same time a good method for 'keeping the doctor away' and for training the mind in philosophical speculation – constitutes for Renaissance readers an essential aspect of Porphyry's doctrine, starting with the author of the first published translation, Giovanni Bernardo Feliciano.[22]

19 See on this topic G. Clark, "Fattening the Soul: Christian Asceticism and Porphyry on Abstinence", in: *Studia patristica*, vol. 35: Papers presented at the Thirteenth International Conference on Patristic Studies held in Oxford 1999, ed. by M. F. Wiles and E. J. Yarnold, Leuven 2001, pp. 41–51.

20 *On Abstinence*, pp. 49–50.

21 *De l'abstinence*, vol. 1, p. liii.

22 The connection and parallelism between the care of the body and the care of the soul is, of course, not an invention of the Renaissance readers of Porphyry, but in the Middle Ages the emphasis lies strongly in the combination of medical and religious practises. See on this topic: P. Biller – J. Ziegler (eds.), *Religion and Medicine in the Middle Ages*, Woodbridge 2001, in particular the following essays: W. J. Courtenay, "Curers of Body and Soul. Medical Doctors as Theologians", pp. 69–75 (focussing on medical doctors who also obtained a degree in theology, especially between 1330 and 1349); J. Bird, "Medicine for Body and Soul: Jacques de Vitry's Sermons to Hospitallers and Their Charges", pp. 91–108 (see for instance p. 103). In the same volume, M. R. McVaugh contributed an essay dealing in particular with Arnau de Vilanova's parallel careers – "[…] one, that of an academic physician pursuing medical learning […] and the other, that of a lay theologian and prophet" (p. 47) – addressing the question whether they were differentiated or intertwined, especially in the 1290s ("Moments of Inflections. The Careers of Arnau de Vilanova", pp. 47–67). Specifically on the interconnection be-

2. RENAISSANCE READERS AND TRANSLATORS OF PORPHYRY'S *DE ABSTINENTIA*

2.1 Giovanni Bernardo Feliciano and the Latin translation of *De abstinentia*

Not very much is known about Feliciano apart from the fact that as a translator he was very successful.[23] The titles of the works he translated show exemplarily the focus of his interest. On the one hand he composed translations of Alexander of Aphrodisias' *In Aristoteles Analytica priora*, of Porphyry's *In categorias Aristoteles*, and especially of Aristotle's *Nicomachean Ethics*, which was published several times between 1542 and 1662[24]; on the other hand, he dedicated himself to the translation of medical and especially surgical treatises, such as *De Chirurgia liber* by Paulus Aegineta (a translation of *De re medica*, book 4)[25] in 1533, and two years later Galen's *De Hippocratis et Platonis decretis opus eruditum, & philosophis & medicis utilissimum nouem libris*.[26] It is probable that Feliciano himself practised as a doctor, having studied philosophy and medicine in Padua.[27]

In the dedication which opens his translation of Porphyry's book (the title of which he rendered as *De abstinentia ab esu animalium*), he directly focuses on the

tween medicine and religion in the work of Arnau de Vilanova, see J. Ziegler's monograph *Medicine and Religion c. 1300: The Case of Arnau de Vilanova*, quoted. Ziegler argues: "The symbiotic relationship between medicine and religion also has a practical dimension. One of its facts is the input of physicians (directly or through the diffusion of medical knowledge) to clerical debates on moral, philosophical, or theological questions. Arnau provides us with such a case in his "On the Eating of Meat" (*De esu carnium*) – the first full-length treatise in the Latin West devoted to the vegetarian diet (ca. 1302–1305), and an example of the use of medical knowledge in support of one party in a religious conflict between monastic orders" (p. 157).

23 See especially D. A. Lines' introduction to Eustratius, Aspasius, Michel Ephesius et al., *Aristotelis Stagiritae Moralia Nicomachia*, trans. by G. B. Feliciano, Stuttgart-Bad Cannstatt 2006 (reprint of the edition Paris 1543).

24 Eustratius, Aspasius, Michel Ephesius et al., *Aristotelis Stagiritae Moralia Nicomachia*, quoted, p. v.

25 See E. Rice, "Paulus Aegineta", in: P. O. Kristeller (ed.), *Catalogus translationum et commentariorum*, quoted, vol. 4, pp. 146–191, especially p. 165: "Albanus Torinus had omitted Book VI from his translation of *De re medica* published in Basel by Cratander and Bebel in March 1532. Thomas Giunta asked Giovanni Bernardo Feliciano to translate the missing book so that the Venetian firm could bring out a Latin translation of Paul's complete work. After some hesitation Feliciano agreed, completing his assignment before August 1532, the date of the colophon."

26 In the context it is interesting to note that Cod. graec. 39 of the Bayerische Staatsbibliothek München (XVI century) contains a copy of Porphyry's *De abstinentia ab esu animalium* together with texts (inspired) by Galen (for instance: *Ex Galeno de venae sectione; Galeni prooemium de alimentorum facultatibus ordine alphabetico; Synopsis de alimentis, Galeni*).

27 See the introduction by A. Heilmann and C. Lohr in *In defensionem praedicamentorum Aristotelis adversus Plotinum*, trans. by G. B. Feliciano, Stuttgart-Bad Cannstatt 2008 (reprint of the edition Paris 1549), p. xxii.

effects that Porphyry's concept of abstinence from eating flesh would have not just on the soul but also on the body. He writes:

> Quamvis enim & de animalium iniuria, & de daemonum immundorum vi, quae ex huiuscemodi cruentis dapibus latenter attrahitur, ex pythagoricae, & Platonicae disciplinae decretis, quibusdamque aliis huiusmodi nonnulla persequatur: omnia tamen eo spectant, sicut ipse etiam quasi videtur interpretari, ut & nutrimento imminuto vinculum animae, quod est corpus, extenuetur, ac debilitetur, quo mens ab affectuum perturbationibus relaxata ascendere ad contemplanda & fruenda divina liberius queat: & subtractis delicatioribus epulis tum parabilior victus curam a gravioribus rebus non avocet, tum omnis gulae occasio circumcidatur. Id quod nihil aliud argumenti habet, nisi ut ieiunii & abstinentiae ratio non solum divina, sed naturali etiam lege comprobata esse demonstretur.[28]

Despite the fact that the body is considered to be the prison of the soul, from which the soul must be set free through the practice of abstinence, Feliciano recollects Porphyry's principle according to which abstinence (in particular, but not exclusively, from meat) is at the same time commanded by divine and by natural law. In other words, abstinence allows the soul to escape its bodily chains and aspire to the contemplation of the divine; this it does, however, not in contradiction with the natural law, but in full accordance with it. This duplicity that Feliciano detects in Porphyry's text has a particular significance from the point of view of a translator who was at the same time engaged in the editing of medical and of ethical treatises.

It is important to notice that in the passage quoted above Feliciano uses the words abstinence and fasting (*abstinentia et ieiunium*) in a generic way, not referring specifically to the consumption of animals: and this is indeed the point. The abstinence from eating meat is understood in the context of Porphyry's instruction to elevate the soul, or rather the mind, above the perturbations caused by life in the body, so that Feliciano reports Porphyry's claim that eliminating the desire for food is not in contraposition to the natural laws, because it preserves rather than undermines health. In other words, the ethical element – that is the abstinence from *killing* for food – is present but is not the only one in Feliciano's account. Abstinence is rather interpreted as a form of conduct which is beneficial to contemplation without transgressing the natural law of the preservation of the body.[29] Indeed Feliciano states that Porphyry's text considers various arguments in favour of abstinence, such as for instance *animalium iniuria*. The ethics of sacrifice is also briefly mentioned: the act of shedding blood through slaughtering is supposed to summon bad demons. In neither case does Feliciano consider these aspects in detail: the role of abstinence in the balance between soul and body seems to be for him the crucial point in Porphyry's argument.

28 Porphyry, *De abstinentia ab esu animalium libri IV*, trans. by G. B. Feliciano, Venice 1547, "Aloysio Michaelio Ioannes Bernardus Felicianus" (without page numbers).

29 Ibid.: "Opus autem ipsum varia ac multiplici refertum eruditione est."

2.2 Abstinence Between Cannibalism and Vegetarianism: Piero Vettori

In the *Praefatio* to his edition of the Greek text, Piero Vettori takes up a similar position when he writes that Porphyry's teaching consists in the fact that he was an enemy of the vices connected with indulging in the pleasures of the stomach. He was thus aiming at the liberation from the prison and chains of the body.[30] In this sense, his doctrine agrees perfectly with our institutions and customs – declares Vettori – even if Porphyry famously opposed Christian doctrine: it is the *temperantia* of the author which constitutes a basis for appreciating Porphyry's books on abstinence.[31] Also in this case vegetarianism is interpreted as consisting of a multiplicity of factors, where the idea of purification has the primacy over the strictly ethical aspects regarding animal suffering. And yet the concept of vegetarianism emerges form a cluster of these different aspects.

Indeed the title that Vettori gives to Porphyry's text seems to suggest the brutality of consuming meat, hinting towards an acknowledgment of the ethical problems involved in slaughtering animals: *De non caedendis devorandisque animantibus*[32], where the accent falls on the actions of killing and devouring, rather than on the practice of abstinence. Indeed Porphyry's text circulated between the fifteenth and sixteenth centuries under different titles, which reflect the variety of attitudes and approaches to its content.[33]

In a chapter of his *Variarum lectionum libri XXV* entitled "Diversa historia de Annibale memoriae prodita declaratur", Vettori also mentions another strictly ethical problem in quoting from Porphyry's book: what is the nature of the link between eating humans and eating animals? And moreover: does the condemnation of the atrocity of cannibalism actually prove Porphyry's doctrine of the necessity to avoid all meat, animal and human? Vettori refers directly to Porphyry's argument in book two of *De abstinentia*, where the connection between eating animals and eating human beings is addressed as follows:

30 Porphyry, *De non necandis ad epulandum animantibus* (1548) (final address "to the learned", without page numbers): "[...] tenuique admodum victu contentus fuit: nam ventris, ac gutturis vitiorum ipsum inimicum, acerrimumque reprehensorem extitisse, viventemque adhuc e corporis carcere, vinculisque evolavisse, vere dicere possumus."

31 Ibid.: "Fuit enim Porphyrius nostrae pietati, late iam patenti, firmasque radices agenti, parum aequus, ac Christiano denique nomini valde infensus, quamvis in his libris nihil tangat, quod eam laedat: ac potius nostris institutis, moribusque mirifice congruat. Ut enim traditam a patribus religionem toto animo probabat, & ab illa fortiter contra adversarios stabat, ita temperantissimum hominem se praebuit [...]."

32 Moreover, in his *Commentarii In tres libros Aristotelis de arte dicendi* (Florence 1579), Vettori first refers to *De abstinentia* as "[libri], quibus disputavit, oportere sibi homines temperare a vescendis animantibus" (p. 111), and then as "de non necandis ad vescendum animantibus" (p. 232).

33 Particularly interesting is a note written in the margin of the manuscript version of the text contained in Cod. graec. 91 at the Bayerische Staatsbibliothek in München, stating that there is *koinônia*, kinship, or affinity, between the souls of the animals and of humans. The note is to be found in the margin on a page from book 3 of *De abstinentia* (fol. 292v).

> After the first war between Rome and Carthage over Sicily, the Phoenician mercenaries defected and brought the Lybians to join them. Hamilcar Barca marched against them, and so reduced them to starvation that when all supplies failed they ate first those who fell in battle, then prisoners of war, then slaves and finally they fell upon one another and, drawing lots, ate their fellow-soldiers. When Hamilcar had them in his power, he had the elephants trample them to death, saying that it was not holy for them to mix with other people. He did not accept cannibalism because some people had brought themselves to do it, nor did his son Hannibal, who was advised when he marched on Italy to accustom his army to cannibalism, so that they would not be short of food. Now it does not follow that, because famine and war cause the eating of other animals, we must also accept doing so for pleasure: we have not agreed to cannibalism.[34]

Porphyry sketches a *crescendo* of atrocities, leading the soldiers from the consumption of human corpses to killing humans with the purpose of eating them. And yet Porphyry reports that Hamilcar and Hannibal did not approve of cannibalism, even if under certain circumstances it could have been a useful strategy to provide food for their own armies. According to Vettori, Porphyry made use of this account in order to encourage abstinence from eating all creatures, animal and human: indeed Vettori writes that Titus Livius refers to the same story but frames it in a context which suggests that anthropophagy was really performed by Hannibal's troops.[35] Vettori thus points out that Porphyry possibly insisted on the connection between cannibalism and eating animals (and especially on Hamilcar's and Hannibal's condemnation of the former) with the sole purpose of proving that it is not right to kill any living being in order to eat it. Indeed it may be that "[...] Porphyrius in ea re tradenda, quae falsa foret, proposito illi suo servivit: qui non solum ab humanis corporibus abstinendum putabat, sed necare animantes ullas epularum causa rectum esse non existimabat."[36]

If cannibalism can't be accepted under any circumstances, not even when death by starvation is imminent, then why should it be considered normal to eat animals? Vettori argues that this is precisely the key question to which Porphyry wants to lead the reader – and the answer is of course that it is not morally right to kill for food.

This chapter from the *Variarum lectionum libri XXV* is not the only instance of Vettori's engagement with Porphyry's radical moral question: is it always wrong to kill a living creature? Vettori discusses the same topic in his commentary to Aristotle's *Rhetoric*, where he refers to Porphyry in connection with a statement by Empedocles reported in the Aristotelian text. The passage reads: "Et ut Empedocles inquit, ostendere volens, non esse caedenda animantes: hoc enim non huiuscemodi est, ut quibusdam quidam iustum sit: quibusdam autem non iustum."[37]

34 *On Abstinence*, pp. 77–78 (book 2, § 57). In *Variarum lectionum libri XXV* (Firenze 1554, p. 233), Vettori renders the passage as follows: "Porphyrius Tyrius in secundo libro περί ἀποχή ἐμψύχων, narrat quendam extitisse, qui Annibali cum exercitu in Italiam venienti, suaserit ut assuefaceret eum humana carne vesci, ne penuria cibi unqueam laboraret [...]."

35 P. Vettori, *Variarum lectionum libri XXV*, quoted, p. 233.

36 Ibid.

37 P. Vettori, *Commentarii in tres libros Aristotelis de arte dicendi*, quoted, p. 231.

Vettori comments on it by reminding the reader that even if Porphyry doesn't quote the same verses from Empedocles, he nevertheless refers to other poems to support the same theory, that is that it is necessary to abstain from animal food. The abhorrence at killing animals emerges again in Vettori's remark, which also points to the Pythagorean custom of avoiding animal sacrifices.[38]

The presence of these references to Porphyry in Vettori's works shows clearly that the interest of the first editor of *De abstinentia* was focused on crucial ethical aspects connected with the doctrine of vegetarianism. Ethical questions were thus not neglected in this reception of Porphyry but simply intertwined with other factors which at times seem to emerge more strongly, such as the medical relevance of vegetarianism, especially with regard to the ambivalent concept of abstinence. Indeed in the *Praefatio* to his edition, Vettori defines Porphyry as *temperatissimus*: the vegetarian philosopher was satisfied with a very frugal diet, which is presented also as the key to an ethical mode of behaviour, based on the rejection of all vices that promote the excesses of the body – and indulging in meat-eating is then one of these vices.

2.3 Curing the Body, Healing the Soul: Porphyry's Abstinence According to Marsilio Ficino

In a letter addressed to Braccio Martelli, Marsilio Ficino also insists on the *temperantia* and *prudentia* which are characteristic of those who reject the consumption of meat. The letter is particularly important in the context of the reception of Porphyry's *De abstinentia* which I have been sketching: Ficino imagines that Plotinus visits him while he is "staying at the home of Filippo and Niccolo Valori and investigating the nature of daemons".[39] Because of the obscurity of Plotinus' teaching, his disciple Porphyry was summoned: Porphyry was indeed "committed to the investigation of daemons" – writes Ficino – so that he appears to work as an interpreter of the Neoplatonic doctrine on this matter.[40] It is in this context that Porphyry expounds to Ficino his doctrine of abstinence, understood

38 Ibid., p. 232: "Porphyrius in ii. libro de non necandis ad vescendum animantibus, hos sane Empedoclis versus non citat, alios tamen eiusdem poëtae adducit, qui declarant eum valde ab ipsis caedendis abhorruisse, quod faciebat ille judium Pythagorae secutus: cuius disciplinam probabat. nam in iisdem illis versibus continetur ratio, qua prisci deos placare soliti essent: & quibus ritibus in sacrificiis uti." See also ibid, p. 111, where Vettori again mentions Porphyry's *De abstinentia* in a passage also dealing with the practice of sacrificing.

39 *Letters*, vol. 7, p. 33.

40 Ficino's letter refers to the fact that he had interrupted his work on Plotinus to dedicate himself to the translation of a series of Neoplatonic texts on daemons (between 1486 and 1489), including a selection from Porphyry's *De abstinentia*. The selection was published for Aldus Manutius in 1497. The extracts in the letter to Martelli are included, though with a different subdivision, in the translation he prepared for publication (see S. Gentile - S. Niccoli - P. Viti (eds.), *Marsilio Ficino e il ritorno di Platone. Manoscritti, stampe e documenti 17 maggio - 16 giugno 1984*, Florence 1984, p. 123). On the mediatory role of Porphyry see also *Epistolae*, p. 6r: De laude platonicorum interpretum (*Letters*, vol. 1, pp. 52–53).

as a necessary practice for the theologian and for the philosopher. Since Porphyry spoke Greek – so Ficino – he had to translate his words into Latin: this letter thus becomes also an attempt to mediate Porphyry's vocabulary into another language and therefore another culture, openly interpreting and adapting the content of Porphyry's fictional speech.[41] Ficino declares that the aim of the summary he provided to Braccio Martelli is to show that the doctrine of Plato and his followers in fact agrees with "our religion", thus highlighting again an aspect to which Piero Vettori had drawn attention: the fundamental agreement between Porphyry's concept of abstinence and the teaching of the Christian religion.[42]

The following part of the letter mainly contains extracts from book two of *De abstinentia*, which Ficino breaks up with titles inserted to explain the content of the text quoted, often merging several paragraphs into one, making it very difficult to detect where the translation ends and where Ficino's own insertions begin. In this way, his reading and translating of Porphyry also highlight the crucial points of his reception, providing the reader with a summary of Neoplatonic demonology in the context of the conception of abstinence and the problem of vegetarianism as they are presented in Porphyry's four books.[43]

As I have said before, book two of *De abstinentia* is mainly concerned with a discussion of sacrifice, and indeed this topic occupies a central place in Ficino's translation in the form of a letter. The main problem that Porphyry seems thus to present to Ficino, according to this narration, is whether sacrificing animals, and then eating their flesh, be an appropriate way to venerate the gods. Glossing Porphyry, Ficino first writes: "Purity and abstinence protect us from the evil daemons to whom contemplatives ought not to sacrifice anything."[44] Abstinence is thus the conduct appropriate for the contemplative, while Ficino insists on the fact that sacrificing animals will evoke bad demons, hungry for bloody meat.[45] For this reason the "followers of Plato offer nothing but contemplation as a sacrifice to God and to the soul of the world, but to the souls that move the stars they offer flowers and the fruits of the earth and of trees".[46] In other words, instead of sacrificing animals, one should "consecrate inanimate things only".[47] *Abstinentia* is therefore a protection against the impurity that derives from killing, and indeed in his Latin translation Ficino often uses the words *puritas* and *castitas* to define the

41 *Letters*, vol. 7, p. 33: "Now Porphyry spoke with us in Greek, but I shall interpret for you in Latin the essence of what he said." (*Epistolae*), p. 148r.

42 *Letters*, vol. 7, p. 33: "If you take the summary with the letter which I dedicated to you in the harmony of Moses and Plato, you will clearly realise how much Plato and also his followers are in agreement with our religion." *Epistolae*, p. 148r.

43 On Ficino's translation of Porphyry see also G. Corsi, "The Life of Marsilio Ficino", in: *Letters*, vol. 3, p. 142.

44 *Letters*, vol. 7, p. 38; *Epistolae*, p. 149v: "Puritas & abstinentia a malis demonibus nos tuetur quibus contemplatores sacrificare nihil debent."

45 Cfr. *Letters*, vol. 7, p. 37; *Epistolae*, p. 149r.

46 *Letters*, vol. 7, p. 33; *Epistolae*, p. 148r: "Platonici deo & animae mundi nihil praeter contemplationem sacrificant: animabus autem stellas moventibus flores sacrificant atque terrae arborumque fructus."

47 *Letters*, vol. 7, p. 37; *Epistolae*, p. 149r.

conduct of the abstinent philosopher. In this context Ficino also adapts the argument often repeated by Porphyry in *De abstinentia* that even if it were necessary to sacrifice animals, it would still remain impermissible to consume their flesh.[48] In his selection Ficino insists on the fact that abstinence from killing animals preserves the purity of the body and of the soul:

> If, then, the theologians ever allow you to sacrifice animals to the evil daemons in order to avoid the evils which they would inflict, at the same time they forbid you to taste such sacrifices. Moreover, before you sacrifice in this way, they command you to cleanse the soul by fasting and especially by abstaining from the flesh of animals.[49]

Despite the distinction drawn between the eating and the sacrificing of animals, Ficino makes clear that Porphyry's doctrine points towards abstinence from both actions. The concluding paragraph in the letter, merging together several quotations from Porphyry, bears the following title: "a wise man will abstain from eating the flesh of animals and from sacrificing them, for through these practices evil daemons are summoned to us."[50]

Given his insistence on the effects that slaughtering would have in terms of summoning bad demons, one might ask whether Ficino's interest is therefore only in the killing of animals to the extent that this is a violent act that burdens the soul of the perpetrator, pulling him down, away from the quietness of contemplation, and therefore causing a traumatic loss of balance in the Neoplatonic structure of the universe. But are there also ethical aspects, concerned with the nature of animals, and medical aspects, which may bring us back to the themes of Feliciano's reception of Porphyry?

Ficino indeed translated not only passages from the second book of Porphyry's *De abstinentia*, which he adapted in the letter to Braccio Martelli: he also translated extracts from the other three books which constitute Porphyry's text.[51] Considered altogether, Ficino's translations therefore reflect the variety of

48 Cfr. for instance *On Abstinence*, p. 55 (book 2, § 2): "[...] the same fallacy goes unobserved in relation to killing animals. It does not follow that if we must kill some, we must kill all, just as it does not follow that if we kill irrational animals, we must therefore kill people."

49 *Letters*, vol. 7, p. 38; *Epistolae*, p. 149v: "Quapropter theologi siquando permittunt demonibus improbis vitandorum gratia malorum quae illaturi sint animalia mactare vetant simul talia sacrificia degustare, preterea iubent antequam ita sacrifices purgare animum ieiunio ac praecipue animalium abstinentia."

50 *Letters*, vol. 7, p. 39; *Epistolae*, p. 149v: "Sapiens abstinebit tum cibo tum sacrificio animalium: per haec enim mali ad nos demones advocantur."

51 On Ficino's translations from Porphyry see also *Letters*, vol. 8, p. 10 (to Francesco Bandini, 6 January 1489): "You knew that I had translated all the books of Plotinus into Latin a long time ago and soon afterwards began to write commentaries on them. I have now finished half of these commentaries. Perhaps I would have completed all of them if, in the midst of writing them, I had not been compelled, in addition, to translate into Latin the Platonist Psellus on daemons, Synesius on dreams, part of Porphyry's work on abstinence [...]". Cfr. *Epistolae*, p. 158r. On the dating of Ficino's translations from *De abstinentia*, as well as on the manuscript versions of the text he translated from, see S. Gentile – S. Niccoli – P. Viti (eds.), *Marsilio Ficino e il ritorno di Platone*, pp. 122-123. On Ficino's translation of Porphyry in the context of his engagement with Neoplatonic texts on daemons see M. Vanhaelen's seminal study: M.

arguments which Porphyry had used in his text in favour of vegetarianism, including the theory about animals' rationality, which Ficino reports in a long passage taken from book 3, entitled: "Quod animae sensuales sint, & rationales, atque immortales".[52] Here Ficino writes that in the third book of *De abstinentia* Porphyry reports the Pythagorean doctrine, according to which: "[...] omnem scilicet animam sensibus, & memoria praeditam, esse rationalem, haberetque rationem, orationemque, tum interiorem, tum exteriorem [...]."[53]

This of course does not mean that Ficino himself agreed with Porphyry's interpretation of animals' rationality. In fact in his *Theologia platonica* he stresses the hierarchy of beings and the differences between the way animals and humans perceive the world.[54] Nevertheless, the selection of this extract shows clearly that Ficino considered the question of animals' rationality to be an important aspect of Porphyry's argumentation. And in fact Ficino also selected a passage from Porphyry's *Sententiae* (translated by him under the title *De occasionibus*) where the topic of animals' intelligence is further discussed with regard to the role of

Vanhaelen, "L'entreprise de traduction et d'exégèse de Ficin dans les années 1486-1489. Démons et prophétie à l'aube de l'ère savonarolienne", *Humanistica* 5.1 (2010), pp. 125-138. See also M. Vanhaelen, "Ficino's Commentary on St Paul's *First Epistle to the Romans* (1497): An Anti-savonarolan Reading of Vision and Prophecy", in: J. Hankins - F. Meroi (eds.), *The Rebirth of Platonic Theology: Proceedings of a Conference held at The Harvard University Center for Italian Renaissance Studies (Villa I Tatti) and the Istituto Nazionale di Studi sul Rinascimento (Florence, 26-27 April 2007)* (Atti di Convegni; 27), Florence 2013, pp. 205-233.

52 Marsilio Ficino, *Opera omnia*, Basel 1576 (reprint Paris 1999), p. 1917. Porphyry's theory on the rationality of animals is mentioned also in the Latin edition of Claudius Elianus' *De vi & natura animalium*, edited by P. Gyllius (P. Gilles) and published in 1533 in Lyon (see p. 14 of the dedication). Gyllius also refers directly to Porphyry's text *De abstinentia ab usu [sic] carnium* (cfr. ibid., p. 144).

53 Ibid., p. 1917.

54 See for instance Marsilio Ficino, *Platonic Theology*, vol. 3, ed. by J. Hankins, trans. by M. J. Allen, Cambridge (Mass.) / London 2003, pp. 154–157 (book 10, chapter 5, §§ 3–5). Cfr. on the same topic P. O. Kristeller, *Die Philosophie des Marsilio Ficino*, Frankfurt a. M. 1972, pp. 368–369: "Die rationale Seele wird von Ficino gern mit den Engeln und auf der anderen Seite mit den Seelen der Tiere verglichen. [...] Die Tiere dagegen besitzen zwar zugleich mit dem Körper auch die auf den Körper bezüglichen Lebensfunktionen sowie Wahrnehmung und Phantasie, aber weder kontemplative Erkenntnis noch diskursives Denken. Es wird ihnen daher lediglich eine sog. irrationale Seele zugeschrieben, welche offensichtlich nicht nur der *natura*, sondern auch dem unteren Seelenteil des Menschen, dem sog. *idolum* entspricht, sofern dieses ja ebenfalls als Träger der Wahrnehmung und Phantasie angesehen wird. Diese irrationale Seele der Tiere erhebt sich nicht über den Bereich des Körperlichen und ist daher auch im Gegensatz zur menschlichen Seele nicht unsterblich. Sie wird aber gelegentlich ähnlich wie der irrationale Teil des Menschen als Schatten der rationalen Seele bezeichnet und nach neuplatonischem Vorgang in ihrem Bestand auf die Weltseele bzw. die Seele ihres Elements zurückgeführt." For much information concerning the place of animals in Ficino's *Theologia platonica* I am indebted to Maria-Christine Leitgeb, who conducted on this topic a session of the reading seminar I organised at the Ludwig-Maximilians-Universität München, 19–20 November 2010 (see the conference report published in *Bruniana & Campanelliana* 17 (2011), n. 1, pp. 325–327).

imagination.[55] Quoting again from book 3 of *De abstinentia*, Ficino inserts the heading "nefas est animalia caedere" (it is malign to kill animals), summarizing Porphyry but also giving a precise indication of the ethical conclusion which emerges from the passages translated.

Like Feliciano, Ficino insists on the word *abstinentia* in his reception of Porphyry – and this word takes us back to an important feature of the Renaissance reception, that is the merging of medical and ethical aspects. To a translation of several passages from book 1, indeed, Ficino gives the title "de abstinentia". A crucial passage from this translation reads: "Praeterea usus carnium ad sanitatem minimi consert, sed sanitatem potius impedit: quoniam per quae recuperatur sanitas, per eadem perseverat, recuperatur aut per victum tenuissimum, & carnibus abstinentem, quapropter & hoc sanitas conservatur."[56] Ficino thereby acknowledges the importance of the medical aspect of *abstinentia*, understood as a cure for the body as well as a means to keep that balance of the soul which sacrificing animals would endanger. In a letter to Bernardo Bembo, Ficino mentions the fact that the Pythagorean diet, based on "fruits, cabbages and apples" proves to be particularly suitable to promote health: indeed "there is no easier nor healthier table than that which bountiful nature provides for us", he argues.[57]

This connection between the care of the body and the care of the soul, as presented in Porphyry, assumes a particular significance in Ficino's reception through the mediation of the word *abstinentia*, a word with a religious resonance but also crucial in the medical tradition (as for instance in the saying "abstinentia est summa medicina").[58] Further, Ficino refers to Porphyry in *De vita libri tres* (book two), where he writes that eating meat on a daily basis would endanger health, and he adds: "Quanquam medici non tam carnium usum vetant, quam abusum".[59] Abstinence from (excessive) consumption of meat is seen in this context from a strictly medical point of view. At the same time, one should not forget that the care of the body and of the soul cannot be separated from one another. Indeed, in a letter to Riccardo Angiolieri Ficino describes as follows the consequences emerging from the behaviour of those who don't properly consider this connection of body and soul: "I can only judge it the most foolish act of all, that

55 Ficino, *Opera omnia*, p. 1929–1932, especially the section entitled "Sensus, imaginatio, memoria, intelligentia" (ibid., p. 1930).

56 Ibid., p. 1934 (cfr. book 1, § 52 in *On Abstinence*). See also ibid., p. 1933: "Vir autem cautus, & qui naturae veneficia suspicatur, cognoscitque naturam corporis, quemadmodum videlicet instrumenti more ad animi vires contemperatur est, intelligit sane quantum passio sonare parata est velis, nolisve, quoties ab externis pulsatur corpus, pulsatoque inceptionem pervenit, perceptio enim ipsa, animadversioque sonus ipsi es" (cfr. *On Abstinence*, book 1, § 43).

57 *Letters*, vol. 2, p. 53: "Certainly we have no desire for the over-fat and oily banquets of Sardanapalus. But we do not want by any means to lack the Pythagorean fruits, cabbages and apples, for there is no easier nor healthier table than that which bountiful nature provides for us." *Healthier* translates the Latin *foelicior* (cfr. *Epistolae*, p. 74r).

58 See for instance Thomas Aquinas' *Scriptum super Sententiis* (liber 4, distinctio 15, quaestio 3, articulum 1, quaestiuncula 2): "[…] unde etiam Galenus dicit quod summa medicina est abstinentia" (available online: http://www.corpusthomisticum.org/).

59 Ficino, *Opera omnia*, p. 513.

many people most diligently feed a beast, that is their body, a wild, cruel and dangerous animal; but allow themselves, that is, the soul, in so far as they have one, to starve to death."[60] And he continues: "[...] we foolishly over-feed the body and neglect the soul, the body becomes fat and robust and the soul tiny and puny".[61] Even if the vegetarian diet is not directly recommended in this letter, the translations of Porphyry as well as the letters previously quoted show that abstinence from animal food plays a role in this context, since Ficino presents it as a remedy for averting precisely such a lack of balance between the soul and the body.

For Ficino, who regarded medicine and philosophy as profoundly connected - as Teodoro Katinis has convincingly argued[62] – this insistence on Porphyry's conception of abstinence can be interpreted as part of his active reception of the text, and not just of translation.[63] In *Oratio de laudibus medicinae*, a short text which Ficino coupled with an *Oratio in laudibus philosophiae*[64], he writes for instance: "[...] Phoebus, as may be read in the *Letters of Hippocrates*, considered the care of the soul and of the body to come together in one."[65] If we interpret Ficino's interest for Porphyry's four books in this frame, focusing also on his translation of *apochê* with the word *abstinentia*, the polymorphic character of the Renaissance reception of this text emerges even more clearly. Indeed the intersection between different levels of the argumentation was at the basis not only of Ficino's reception, but also of the interest of other readers who dedicated themselves to the transmission of Porphyry's book between the end of the fifteenth and the beginning of the sixteenth century.

If we ask, then, what is the role of reflections on the ethical status of animals in this phase of Porphyry's reception, it appears that these interpreters and translators of *De abstinentia* point if not to an answer to the question, at least to a different way of posing the problem. The cluster of aspects considered by Feliciano, Vettori and Ficino – medical, ethical, religious – indicate that concern about the health of the human body, about the best way to promote the human mind, and *also* about the place of animals in the world, were considered in the Renaissance-reception of this text as parts of one and the same problem, to which abstinence was suggested as a possible answer. From Feliciano's medical perspective, to Vettori's interest in the link between vegetarianism and cannibalism, to Ficino's Porphyrian daemonology, one encounters a variety of conceptions of abstinence inspired by Porphyry and including ethical questions regarding the status of animals. This proves an important starting point not only for reconsidering the rea-

60 *Letters*, vol. 1, p. 103; *Epistolae*, p. 16v.

61 Ibid.

62 T. Katinis, *Medicina e filosofia in Marsilio Ficino. Il Consilio contro la pestilentia*, Rome 2007. See also G. Baader, "Die Antikenrezeption in der Entwicklung der medizinischen Wissenschaft während der Renaissance", in: R. Schmitz – G. Keil (eds.), *Humanismus und Medizin*, Weinheim 1984, pp. 51–66, especially pp. 53–54.

63 On Ficino's theory of translation see J. Hankins, *Plato in the Italian Renaissance*, Copenhagen 1990, p. 314 ff., especially p. 317.

64 For further details see T. Katinis, *Medicina e filosofia*, quoted, p. 72.

65 *Letters*, vol. 3, p. 24; *Epistolae*, p. 84v.

sons for the rising popularity of Porphyry's *De abstinentia* in the fifteenth and sixteenth centuries, but also, and more fundamentally, for understanding how to frame speculations on vegetarianism in the Renaissance, more than a thousand years after Porphyry's appeal to Firmus Castricius, who had made a choice unworthy of a philosopher: eating animals.

LA MEDECINE MORALE DE LUIGI LUISINI. LE PREMIER TRAITEMENT MEDICO-PHILOSOPHIQUE DES PASSIONS DE L'AME

Roberto Poma

L'idée selon laquelle les facultés intellectuelles et physiques d'un être humain pourraient être affaiblies, altérées voire anéanties par la force des émotions est un *topos* de la tradition médicale occidentale depuis Hippocrate.[1] L'expérience personnelle de tout un chacun confirme l'intérêt de cette idée pour la santé humaine. Il suffit d'avoir connu au moins une fois le trac avant de se produire en public ou les effets pathogènes de l'annonce d'une mauvaise nouvelle ou de la perte d'un être cher pour savoir que les frontières entre les organes sensoriels, l'imagination, les processus physiologiques et la pensée sont loin d'être infranchissables. Le constat que les émotions ont un effet sur la santé a induit des discours savants à cheval entre les sciences morales et médicales. C'est pourquoi, depuis le Ve siècle avant J.-C., les émotions et la santé constituent des sujets d'enquête à la fois philosophique et médicale. D'une part, dans les écrits de Platon, d'Aristote et des écoles hellénistiques, les émotions, conçues comme des « passions de l'âme », sont traitées comme des mouvements corporels à harmoniser, à modérer ou à extirper.[2] Dans certains cas, il est même recommandé d'exprimer ses émotions/passions de l'âme, notamment la colère.[3] D'autre part, les auteurs de la grande tradition hippocratico-galénique ainsi que les médecins empiriques, de l'Antiquité grecque à la Renaissance, malgré les discordances théoriques de fond, s'accordent tous sur un point : les perturbations de l'âme affectent l'équilibre physiologique et peuvent engendrer des maladies de toutes sortes. Par ailleurs, à la faveur de la théorie des tempéraments, qui s'impose au Moyen Âge, à partir du XVIe siècle on tend à assimiler une attitude émotionnelle avec les mouvements d'une humeur corporelle (sang, phlegme, biles blonde et noire). Par conséquent, la signification physiologique du terme « humeur » s'élargit peu à peu au sens moral

1 La littérature critique sur ce sujet est abondante, notamment depuis la publication de l'ouvrage pionnier de J. Pigeaud, *La Maladie de l'âme. Étude sur la relation de l'âme et du corps dans la tradition médico-philosophique antique*, Paris 1981, pp. 31-138, pp. 245-371.

2 Pour un bon aperçu général, Cf. J. Fillion-Lahille, *Le De Ira de Sénèque et la philosophie stoïcienne des passions*, Paris 1984, pp. 17-28. Sur l'histoire des termes « passion » et « émotion », cf. T. Dixon, *From passions to emotions : the creation of a secular psychological category*, Cambridge, 2003.

3 Cf. G. Mathieu-Castellani, *Éloge de la colère. L'humeur colérique dans l'Antiquité et à la Renaissance*, Paris, 2012.

de « disposition de caractère »[4]. L'« humeur pindarique » de Pierre de Ronsard (*Nouvelle Continuation des Amours*, 1556, XLIV) montre la voie vers le sens psychologique moderne du terme « humeur ». Les plus anciens ouvrages de diététique comme le traité hippocratique *Du régime* (V[e] av. J.-C.), l'*Epître sur la vie saine* (IVe av. J.-C.) de Dioclès de Caryste, les *Préceptes de santé* (Ier apr. J.-C.) de Plutarque ou le traité sur l'*Hygiène* de Galien ont mis l'accent sur les maladies dues à de mauvaises habitudes, aux états d'âme et au tempérament individuel.[5] De nombreux auteurs médiévaux s'exprimant en langues arabe et latine s'inscrivent dans ce courant tout en ajoutant une multitude d'éléments nouveaux.[6] De surcroît, les histoires de mères qui expirent soudainement en voyant leur fils revenir d'une bataille[7], des professeurs de philosophie mourant littéralement de honte pour ne pas avoir su réponde à une question, de cavaliers morts dans l'acte vénérien[8] ou le récit d'hommes muets de naissance qui retrouvent la voix après une grande frayeur[9] alimentent au fil des siècles une véritable histoire naturelle de la force des émotions.

Une véritable physio-pathologie ainsi qu'une sémiotique des émotions, avec des résonances éthiques et politiques en philosophie et des visées thérapeutiques en médecine, sont disséminées dans un corpus de textes médicaux et philosophiques anciens et médiévaux. Dans le prolongement de cette littérature assez hétérogène, un obscur médecin italien du XVIe siècle, Luigi Luisini, apporte selon

4 Cf. J. Pigeaud, « L'humeur des Anciens », dans *Poétiques du corps*, Paris, pp. 149-173.

5 Cf. P. Gil-Sotres, « Les régimes de santé », dans M. Grmek (éd.), *Histoire de la pensée médicale en Occident*, vol 1, *Antiquité et Moyen Age,* Paris, 1995, pp. 255-281.

6 Dans le cadre de la médecine arabe, la *Médecine spirituelle* de Razi (trad. fr., intr. et notes par R. Brague, Paris 2003) mérite une mention particulière. Cf. P. Koetschet, « Médecine de l'Âme, médecine du corps », dans *Bulletin d'études orientales* 57 (Janvier 2008), pp. 155-167 [mis en ligne le 13 novembre 2009, consulté le 06 juin 2012 : http://beo.revues.org/132].

7 Tite-Live, *Ab urbe condita*, XXII, 7 : « L'une d'elles, à la porte même, se trouvant soudain en face de son fils sauvé, mourut, dit-on, dans ses bras ; une autre, à qui l'on avait annoncé par erreur la mort de son fils, et qui était tristement assise chez elle, dans sa première émotion, en voyant son fils de retour, expira d'un excès de bonheur » (trad. fr. E. Lasserre, Paris 1937).

8 Pline, *Historia naturalis*, VII, 54 : « (1) Diodore, professeur de philosophie dialectique, mourut de honte pour n'avoir pu se résoudre sur-le-champ, sous les interrogations de Scipion, une question qui n'était pas sérieuse ; … (5) P. Quinctius Scapula, en dînant chez Aquilius Gallus; Décimus Saufeius, scribe, en déjeunant chez lui; Cornélius Gallus, qui avait été préteur, et Q. Haterius, chevalier romain, moururent dans l'acte vénérien, ainsi que deux individus de l'ordre équestre dont on a parlé de notre temps, et qui expirèrent ayant affaire au pantomime Mysticus le plus bel homme d'alors » (trad. fr. E. Littré, Paris 1848-1850).

9 Hérodote, *Histoires*, I, 85 : « Après la prise de la ville, un Perse allait tuer Crésus sans le connaître. Ce prince [muet de naissance] le voyait fondre sur lui ; mais, accablé du poids de ses malheurs, il négligeait de l'éviter, et peu lui importait de périr sous ses coups. Le jeune prince muet, à la vue du Perse qui se jetait sur son père, saisi d'effroi, fit un effort qui lui rendit la voix : « Soldat, s'écria-t-il, ne tue pas Crésus ! » Tels furent ses premiers mots ; et il conserva la faculté de parler le reste de sa vie » (trad. fr. P.-E. Legrand, Paris 1932).

moi une dimension nouvelle : il réunit et articule en un seul ouvrage de multiples savoirs anciens sur les passions de l'âme.[10]

LA FIGURE DE LUIGI LUISINI

Luisini est un compilateur de textes anciens. En vain rechercherait-on dans l'ouvrage que nous allons étudier un quelconque remède pharmaceutique, une théorie philosophique ou un précepte de santé qui ne soient pas présents dans la tradition philosophique et médicale. C'est essentiellement pour cela que son nom ne figure pas dans les manuels et les ouvrages généraux. Seuls les historiens de la médecine, ainsi que les lecteurs de Ludwig Fleck[11], se souviennent sans doute de lui en tant qu'éditeur du premier recueil de textes importants sur la syphilis[12] publié à Venise en 1566-67, augmenté et réédité dans la même ville en 1599[13], puis à Leyde en 1728 par Hermann Boerhaave.

Nous avons très peu d'informations sur sa vie.[14] Il existe quatre graphies différentes de son nom de famille – Luisini (Luisinus), Luigini, Lovisini et Luvigini – et deux de son prénom : Aloisio (Aloysius) et Luigi. Né en 1526 à Udine, dans le Frioul, de parents aristocrates – Bartolomeo Luigini et Paola Manini – il se forme d'abord dans sa ville natale, puis à Padoue, où il étudie la philosophie et la médecine. Il suit les cours de Bernardino Tomisano.[15] Jusqu'en 1554, il pratique la médecine à Venise sous le regard bienveillant de Giovanni Antonio Sicco, auteur d'un important traité de déontologie médicale.[16] Luigi Luisini est très apprécié par ses patients dans l'exercice de l'art médical.[17] Son premier ouvrage est une traduction versifiée des *Aphorismes* d'Hippocrate.[18] En 1562, il publie son premier traité de médecine : *La répression des passions de l'âme par la philosophie*

10 Nous allons utiliser le mot « passion » en tant que terme technique le plus souvent employé par les médecins et les philosophes de la Renaissance pour traduire le grec *pathos* et le latin *affectus.*

11 L. Fleck, *Genèse et développement d'un fait scientifique*, Paris 2005 [1935[1]], pp. 5-14.

12 L. Luisini, *De morbo gallico omnia quae extant apud omnes medicos cujuscumque nationis*, 2 vols. Fol., Venise 1566-67.

13 L. Luisini, *Aphrodisiacus sive de lue venerea*, Venise 1599.

14 Dans le *Dizionario Biografico degli Italiani* (Treccani), Fiammetta Cirilli se penche surtout sur la figure de son frère Francesco sans donner sur Luigi plus d'informations que la *Biographie universelle ancienne et moderne* (Michaud), publiée au XIXe siècle.

15 Cf. G.-G. Liruti, *Notizie delle vite ed opere scritte da' letterati del Friuli*, vol. II, Venise 1762, p. 148.

16 G. A. Sicco, *De optimo medico,* Venise 1551.

17 G.-G. Liruti, *Notizie delle vite ed opere scritte da' letterati del Friuli*, vol. II, Venise 1762, p. 148 : « In questa sua professione di medico egli è certo che fu molto stimato, ed acquistò un assai glorioso nome nella Città suddetta ; come siamo assicurati da Ottaviano Manini suo contemporaneo nelle mentovate Memorie MSS. Che presso di me conservo, con queste parole : *Alvise Luisino fu medico molto stimato in Venezia...* ».

18 L. Luisini, *Aphorismi Hippocratis hexametro carmine conscripti*, Venise 1552.

morale et l'art médical[19] dédié à Giovanni Antonio Sicco, qu'il tenait en haute estime.[20] Luisini peut donc être considéré comme un médecin érudit et un clinicien, davantage intéressé par les multiples enjeux éthiques de la pratique médicale que par les sciences de son temps. En témoignent deux autres ouvrages, l'un sur la confession des malades,[21] l'autre, un dialogue en vulgaire sur la cécité, dans lequel il fait l'éloge du philosophe vénitien Niccolò Massa, adepte du stoïcisme, qui finit sa vie aveugle mais heureux.[22] Le lieu et la date de sa mort demeurent dans l'ombre. La renommée du *De morbo gallico* d'une part, son intérêt pour la pratique médicale au détriment des recherches anatomiques et de l'enseignement théorique à l'Université de l'autre, expliquent en grande partie l'oubli du reste de son œuvre.

Son traité sur « La répression des passions de l'âme » (dorénavant : *De compescendis*) présente cependant une originalité certaine et met en lumière les rapports complexes que la médecine entretient avec la philosophie au XVIe siècle. Cette étude tentera de définir sa place dans l'histoire de la psychopathologie et de l'éthique médicale.

PASSIONS, ERREURS ET MALADIES : UNE ETHIQUE DE LA FAILLIBILITE

La contribution de Luigi Luisini à l'histoire de l'éthique et de la thérapeutique médicale s'inscrit délibérément dans le paradigme galénique. Dans le *De compescendis*, la source médicale la plus fréquemment exploitée est le traité galénique sur *Les passions et les erreurs de l'âme*[23] centré sur l'étude de la relation que les erreurs de jugement entretiennent avec les passions de l'âme. « L'erreur (*amartê-*

19 L. Luisini, *De compescendis animi affectibus per moralem philosophiam et medendi artem, tractatus in tres libri divisus*, Bâle 1562. Pour rester fidèle à l'original latin, on pourrait traduire le titre de la manière suivante : « Traité en trois livres sur les passions de l'âme qui sont à réprimer par la philosophie morale et l'art médical ».

20 Cet ouvrage sera réédité à Strasbourg en 1713 avec des notes renvoyant aux sources classiques et bibliques. Tout en disposant des deux éditions (1562 et 1713) en version électronique, je vais citer le *De compescendis* à partir de l'édition strasbourgeoise (Dulsekker, 1713), plus lisible et identique à la première, sauf pour la pagination et pour les références ajoutées par l'éditeur. Gian-Giuseppe Liruti (*op. cit.*, p. 149) fait mention d'une première édition du *De compescendis* publié à Venise en 1561 dont tous les exemplaires auraient été vendus en si peu de temps qu'une deuxième édition (Bâle 1562) s'imposa. N'ayant trouvé nul part cette édition de l'ouvrage, nous sommes enclins à croire qu'il s'agit d'une histoire inventée par Liruti pour mettre en valeur l'œuvre du médecin frioulan.

21 L. Luisini, *De confessione ægrotantium a die decubitus instituenda*, Venise 1563.

22 L. Luisini, *Dialogo intitolato La cecità*, Venise 1569.

23 Ce traité est imprimé en traduction latine dès le début du XVIe siècle. Nous allons citer la traduction française publiée dans Galien, *Les passions et les erreurs de l'âme*, dans *L'âme et ses passions*, intr., trad. fr. et notes par V. Barras, T. Birchler et A.-F. Morand, Paris 1995. Pour le texte grec (*peri diagnôseôs kai therapeias tôn en tê ekastou psuchê idiôn pathôn*) et latin (*De propriorum animi cuiusque affectuum dignotione et curatione*), nous avons consulté l'édition Kuhn (Leipzig 1825, V, pp. 1-57).

ma) – dit Galien – provient d'une opinion fausse (*pseudê doxa*), tandis que la passion (*pathos*) provient d'une force irrationnelle (*ormê*) en nous qui désobéit à la raison ».[24] L'erreur dérive d'une opinion, c'est-à-dire d'une représentation mentale qui n'est pas en adéquation avec la réalité. C'est une pensée inadéquate qui se traduits en jugements et en actes inadéquats, préjudiciables et mauvais. En revanche, la passion (lat. *affectus*) n'est pas une représentation, ni une pensée. C'est avant tout une force corporelle désordonnée, floue et opaque, une énergie débordant du vase des représentations, qu'elle charge de toute sa violence. Elle se présente comme un mouvement interne ou une impulsion corporelle primaire comme la peur ou la colère, la tristesse ou la joie et s'oppose à l'ordre rationnel qui est censé discipliner les activités humaines. L'erreur et les passions ont des statuts ontologiques hétérogènes, la première relevant de l'activité mentale, les secondes de l'élan physique. Quelle relation pourrait donc les unir ? Pour la cerner nous devons changer de point de vue et nous placer sur le plan de l'intentionnalité, car l'erreur (de jugement) et la passion se produisent toutes deux involontairement.

Il est inconcevable pour Galien, et pour bien d'autre philosophes contemporains, de vouloir se tromper ou de produire intentionnellement une passion/émotion. On se trompe de la même manière qu'on se laisse dominer par une passion. Il y a une similarité causale, car les erreurs et les passions dérivent d'un affaiblissement des facultés rationnelles. L'âme entière se soumet ainsi aux opinions infondées et à la force des impulsions corporelles. C'est un cercle vicieux ! L'erreur de jugement est causée par un aveuglement intellectuel causé lui-même par l'emprise d'une passion liée soit au tempérament naturel, soit aux habitudes comportementales. Nous tombons dans l'erreur à cause d'un élément que nous n'avons pas vu ou que nous n'avons pas pris en considération dans notre jugement. Par conséquent, notre faculté de juger s'exerce sur des données partielles. Comment cela peut-il arriver ? Qu'est-ce qui trouble notre vue ? Qu'est-ce qui altère l'activité normale des fonctions naturelles comme la sensibilité et le jugement ? Qu'est-ce qui nous rend aveugles à l'égard de nos propres erreurs ? Ce sont les passions, répond Galien. Leur pouvoir aveuglant est à l'origine de nombreux malheurs. Elles entravent lourdement la capacité de se connaître soi-même qui devrait caractériser l'*optimus medicus*. Mais une passion en particulier s'avère extrêmement néfaste : le sentiment d'être infaillible ou de ne pouvoir se tromper que sur des points mineurs. Cela freine lourdement le perfectionnement moral et intellectuel du futur médecin.

Par amour excessif de soi, l'apprenti médecin ne voit pas ses propres erreurs et *a fortiori* ne peut pas les éviter. « Il est probable de tomber dans l'erreur même si nous n'avons pas l'impression de nous tromper »,[25] affirme Galien, conscient que l'auto-critique est une attitude aussi féconde qu'ardue à mettre en pratique. S'il est extrêmement difficile de voir ses propres erreurs et de s'en détacher, il est tout aussi difficile de changer et de s'améliorer par soi-même, quand bien même nous connaissons et reconnaissons nos limites et erreurs. Car l'intempérance fon-

24 Galien, *Les passions*, p. 4.
25 Ibid.

damentale de la nature humaine, les vives émotions et le mauvais caractère peuvent troubler l'exercice de la faculté rationnelle. Galien met donc sérieusement en doute notre capacité d'auto-critique et d'auto-changement. « Quiconque en effet désire devenir un homme de bien doit comprendre ceci : il ignore nécessairement une grande partie de ses erreurs ».[26] Platon (*Lois*, 731e) a eu bien raison de soutenir que « celui qui aime est aveugle face à l'objet aimé », car, selon Galien, l'amour pour soi-même fait de la recherche de ses propres erreurs une quête désespérée. L'amour pour soi-même rend l'amant aveugle face à ses propres erreurs. Ces dernières ne peuvent éventuellement devenir visibles qu'à la faveur du détachement de soi. D'où la nécessité de s'en remettre à « l'appréciation d'excellents hommes » pour reconnaître ses propres erreurs. Il faut apprendre à se concevoir soi-même comme un objet d'étude et non pas d'adoration ou de commisération pour commencer à se libérer d'abord des passions immodérées, puis des fausses opinions. L'antériorité des passions dans le rapport causal qui les associe aux erreurs marque la priorité de l'éthique – d'une éthique appliquée – dans la formation médicale.

L'apprenti médecin doit assimiler une éthique de la faillibilité. Il doit apprendre à se concevoir soi-même comme étant un sujet faillible usant d'un savoir solide. Un savoir qui, bien qu'il soit ancré dans la logique la plus sûre et dans l'expérience la mieux attestée, s'applique à une matière aussi vivante que protéiforme. De ce fait, dans l'art du diagnostic, l'incertitude règne souveraine. L'éthique de la faillibilité, fondamentale pour l'apprentissage de l'art (*téchnê*), s'avère tout aussi capitale pour la science (*epistêmê*). Dans cette perspective, une sorte d'épistémologie de la faillibilité découlerait de l'éthique. Pour s'engager dans la voie de la science et de la sagesse, pour prévenir et remédier aux erreurs nécessairement liées à la pratique de la médecine, il faut développer des vertus épistémiques, c'est-à-dire des qualités morales comme la tempérance (*sôphrosúnê)* et la prudence (*phrónêsis*).[27] Galien prône une éthique et une épistémologie fondées sur les vertus (*virtue-based Ethics and Epistemology*), la vertu étant le terreau de la science. La tempérance donne la lucidité qui éclaire l'action, tandis que la prudence guide la pensée, conseille la parole et dirige la main. Dès lors, ces deux vertus deviennent fondamentales dans la réflexion éthique et épistémologique, car elles inspirent les meilleures attitudes épistémiques et morales. Meilleures, puisqu'elles permettent de traquer et juguler les erreurs de toutes sortes.

Nous pourrions nous étonner, aujourd'hui, de voir jusqu'à quel point un *êthos*, une disposition psychique bien déterminée, a pu être considéré aussi important dans la transmission d'un savoir. La raison en est peut-être que nous pensons tacitement que la personnalité du savant n'influence que marginalement l'élaboration ou la vérification d'une théorie. Malgré la validité très circonscrite de cette opinion, nous demeurons profondément imprégnés par une attitude de pensée positiviste, qui n'accorde aucune place au *psychologisme* dans l'étude du processus de formation d'une théorie scientifique. Au contraire, pour Galien, il est évident que,

26 Galien, *Les passions*, p. 6.
27 Ibid., p. 24.

par la rapidité de sa manifestation, la passion est un mouvement psycho-physiologique primaire, antérieur à l'erreur. Elle en est la cause.

> Du fait que les erreurs proviennent d'une opinion fausse, alors que les passions proviennent d'un élan irrationnel, j'ai considéré qu'il fallait me libérer moi-même d'abord des passions. Il est vraisemblable qu'à cause de celles-ci nous nous forgeons en quelque sorte de fausses opinions[28]

affirme Galien avant de proclamer le principe de la « juste mesure » comme critère du beau et du bien. L'accent mis sur l'*êthos* et sur la morale du *mêdèn ágan*, loin de signifier un quelconque rapport hiérarchique entre la médecine des anciens et celle des modernes, témoigne de la conscience aiguë, chez Galien, du caractère éminemment « artistique » de la médecine conçue comme *téchnê.*

Mais revenons à la question de la relation entre la passion et l'erreur. Dans l'usage des passions, l'excès est une erreur qui, à force d'être réitérée, conduit tout droit à la maladie. La maladie est le fruit malheureux des erreurs de l'âme. En ce sens, la recherche de la *medietas* rapproche le médecin du philosophe et, en parallèle, le savant accompli du citoyen responsable. S'agit-il d'un idéal atteignable ? Le parfait médecin doit-il atteindre la tempérance ? Ou bien devrait-il cultiver l'apathie ? Considérer les passions comme la principale cause d'erreur, conduit Galien à soutenir qu'il faudrait les éradiquer afin d'éliminer toutes les erreurs : « [après avoir trouvé un vieillard, capable de discernement, qui voit et dénonce nos moindres défauts, il faut] s'efforcer d'extirper la passion non seulement jusqu'à ce qu'elle ne soit plus visible aux autres, mais au point de ne pas même en laisser la racine dans son âme. Sinon elle repousse, abreuvée par la méchanceté des passions conjointes ».[29] Toutefois, puisqu'il « est difficile, pour celui qui s'est habitué pendant longtemps à l'erreur, d'effacer la trace de ses passions »[30], la passion s'avère être le plus souvent indéracinable. A propos de la colère, par exemple, Galien affirme qu' « il est impossible de devenir exempt de colère aussitôt qu'on le désire ; tu peux en revanche contenir l'inconvenance propre à cette passion »[31]. Galien prône donc la modération, l'éradication des passions étant une entreprise le plus souvent vouée à l'échec, surtout chez les jeunes, fougueux par nature. Dans l'apprentissage de la modération, l'éthique de la faillibilité fournit un grand soutien. Des déclarations incitant le néophyte à prendre conscience de sa propre faillibilité se multiplient tout le long de l'ouvrage : « Ne crois pas être devenu exempt d'erreurs »,[32] « il t'est impossible de ne point commettre d'erreurs »,[33] « j'affirme que personne n'est exempt de passions ni d'erreurs, fût-il très doué ou élevé dans les meilleures manières, mais que l'on se trompe de toutes façons, surtout lorsqu'on est encore jeune ».[34] La réflexion sur les erreurs

28 Galien, *Les passions*, p. 7.
29 Ibid., pp. 27-28.
30 Ibid., pp. 19-20.
31 Ibid., pp. 13-14.
32 Ibid., p. 9.
33 Ibid.
34 Ibid., p. 12.

s'entremêle constamment avec celle sur les passions. Nous avons vu de quelle manière l'erreur et la passion, en dépit de leurs sources différentes – d'une part une opinion (*doxa*), de l'autre un élan irrationnel (*ormê*) – sont souvent jumelées en raison du lien causal qui les unit. Asservis aux passions excessives, véritables maladies de l'âme et sources de nombreuses erreurs, ni le philosophe et ni le médecin ne pourraient se connaître eux-mêmes. C'est ainsi que leurs possibilités de perfectionnement s'amenuisent, car dans le cadre de ce paradigme, puisqu'il est « impossible de dissocier le jugement de la manifestation physiologique qui l'accompagne » et que « la passion est constituée de ce *recto-verso* indissociable du jugement et du mouvement de la contraction, ou de la dilatation »[35], un jugement erroné peut se cristalliser dans l'esprit au fur et à mesure qu'un nouveau processus physiologique lié à la manifestation d'une passion se normalise. Dès lors l'opinion, la représentation erronée, s'enracine durablement dans le corps.[36] Au bout d'une argumentation circulaire, qui décrit l'emprisonnement de l'âme dans la tension existentielle entre les passions et les opinions fausses, Galien indique de nouveau la seule voie de sortie de l'état d'erreur et d'aveuglement :

> Pour observer leurs erreurs, les jeunes gens désirant être sauvés doivent donc recourir à d'autres qu'eux-mêmes, des personnes d'un certain âge, qui ont donné, leur vie durant, une preuve suffisante de leur liberté d'opinion ; des personnes qu'il ne convient pas de contredire ou de haïr lorsqu'elles font des reproches, mais envers lesquelles il faut être reconnaissant et qu'il faut prier de toujours dire la vérité.[37]

Selon Galien, nous sommes incapables de nous libérer par nous mêmes des chaînes des passions. Dépouillé de son orgueil, le jeune fougueux doit accepter une autorité autre que soi-même pour que la contemplation, l'analyse et l'acceptation de ses passions et ses erreurs l'incite à aimer la tempérance.[38] Sans connaissance, pas de maîtrise des passions. Sans maîtrise de soi, pas de sortie de l'erreur et des maladies (de l'âme/corps) causées par les excès.

Nous avons analysé jusqu'ici l'argumentaire de Galien en faveur de la modération des passions. Le médecin de Pergame met en évidence un sujet qui concerne à mesure égale le médecin et le philosophe, c'est-à-dire la relation qu'un homme bon et sain devrait entretenir avec ses propres passions. Toutefois Galien ne s'efforce pas d'en décrire le processus psycho-physiologique sous-jacent, ni de proposer une méthode médicale pour les contrer, doublée d'une méthode philosophique adaptée à chaque passion. Son propos relève de l'éthique. Il faudra attendre Luigi Luisini avant de réaliser, dans le cadre de la tradition galénique, une synthèse médico-philosophique bien ordonnée des savoirs sur les passions qui s'étaient sédimentés dans la culture du Moyen-Âge.

35 Cf. J. Pigeaud, *Les maladies de l'âme*, Paris 1989, p. 267 et 297.

36 Ce sujet se prête à controverse. Pour Chrysippe et Cicéron, la passion et le jugement sont deux aspects d'un seul et même acte, tandis que pour Galien il s'agit deux actes distincts, bien qu'ils soient analogues, parallèles ou simultanés.

37 Galien, *Les passions*, pp. 40-41.

38 Ibid., p. 24.

UNE SYSTEMATISATION ORIGINALE

Dans le *De compescendis*, Luigi Luisini ordonne un ensemble relativement important de théories et de pratiques, d'*exempla* et de conseils à propos des passions de l'âme.[39] Il le fait en s'appuyant sur une méthode déjà utilisée dans l'étude d'une passion particulière comme la colère[40] ou de maladies comme la mélancolie ou le mal d'amour.[41] Sa dette intellectuelle à l'égard de Cicéron (*Tusculanes*, III-IV) et de Galien (*Les passions et les erreurs de l'âme* et *Les facultés de l'âme suivent les tempéraments des corps*) est immense. Le traité tout entier repose sur le raisonnement suivant : puisque les passions de l'âme causent de nombreuses affections corporelles et qu'elles peuvent être neutralisées par la philosophie morale, on peut donc se servir de la philosophie morale pour agir efficacement contre les affections corporelles causées par les passions de l'âme. Le traitement médical classique contre les effets morbides des passions était fondé sur une hygiène de vie, une pharmacopée et éventuellement une intervention chirurgicale (la saignée) adaptées au tempérament du patient. En effet, les passions de l'âme agissent sur le corps comme un poison. A la manière d'un poison, elles corrompent les humeurs, perturbent plus ou moins gravement la complexion individuelle et engendrent des maladies corporelles.[42] Pour Luisini, la philosophie morale en est le contrepoison naturel ainsi que le vaccin *ante litteram*. Le traitement « philosophique » doit *a fortiori* précéder le traitement médical, comme la cause précède l'effet. *Per moralem philosophiam* le médecin cherche à agir sur les causes profondes (liées au contexte socio-culturel de l'individu) des maladies de l'âme dans l'espoir de renforcer l'action des remèdes médicaux et de traiter le patient de manière globale. L'entrelacement de médecine et philosophie atteint des sommets. Pour le mettre en exergue, nous allons présenter brièvement la structure de l'œuvre avant d'étudier de façon détaillée la notion d'erreur et le traitement de quelques passions particulières.

Dans le premier livre, Luisini s'attache à définir et à légitimer son propos ainsi que la méthode utilisée. Il fonde la légitimité et la finalité de la médecine sur sa conception de la dignité de l'homme. En raison de sa double nature, céleste et terrestre, l'homme se tourne vers la contemplation (ciel) et vers l'action (terre). De même que les corps inférieurs (terrestres) imitent les corps supérieur (soleil,

39 Nous traduisons *affectus* par « passion » parce que les termes « affection », « affect » ou « état d'âme » pourraient prêter à confusion. Nous nous conformons ainsi à une tradition médico philosophique bien établie depuis le XVIe siècle.

40 Cf. J. Fillion-Lahille, *Le « De Ira » de Sénèque et la philosophie stoïcienne des passions*, Paris 1984.

41 Cf. Galien, *De la bile noire*, trad. fr., introduction et notes par V. Barras, T. Birchler et A.-F. Morand, Paris 1998 ; M. F. Wack, *Lovesicknes in the Middle Ages*, Philadelphia 1990, pp. 3-30.

42 Luisini, *De compescendis*, « dedicatio », p. 3r-v : « Quae vero in humoribus aggregentur venena in corporum perniciem ob animi affectus, quibus omnes solutis (ut aiunt) habenis nunc inserviunt, cum alioqui summopere ab his cavendum sit, cuiusmodi sunt hæc ira, furor, invidia, metus, tristitia, neminem profecto esse, quem lateat, puto. ».

lune et étoiles), de même les actions humaines doivent se modeler sur les visions intellectuelles et les passions sur la raison.[43] La *dignitas hominis* réside dans le bon usage de la faculté rationnelle, qui marque la supériorité de l'homme sur le reste de la Création. Le médecin doit être lui-même disciple et imitateur de la nature (*naturæ famulus et æmulator*)[44], d'une nature ordonnée de façon telle que les passions font allégeance à la raison. L'ordre naturel est bon et sain. Il est donc naturel et salutaire pour un homme d'utiliser l'énergie des passions pour suivre la « juste norme de vie » (*recta norma vivendi*) dictée par la raison. Il serait malsain de s'en écarter. Dans ce contexte, où la cosmologie sert de modèle pour l'anthropologie et pour l'éthique, le savoir et l'art du médecin visent essentiellement à rétablir l'ordre naturel.[45]
Pour atteindre un bon état de santé général, il ne suffit pas de prescrire de simples règles de conduite. Ce serait superficiel et inefficace. Il faut que le médecin et le patient travaillent de conserve sur leurs propres émotions à l'aide d'une discipline intérieure, pour faire en sorte que la partie rationnelle de l'âme devienne le véritable guide de leurs dispositions internes et de leurs comportements.[46] Luisini affirme dès les premières pages que non seulement la philosophie morale doit éclairer la conduite du médecin pour une plus grande efficacité du traitement, mais surtout qu'il est nécessaire de prescrire de nouvelles règles de gestion des passions comme on prescrit un régime adapté ou un remède pharmaceutique.

Il passe ensuite à la définition de l'*affectus animi* en soulignant que si dans le domaine de la rhétorique l'*affectus* représente le moment d'un discours où l'orateur cherche à émouvoir les juges,[47] la philosophie se sert des *affectus* pour la perfection de l'âme et la médecine pour la santé du corps.[48] Luisini fonde sa description des passions sur les définitions et classifications stoïciennes. Les positions des péripatéticiens seront étudiées dans un deuxième temps.[49]

Dans le sillon des analyses stoïciennes, la question des affections de l'âme relève de la physique des qualités. On doit pouvoir étudier n'importe quel *affectus* sous le prisme des quatre qualités fondamentales (chaud, froid, sec, humide). Mais

43 Luisini, *De compescendis*, p. 1 : « Si enim ratione utatur qua solus potest inter omnia animantia uti, inveniet profecto sese coelestis, terrestrisque participem esse naturae, duplicemque finem sortitum, speculationem nempe et actionem, ut illa inferiores hac vero superiores imitaretur naturas ».

44 Ibid., p. 3.

45 Cette représentation de l'ordre naturel puise à la philosophie de Pic de la Mirandole et plus généralement à l'Hermétisme de la Renaissance. Cf. E. Garin, *L'Ermetismo del Rinascimento*, Rome 1988 (trad. fr. par B. Schefer, Paris 2001).

46 Comme chez Galien, la notion d'exercice (*askêsis* ou *exercitium*) revient très souvent. Cf. M. Foucault, *Histoire de la sexualité II, L'usage des plaisirs*, Paris 1984, p. 97-105.

47 Luisini, *De compescendis*, p. 14 : « Affectus significant partem illam perorationis, in qua orator conatur movere iudicum animos ».

48 Ibid. : « Sed nos de affectibus instituimus agere, non ad persuadendum, ut Rhetores, sed ad animi perfectionem, ut Philosophi, et ad corporis sanitatem, ut Medici ».

49 Ibid., p. 15 : « Utamus tamen in his describendis affectibus Stoicorum definitionibus, et partitionibus, qui mihi videntur in hac quaestione uberrime versari, postea et quid sentiant de his Peripatetici, videbimus ».

qu'est-ce qu'est précisément un *affectus* ? Pour le définir, Luisini reprend les termes du philosophe Zénon : « *Affectio* (*pathos* inquit ipse) *est aversa a recta ratione contra naturam animi commotio* »[50] et de Galien, qui souscrit à la définition de Zénon tout en ajoutant qu'une passion est un mouvement de l'âme qui désobéit à la raison.[51] Ainsi le définit-il comme un mouvement intérieur qui trouble l'équilibre naturel de l'âme.

L'*affectus* s'oppose à la *ratio*. Il en est, à certains égards, l'ennemi naturel. C'est un mouvement intérieur toujours accompagné d'un jugement (*opinio*) qui peut être bon ou mauvais, tourné vers le présent ou bien vers le futur.[52] Les quatre passions fondamentales sont la joie (*laetitia*) et le désir (*libido*) immodérés, la tristesse (*aegritudo*) et la peur (*metus*). En fonction de l'objet sur lequel elles s'exercent, ainsi que de leur intensité, elles génèrent des passions subsidiaires. La joie se décline en malveillance (*laetans alieno malo*), plaisir (*delectatio*) et vantardise (*iactatio*) ; le désir, en colère (*ira*), susceptibilité (*excandescentia*), haine (*odium*), inimitié (*inimicitia*), discorde (*discordia*) et besoin insatiable (*indigentia*) ; la tristesse, en envie (*invidia*), jalousie (*aemulatio*), tendance à dénigrer (*obtrectatio*), pitié (*misericordia*), angoisse (*angor*), chagrin (*luctus*), affliction (*moeror*), peine (*aerumna*), douleur (*dolor*), lamentation (*lamentatio*), inquiétude (*sollicitudo*), accablement (*molestia*), detresse (*afflictatio*) et désespoir (*desperatio*) ; la peur, en paresse (*pigritia*), pudeur (*pudor*), terror (*terreur*), crainte (*timor*), effroi (*pavor*), épouvante (*exanimatio*), affolement (*conturbatio*), frayeur (*formido*). Cette classification des passions de l'âme permet à Luisini de structurer le deuxième livre. Mais par-delà la multiplicité de leurs manifestations, les différentes passions s'abreuvent toutes à la même source : l'intempérance. Cette dernière constitue leur substrat psychophysiologique, leur réservoir énergétique d'élection. Un individu tempérant demeure impassible lorsqu'il se juge plus pauvre que son frère, tandis que le même jugement (*opinio*) pourrait produire un *affectus* (l'envie) dévastateur chez l'intempérant. L'intempérance est une disposition, une fragilité physique et mentale qui rend les individus vulnérables aux passions. Le médecin peut aider l'intempérant à lutter contre ses dispositions hautement pathogènes grâce à la philosophie morale et à l'art médical, les deux disciplines étant complémentaires.[53]

50 Luisini, *De compescendis*, p. 15.

51 Ibid. : « […] animi motum, rationi non obedientem ».

52 Ibid. : « Quoniam vero omnis affectus est animi motus vel rationis expers, vel rationem aspernans, vel rationi non obediens, isque motus aut boni aut mali opinione citatur tam praesentis quam futuri, bifariam quatuor affectus aequaliter distributi sunt. Duo enim sunt ex opinione boni, utpote vel [p. 16] praesentis, vel futuri : totidem ex opinione mali, similiter vel praesentis, vel futuri. Affectus ex opinione boni praesentis laetitia est, futuri vero libido. Affectus autem ex opinione mali praesentis aegritudo est, futuri vero metus : quae enim venientia metuuntur, eadem efficiunt ægritudinem instantia ».

53 Ibid., p. 17 : « Omnium porro affectuum fontem esse dicunt intemperantiam, quae est a tota mente, & a recta ratione defectio, sic aversa a praescriptione rationalis, ut nullo modo appetitiones animi nec regi, nec contineri queant. Inflammat haec, conturbat, incitat omnem animi statum inimica temperantia […] ; sic conturbatus animus ab intemperantia, non est aptus ad

Sur un point Luisini s'éloigne des stoïciens (Chrysippe) pour suivre Aristote : les *affectus* ne sont pas *contra naturam.* Ils sont naturels et innés (*ingenitos nobis*).[54] Les passions de l'âme sont neutres, car, prises par elles-mêmes, elles ne sont ni des vices ni des vertus.[55] En effet, quatre arguments montrent le caractère neutre des passions. Premièrement, les passions ne déterminent pas notre bonté ni notre méchanceté, ce sont les vices et les vertus. Deuxièmement, c'est la manière dont un *affectus* se manifeste qui peut être considérée comme blâmable ou pas, vertueuse ou vicieuse. Troisièmement, nous ne choisissons pas les passions, nous choisissons les vertus. Pour finir, les passions créent une disposition (en puissance) et non pas un mouvement (en acte) de l'âme et du corps.[56] Sur ce point, Luisini se range donc du coté d'Aristote et de Galien, mais contre Cicéron : les passions étant innées, il est impossible de les éradiquer. On peut toutefois les modérer grâce à la *ratio*.[57]

Partant de ces prémisses, Luisini définit le périmètre et le but de l'ouvrage : l'étude analytique des passions susceptibles d'altérer considérablement l'état de santé, la prévention de l'excès des passions et la cure de ses effets.[58]

Le deuxième livre est le plus long des trois. Luisini donne une définition de chaque *affectus*. Il analyse les principales passions de l'âme en les décrivant minutieusement sous des angles différents, par la description de l'action des organes et des humeurs puis des esprits et des facultés naturelles. L'étude des causes « proches », comme le tempérament individuel ou l'influence de la nourriture et des boissons, précède généralement celle des causes « lointaines », c'est-à-dire les habitudes de vie, le milieu social et l'éducation reçue. Mais la principale originalité du *De compescendis* consiste à consacrer des sections entières à la manière d'éviter et de traiter les ravages d'une passion singulière (*modus praeservandi et*

exsequendum munus suum ; munus enim animi est ratione bene uti ; atque ob id in morbos incidit ».

54 Luisini, *De compescendis*, p. 18 : « Zeno vocet affectus animi commotiones contra naturam, Aristoteles contra, Peripateticorum princeps, testatur (Ethica, II, 5), eos neque virtutes esse, neque vitia ; quorum quia neutrum naturale est, eoque neutrum a natura inest nobis, ob id velle illum sic loquentem tenendum est, affectus naturales esse, et ingenitos nobis ».

55 Sur l'histoire du concept de « neutrum », cf. M. Van der Lugt, « Neither ill nor healthy – The intermediate state between health and disease in medieval medicine », dans *Quaderni storici*, 136 (2011), p. 13-46.

56 Luisini, *De compescendis*, p. 18-19 : « Primum quidem, quia secundum eos [affectus] non dicimur boni vel mali ; secundum virtutes autem et vitia dicimur. Deinde quia secundum affectus nec laudamur, nec vituperamur, non enim laudatur (inquit ipse) qui timet aut irascitur, sed qui certo modo ; at secundum virtutes et vitia laudamur et vituperamur. Tertio quoniam affectus sunt in nobis sine electione, virtutes autem electiones quaedam sunt vel non sine electione. Demum vero quo secundum affectus moveri dicimur, sed secundum virtutes et vitia non moveri, sed certo modo dispositi nuncupamur ».

57 Ibid., p. 20 : « Rectius itaque tenendum cum Peripateticis affectus innatos nobis esse, neque evelli omnino posse, sed posse resecari : licet enim primi motus affectuum in manu ac potestate nostra minime sint, adest tamen moderatrix illorum paullo post ratio ».

58 Ibid., p. 25 : « Quoniam igitur magni admodum sunt affectus momenti ad corporis humani valetudinem, atque aegritudinem, facturos operae pretium nos arbitramur. Si tractatum de his, [...] ut quomodo praeservari ab his possit et curari doceamus ».

curandi animi affectus) premièrement à l'aide de la philosophie morale (*per moralem philosophiam*), puis par l'art médical (*per medendi artem*). Luisini met en avant la nécessité d'accompagner systématiquement le traitement physique des maladies par un traitement moral s'inspirant ouvertement de la philosophie stoïcienne (Chrysippe, Cicéron et Galien). Les remèdes et le régime renforcent l'action de la philosophie morale, conçue comme une thérapie de l'âme, et vice-versa. Dans l'étude aussi bien que dans le traitement de toutes les passions, les approches morales et médicales sont pour Luisini incontournables et complémentaires.

Dans le troisième livre, Luisini étudie les passions particulières provoquées par l'usage d'un remède ou par l'idée même de devoir recourir à un remède.[59] Chez l'individu sain ou malade, les traitements médicaux peuvent susciter tout un monde de représentations mentales et de passions bien réelles qui influencent l'état de santé et les décisions du patient. D'où l'intérêt de développer jusqu'à la fin de l'ouvrage toute une batterie d'arguments imparables pour préférer les soins médicaux des professionnels aux caprices du hasard et de l'automédication. Cela devient un prétexte pour se livrer à une véritable apologie de l'art médical, notamment de la thérapeutique. Les remèdes sont nécessaires en raison de la faiblesse de la nature du corps humain à l'égard des maladies (*ratione humani corporis suapte natura imbecillis, ægrotabilisque*). Ils sont utiles, parce qu'ils permettent de préserver la dignité du patient (*dignitas subjecti*) et qu'ils lui rendent la vie plus agréable.[60] La majorité des gens se servent avantageusement des remèdes médicinaux (*a maiori sumptum*). Et si même les animaux, qui sont dominés par leurs instincts naturels (*solo naturali instinctu regatur*), ont leur propre médecine naturelle, pourquoi les hommes, qui sont doués d'intellect (*intellectus*), ne devraient pas s'en servir ? Les histoires paradigmatiques (*exempla*) de l'Antiquité attestent bien l'utilité des remèdes.

Par ailleurs, Luisini insiste sur l'importance des croyances personnelles et collectives dans la prise en charge d'un malade. La foi dans le déterminisme astral, notamment, peut rendre la mort acceptable à celui qui y adhère et soulager la souffrance physique et morale. De plus, si les perturbations de l'âme troublent et gâtent les humeurs,[61] certains, ajoute-t-il, recouvrent la santé grâce à une forme particulière de crainte : la peur d'aller voir le médecin. Ils expulsent ainsi des maux passés et futurs. D'autres redoutent l'autorité du médecin et ses manières brutales ou « tyranniques » à un point tel que leurs humeurs se corrompent et la santé

59 Luisini, *De compescendis*, p. 144 : « Id porro est animi affectus quidam in sanis, et aegris circa remediorum usum, quae illis vel praeservandi, vel curandi causa exhibentur a medico : et tria sunt, diaeta, pharmacum, phlebotomia. ».

60 Ibid., p.153 : « Haec ergo utilitas est, vita inquam et vitae commoda, medicinalius remediorum ».

61 Ibid., p. 145 : « Incusant anim aliqui astra, quae ad tantum eos infortunium impulerint, ut ea sibi toleranda sint, quibus mors ipsa levior sit. Nonnulli suam in ante acta vita intemperantiam, imprudentiam, ec temeritatem arguunt, quod multos et pravos humores coacervarint, quod non eo se perventuros praeviderint ».

s'empire.[62] L'attention est concentrée sur les stratégies argumentatives à mettre en œuvre pour vaincre la résistance du patient afin de mieux le convaincre de l'utilité de la médecine. On pourrait considérer ce troisième livre comme un traité d'éducation thérapeutique *ante litteram*.

En conclusion, Luigi Luisini a relevé le défi de présenter une médecine de l'âme offrant l'analyse et le traitement philosophique des passions au même temps que leur analyse et traitement médical. Le *De compescendis* est fort probablement le premier traité moderne entièrement consacré à l'étude systématique de toutes les passions de l'âme.[63] Luisini semble être parfaitement conscient de sa propre originalité.[64] Même un médecin et homme de lettres aussi érudit que Gabriel Naudé le considère comme le premier traité sur les pathologies des passions de l'âme.[65] Bien qu'il ne puisse pas être considéré comme un novateur en médecine ni en philosophie, Luisini introduit dans le discours savant sur les maladies, provoquées ou guéries par les émotions, une approche interdisciplinaire promise à un grand avenir.

62 Luisini, *De compescendis* : « Sunt et qui medicorum severitatem, atque crudelitatem arguant, tanquam lenius hi possent, si velint, vel praesentes, vel futuros morbos expellere, quem vel per pharmacum, vel per diaetam, vel per phlebotomiam, quae tamen imperatorio quodam, atque adeo tyrannico modo, sibi institui conqueruntur, ut nisi aequo animo ea perferas, actum omnino de vita habeas. Ex quo postea animi affectu, tumultuve fit, ut corporis humores maxima exagitatione circumvoluantur, summaque ebullitione conflictentur... ».

63 Cette idée nous est suggérée, entre autres, par la consultation du catalogue de la BNF. La cote T-65 rassemble chronologiquement 211 ouvrages sur le traitement moral et médical des maladies de l'âme, dont la folie, du milieu XVIe au début du XXe siècle. Le premier titre de la liste est bien le *De compescendis* (1562).

64 Luisini, *De compescendis*, 1713 (1562^{1}), « dedicatio », p. 5r-v : « Unum illud minime praetereundum censeo, neminem adhuc neque inter Graecos neque inter Arabos, neque inter Latinos, inventum fuisse, qui ad illud tractandum hoc pacto accesserit, cuius extent monumenta, neque enim ignoro, paucula quaedam obiter a nonnullis tradita esse de compescendis animi affectibus, ab aliis etiam de industria, inter quos Galenus fuit, cuius tamen quaecunque de cognoscendis curandisque animi morbis scripta fuere, uno duntaxat capite a nobis comprehensa sunt. ».

65 G. Naudé, *Bibliographia politica*, Venise 1633, pp. 16-17 : « Pathologiam praeterea animi passionum Germanus aliquis non ita pridem edidit, cuius nomen cum suo libro Parisiis discedens reliqui ; sed eadem materiam prius absoluerat Altisius [sic !] Lusinus elegantissimo opusculo de compescendis animi perturbationibus, & Iustus Lipsius libello de Constantia… ».

EARLY MODERN MEDICAL ETHICS AND MEDICAL HUMOR

Winfried Schleiner

My subject is humor that involves physicians and curing in the early modern period. I take 'humor' in the modern sense, not the humoral one, although both senses are of course related. The topic touches on, and even overlaps with medical ethics, because (first) even in that period physicians thought about the place of humor at the patient's bedside or more generally in curing and because (second) most physicians qua humanists would have agreed that a cure is difficult if the physician considers his patient laughable or ridiculous. Writers like Poggio and Rabelais unquestionably belong to the core of early modern humanists. I have drawn on major Italian and French joke collections such as Orazio Toscanella, *I motti, le facie* (1561), Arlotto Mainardi's *Fazetie* (1565), Poggio's jokes, which circulated in Italian and French translations, collections by Giles Corrozet (1544 and 1603) and Abel Boyer (1700), but also on medical books, and finally also on such books of imaginative literature as those by Rabelais and Cervantes. What role laughter has in curing was of intense interest to the Portuguese physician Roderigo a Castro, who wrote the first extensive book on medical ethics (1614) and to the French physician Laurent Joubert, who devoted an entire book to the subject of laughter, *Le traité du ris* (1579). With the question of what is laughable or causes humor (which Joubert asks and discusses), we are approaching aspects of the topic that are particularly interesting to a new historical consideration of humor, because the question points to the nexus between humor and culture and to changes occurring over time as to what can be laughed at.

After a brief glance at an early modern justification of humor in curing, I will survey verbal humor at the patient's bedside, humor resulting from misunderstanding of medical jargon or medical euphemisms, and humor based on an early modern understanding of the relationship of medicine to other healing professions. Then I will highlight humor based on some specific by-gone notions of medicine, and finally survey humor that for many reasons would now be labeled politically incorrect: because of degrading views of the disabled and offensive notions of gender or of race.

In his treatise on laughter,[1] Joubert asks what good comes from laughter and whether a sick person can be healed by it. To demonstrate that one can, he tells three monkey stories, stories in which patients are healed by the amusement of seeing their monkey act in some way imitating human or even medical action. In the first, the monkey gets hold of a medication a physician has left for the patient,

1 L. Joubert, *Le traité du ris*, bk. 3, ch. 14, Paris 1579.

who observes him drinking it slowly and making faces as he appreciates its bitterness and sweetness. In the second, a man who has lost his speech gains it back by watching his monkey trying to handle the bedpan with the urine the way the physician had done. He puts it on the fire, inspects the contents, but drops the pan because of its hot rim.[2] The third, located in Montpellier, tells of a doctor of law, who is single, seemingly dying, and served by people who are waiting for his demise. As the monkey watches these servants grabbing what they can, it gets hold of the furred red hood that its master had worn on solemn occasions and puts it on. The patient is so amused that he recovers his health. In his *Medicus-Politicus* (1614) Rodrigo a Castro argues that raunchy jokes do not agree with the desirable image of the serious and prudent physician, but to make the point that mild humor is part of the physician's desirable bed-side manners, he tells the presumably admirable case of a Spanish physician, who (to give more emphasis to his medical forecast that the patient's fever would end) said to the patient that if his forecast was correct and the fever disappeared, he would accept a certain silver dish, in Spanish called *plato*. The next day, when touching the patient's arm, he realized that his forecast had been wrong, he said: "Socrates is my friend, Plato is my friend," and as he touched the attractive silver dish with his finger, he added: "But a greater friend is truth".[3] While the wordplay is only possible in Spanish, reverting to Spanish in the context of a medical work in Latin also authenticates the story. Although I am tempted to do so, I will resist the temptation to argue that this story relates to Carpi's accusation that Zerbi purloined two vases from a bishop who was his patient.[4]

Speech, the medical professional's control of a situation by language or the lack of understanding of euphemistic medical language by the uninitiated, is often the source of medical humor. Of course, just like the stories built on puns, these jokes do not translate. *Le courrier facétieux* (1653) gives the case of a spectator injured at a *jeu de paume* or tennis game: a ball hits him on the eye as he watches the game from below the gallery. In pain and also fearing for his sight, he asks the surgeon: "Monsieur, dites-moy ie vous prie, mon oeil est-il perdu? Non, non, Monsieur, repondit le Chirurgien, n'apprehendez rien de ce costé-là, il n'a garde d'estre perdu, ie le tiens dans ma main."[5]

Perhaps this is a bad joke, a joke of bad taste in the early modern as in the modern period, just as bad or regrettable as Marcantonio dalla Torre's remark on his former anatomy teacher Zerbi. According to Giovio, Dalla Torre joked that Zerbi's death (he supposedly was hacked to pieces by the Turks) was a fitting punishment for misleading his students "by cutting up cadavers incorrectly".[6]

In *Le courrier facétieux* there is the story of a physician who asks whether the medication he has prescribed recently has had its effect: "La medicine que ie luy

2 This story is retold in the collection *Le courrier facétieux* , Lyon 1653, p. 296.
3 R. a Castro, *Medicus-Politicus*, bk. 4, ch. 8, Hamburg 1614, p. 250.
4 J. Berengario da Carpi, *Commentaria* [...] *super anatomia Mundini*, Bologna 1521, fol. 17v.
5 *Le courrier facétieux*, p. 69.
6 P. Giovio, *Elogia*, Basel 1577, p. 86.

ay fait bailer, l'a-t-elle bien fait aller du ventre?" using what is most likely a euphemism for 'having one's stool'. The servant, identified as a Gascon, (perhaps willfully) does not understand and replies: "Comme voulez-vous que mon Maistre aille du ventre, il ne sçauroit se soutenir des pieds!"[7] In another anecdote, when the physician requests that the patient's urine be brought for inspection, the servant is not familiar with the word and asks whether he means the *pissat*, a word at which the physician bristles: "Il ne faut pas dire ainsi; c'est que vous m'apportiez de l'eau qu'il a fait." But the servant, naïve or beholden to his direct or non-euphemistic language, argues: "How can I do that if he only drinks wine?"[8]

Witty repartee in some medical anecdotes may rely on specific principles of Renaissance medicine, abandoned longtime ago and little known today. When Henri IV hears that a famous Protestant physician has converted to Roman Catholicism, he says to the Duc de Sully, who happens to be with him: "Mon ami, ta Religion est bien malade, car elle est abandonee des Medecins."[9] Here Henri IV speaks as a Catholic (it is well known that he converted to become King of France – "Paris vaut bien une messe") and one may easily deduce that Sully is a Protestant. The wit of the king's comment, however, relies on the addressee and the reader knowing that according to ancient and Renaissance medical ethics physicians were supposed to abandon the incurable or dying – not as a cowardly escape but as an ethical act.

Sometimes the ineptness of physicians is the source of humor, as in the story of the physician who prepared in advance his prescriptions and doled them out haphazardly, saying: "Prega Dio te la mandi buona." (May God have it help you.)[10] Like Rodrigo a Castro in his anecdote about Spanish *plato*, so the Florentine Poggio here gives these words in the 'vulgar' tongue.

In general, early modern medical jokes show the physician at the apex of the medical profession – not uncontestedly, but rivalry of others becomes the source of humor, i. e. is laughable. Abel Boyer tells the story (derived from Poggio) of a physician who has his mule treated by a farrier (French *maréchal*). After the second visit by the farrier, the physician puts some thirty *sous* into his hand. But the farrier returns the money, saying: "Monsieur, nous ne prenons jamais d'argent de ceux de notre profession".[11] Certainly in Europe – and possibly even in the US – there are remnants of the custom that physicians treat each other (including family members) without charge. The medical humor lies in the farrier's attempt to use this custom to elevate his status to the imaginary level of one health profession combining human and veterinary medicine.

Barber surgeons seem at the beck and call of the physicians and work under their guidance, as in the following story told by Orazio Toscanella. Assaulted by a

7 *Le courrier facétieux*, p. 199. The physician asks whether the medication made the patient 'go' *du ventre* (with his belly). The servant replies: "How would you that my master go with his belly; he would not be able to keep himself up with his feet!"

8 Ibid., p. 352.

9 A. Boyer, *Le compagnon sage et ingénieux*, London 1700, p. 140.

10 G. F. Poggio Bracciolini, *Les facéties de Pogge*, II, no. 203, Paris 1878, pp. 168–169.

11 Boyer, *Compagnon*, p. 140.

large crowd of sick people, and unable to get rid of them, a famous physician, a specialist in curing reeking sores, calls all the barbers he can find to come and display their razors. He tells the sick people that he would flay one person from head to foot, soak that person's skin in a special liquor he has, and then put it on the others one after the other, to cure them all. They should determine by lot who would be the first. One after the other, the sick people leave in silence.[12] My interest in the story is to show that the barbers are presented as willing participants in something like a stage-play organized by the physician as stage-manager. If there is humor here, it is not so easily identified, except that the at first so pressing patients are shown to be timorous and self-centered.

What is most interesting to the cultural historian is of course the kind of humor that is dated, that in some way makes us uncomfortable, because it rests on different notions of disability, race, or gender. I begin with a story that is almost modern, almost, but not quite, of a man who, after losing his eyesight in an accident, simply says: "J'ai fait un grand gain; car premierement i'allois seul, maintenant i'auray tousiours compagnie."[13] This good cheer is so exaggerated that it seems to turn into naïveté or even foolishness.

According to Renaissance medical theory, one kind of the condition that was called melancholy was caused by a diseased or injured imagination.[14] The cure called upon an imaginative physician, who would cure the imagination by the imagination. One list of such cures by the famous French physician André du Laurens is prefaced by identifying the following case as the most laughable or ridiculous – a classification of course unimaginable in modern medical discourse: the medical author tells the case of a man who refused to urinate because he feared that, when he did, he would flood the world. Unless he was persuaded somehow to relieve himself, he was going to die within a few days. The inventive physician had a neighboring house set on fire, had the church bells be rung and servants cry "to the fire!". He also had some city officials entreat him to save the city; people would die unless he would help with his unusual prowess. According to the Renaissance translation, they asked

12 O. Toscanella, *I motti, le facetie, argutie, burle*, Venedig 1561, fol. 32v–33: "Assalito un giorno da una turba grandissima d'infermi certo Medico dottissimo, che aveva curato infinita sorte de piaghe fetenti, et altre infermità pericolosissime; & non potendosili staccare dattorno in modo alcuno; mandò a chiamare quanti barbieri erano nella terra; e fece loro portare alla presenza di quegli infermi molti rasoi, poi voltatosi a gl'infermi, disse; fratelli s'io voglio guarivi, conviene, ch'io faccia scorticare uno di voi da capo a piedi; & bagnata quella pelle di certo licore, ch'io tengo; la ponga adosso de gli altri d'un in uno, & cosi risanarete: Mettete le sorte tra voi a chi tocca essere scorticato; & non dimorate più. Ciò vedendo gl'infermi, senza altra riposte l'un dietro l'altro partirono."

13 *Le courrier facétieux*, p. 27: "I have gained a lot. For before, I went alone; now I will always have company."

14 See my *Melancholy, Genius and Utopia in the Renaissance*, Wiesbaden 1991, particularly the subsection "Laesa imaginatio", pp. 98–108. The best source of information on what kind of (usually Galenic) medicine was taught at European and particularly Italian universities are the various books by Nancy Siraisi.

> that he should pisse quicklie and quench the fire. Then this sillie melancholike man which abstained from pissing for feare of loosing his towne, taking it for granted, that it was now in great hazard, pissed and emptied his bladder of all that was in it, and was himself by that means preserved.[15]

It is well known that much of Cervantes' *Don Quijote* is built on the principle of *laesa imaginatio* and cure by the imagination. In the process, the characters about Don Quijote enter into his fiction of medieval knighthood and romance, and they play-act, often ostensibly to cure him. Although thus much of humor in this novel is medical humor, it is at present too large a topic for me to broach. Instead I want to mention one of his *Novelas ejemplares*, the story of Rueda who believes that his body is of glass, clearly a case of what was called melancholy. Cervantes scholars have suggested that Cervantes knew the case of a Parisian who believed he was of glass, a case, however, not recorded in print until 1622 by Alphonso Ponce Santacruz.[16] I will resist entering in the debate, which has been conducted elsewhere, and would only like to point out how differently any humor in the story of the Parisian psychiatric case, if there is any humor at all, is located.[17] Seemingly to ease the patient's fears of shattering his limbs, his physician beds him on straw. But one day the physician has the straw set afire and has the only door of escape locked. Fearing for his life, the patient pounds against the door with his fists but is not let out until he acknowledges that, since his fists do not shatter, his body is not of glass.

If there is humor here, it is overshadowed by cruelty, at least for the modern reader. I mention the medical case only to show that Cervantes was possibly ahead of all the physicians of his time. For the focus of his story of Rueda, the man of glass or Licenciado Vidriera, is different. Cervantes is not interested in cure – Rueda is cured by a charitable monk, we do not learn how. The focus of the story is the cruelty of the inhabitants of Salamanca, young and old, who for their amusement follow the man of glass around to laugh at his pithy sentences and throw stones at him to see him wince. Cervantes shifts the focus of 'humor' and has laughter and amusement be part of an indictment of cruelty.

In the story of Rueda (as in that of *Don Quijote*), humor derives from the reversal of the perspectives of madness and sanity. Rueda loses his ability to coin pithy retorts after he is healed, and in *Don Quijote* many characters regret when in

15 A. du Laurens, *A Discourse of the Preservation of Sight. Of Melancholike Disease, of Rheumes, and of Old Age*, transl. by R. Surphlet, London 1599, p. 103. The french ed. is of Paris 1597. See also the section "The laughable psychotic", in: *Melancholy, Genius, and Utopia in the Renaissance*, pp. 145–147, where the entire case is quoted. It should be said that du Laurens was far from a benighted traditionalist, but was possibly the first physician to critique what has come to be called the 'one-sex model'. See my "Early Modern Controversies About the One-sex Model", *Renaissance Quarterly* 53 (2000), pp. 180–191.

16 A. Ponce Santacruz, *Dignotio et cura affectuum melancholicorum*, Madrid 1622, p. 16. The first scholar to call this medical case to the attention of Cervantes scholars was S. Rivera Manescau, "El modelo del Licenciado Vidriera", in: *IV Centenario de Miguel de Cervantes*, Valladolid 1947, pp. 1–11.

17 See my essay "The Glass Graduate and the Aphrodisiac That Went Wrong. New Light from Old Texts", *Forum for Modern Language Studies* 27 (1991), pp. 370–381.

the end the ingenious melancholic is healed of his delusions. The reversal of the wisdom-folly distinction is of course an early modern commonplace, sometimes (as in the case of Cervantes) supported by the pseudo-Aristotelian Problem XXX,1 and sometimes fleshed out with specific details of treating the insane. Abel Boyer's collection includes the story, deriving from Poggio, of some melancholics or madmen who in the yard of a famous physician are forced to stand in water the depth of which indicates the degree of their insanity. Those who are raving mad are in water up to their chin. (Of course Galenic medicine cures by opposites: the melancholic humor was considered 'dry'.) Each patient is tied to a post.[18] One of them who has been almost healed in this way and is allowed to roam about in the yard looks through the gate and sees a nobleman riding by, with a falcon on his fist and trailed by his dogs. The inmate asks what is the purpose of all this gear and receives the answer that it is to kill certain game. The patient now wants to know what the game he brings home in a year is worth and learns that its price is about nine or ten pounds. Then he insists to know what the yearly upkeep of all the hunting gear costs the nobleman. The answer is four hundred pounds. "Le Malade entendant cela lui dit de s'en aller au plus vite, si son salut lui étoit cher; Car, dit-il, si notre Maitre vient, et vous trouve ici, il vous metra asurément dans son creux avec les Foux jusqu'au Menton."[19]

The cruelty of the treatment of the insane, tying them up and submerging them, is particularly striking to the modern reader. The academic and non-aristocratic perspective on hunting, however, basis for the comic reversal, is more acceptable and less striking than before – and possibly also less comic.

It might be argued that my one example of medical humor in relationship to race is misplaced, since it may not involve race in the modern sense at all, but it is striking none the less. The anecdote from the Spanish physician Juan de San Juan ultimately highlights the difference between a Renaissance understanding of what is a Jew from a modern one. It is from a period of renewed efforts to expel from Portugal and Spain not only Jews but all converts, for fear that they might be Marranos. The context is a discussion of the question whether Jews are the world's best physicians (possibly still because of the effects of the manna the Israelites were fed in the desert?) and whether Egypt is the region most suitable for developing the imagination. Thus the passage relates to what recently has been called philo-Judaism (or Judeophilia), rather than philo-semitism, although it might be argued that, if one were to take seriously Huarte's notion of basing the Jewish physicians' superiority in food consumed by the tribe, the term philo-semitism might apply.[20] From such philo-semitism, the focus in this anecdote shifts to the

18 The water treatment may have been rationalized by the notion that in the Galenic humoral system melancholy was considered cold and dry. For this story, see Poggio, *Les facéties*, I , no. 2, pp. 13–18; Boyer, *Compagnon*, p. 204.

19 Boyer, *Compagnon*, p. 206.

20 On the general context, see D. L. Graizbord, "Philosemitism in Late Sixteenth- and Seventeenth-Century Iberia. Refracted Judeophobia?", *Sixteenth Century Journal* 38 (2007), n. 3, pp. 657–682. Graizbord discusses these terms particularly on p. 657. He does not mention physicians.

French king's philo-Judaism. I am quoting from an Elizabethan translation of Huarte's *Examen de ingenios*:

> But the argument which most over-ruleth me in this behalfe, is that when Francis of Valois king of France, was molested by a long infirmitie, and saw that the Phisitians of his houshold and court, could yeeld him no remedy, he would say every time when his fever increased, It was not possible that any Christian Phisition could cure him, neither at their hands did he ever hope for recoverie: wherethrough one time agreeved to see himselfe thus vexed with his fever, he dispatched a post into Spaine, praieng the emperour Charles the fifth, that he would send him a Jew Phisition, the best of his court, touching whom he had understood, that he was able to yeeld him remedie for his sicknesse, if by art it might be effected. At this request the Spaniards made much game (La qual domanda fue harto reyda en España), and all of them concluded it was an humorous conceit of a man, whose brains were turmoiled with the fever. But for all this, the Emperour gave commandement that such a Phisition should be sought out, if anie there were, though to find him they should be driven to send out of his dominions; and when none could be met withall, he sent a Phisition newly made a Christian, supposing that he might serve to satsfie the kings humour. But the Phisition being arrived in France, and brought to the kings presence; there passed between them a gratious discourse, in which it appeared that the Phisition was a Christian: and therefore the king would receive no phisicke at his hands. The king with opinion which he had conceived of the phisition, that he was an Hebrue, by way of passing the time, asked him whether he were not as yet weary in looking for the Messias promised in the law? The phisition answered; Sir I expect not any Messias promised in the Jews law. You are verie wise in that (replied the king): for the tokens which were delivered in the divine scripture, whereby to know his comming, are all fulfilled manie daies ago. This number of daies (reioyned the phisition) we Christians do well reckon: for there are now finished 1542 yeares; in the end of which he died on the crosse, and the third day rose again, and afterwards ascended into heaven, where he now remaineth. Why then quoth the king you are a Christian? yea, Sir, by the grace of God, I am a Christian (quoth the phisition) then (answered the king) return you home to your own dwelling in good time: for in mine owne house and court I have Christian phisitions very excellent, and I held you for a Jew, who (in mine opinion) are those that have best naturall abilitie to cure my disease. After this maner he licenced him without once suffering him to feele his pulse, or see his state, or telling him one word of his griefe. And forthwith he sent to Constantinople for a Jew, who healed him with onely milke of the she Asse.[21]

To some extent the anecdote reveals the cleft between the inquisitorial culture in Spain and philo-Judaism. It also shows, like a modern sitcom by canned laughter, where its humor lies for the early modern reader, although the word humorous used by the translator in the phrase humorous conceit had of course a very different meaning. (It meant fanciful, fantastic or off-balance because of inordinate prevalence of one of the four humors.) But people at the Spanish court were clearly amused by the French king's request to send him a Jewish physician. Without overtly stating it, the text itself makes clear why: there could not be any Jewish physician at the court. The Emperor's order to look for one will specifically embrace the possibility or, rather, likelihood, that none will be found in his entire domain. Is it surprising that none came forth? Perhaps the French king's reaction

21 J. Huarte de San Juan, *The Examination of Mens Wits*, trans. by R[ichard] C[arew], London 1594, pp. 183–185. The Spanish is quoted from J. Huarte, *Examen de ingenios para las sciencias*, Huesca 1581, p. 229.

to the New Christian physician, who is not even allowed to feel his pulse, is also laughable, because naive, but it certainly is not racial. It has nothing to do with theories just mentioned as to why Jewish physicians were superior, notions one might call philo-semitic, but is based in philo-Judaism. The French king's categories are exclusively religious.

Medical humor relating to gender can be found frequently in the early modern period. But since my impression is that it is quite repetitive, I may restrict myself to just a few examples.

Poggio tells the story of a physician he calls «aussi avisé que ignorant» (just as crafty as ignorant), who asked that the urine of a lady he was treating be preserved and be brought to him. On the way to deliver it, the young female servant, a virgin, somehow spills it and substitutes her own. The physician diagnoses the woman's condition, which includes elevated temperature, as brought on by lack of sex – a diagnosis he does not reveal to her, but to her husband. Naturally she is surprised and even frightened when her husband has sex with her four times at night. The next day her fever is gone. "Ainsi la fraude dont le Médecin avait été la victime fut cause de la guérison."[22]

If the subtext of this story and the source of its humor is the notion that all women need or even crave sex and most of their ills will be healed by it, we are close to Rabelaisian medical humor. Writing about Rabelaisian humor, Ian Maclean, author of what is still one of the best books on early modern women, has suggested that the notion of female frigidity is a recent one.[23] Of course, Rabelais was a physician and wrote several times (for instance at the opening of the Quart Livre in the prefatory letter addressed to Odet, Cardinal de Chastillon) about his intent to trick the enemy (*tromper l'ennemi*) and bring his readers *alaigresse et consolation* by a work that should operate "comme une comédie".[24] Of prime interest for this topic are of course chapters 31 to 34 of the Tiers Livre dealing with the *question de marriage*: Panurge here consults his friends, including the physician Rondibilis (Guillaume Rondelet, a physician at Montpellier, was a friend of Rabelais') as to whether he should marry.

Over pages and pages, the discussion centers on what Rondibilis calls "coqüage", cuckoldry, and particularly the question whether it will be possible for Panurge to find a good-looking woman who will not be unfaithful to him. Of course this is the older, pre-modern, notion of marital unfaithfulness, which invariably is laughable as even the words *cuckoldry* and *cocuage* suggest. For reasons that involve ancient and early modern conceptions of the married woman essentially as property of her husband, a tragic view of the deceived husband does not

22 Poggio, *Les facéties*, I , no. 111, p. 237.

23 On the subject, see I. Maclean, "Dr. Rabelais's 500 Year Old Prescription. Laughter Really is the Best Medicine," *British Medical Journal* 308 (1994), pp. 803–804. The title of the book is *The Renaissance Notion of Woman. A Study in the Fortunes of Scholasticism and Medical Science in European Intellectual Life*, Cambridge 1980.

24 F. Rabelais, *Oeuvres complètes*, Paris 1940, p. 517.

develop until the modern period.[25] Dr. Rondibilis imagines a new deity *cocuage* that will be implored for protection and worshipped by worried husbands on the same day as the goddess Jealousy. Their sacrificial offerings that presumably would assure protection from the deity would be suspicion, doubt, distrust. Carpalim, one of participants in the discussion, laughs outright at the physician's remedy: "Ha, ha, ha" (dist Carpalim en riant). "Voilà un remede encores plus naïf que l'anneau de Hans Carüel."[26]

The ring of Hans Carüel is the remedy most readers of Rabelais remember. It is crude and comes up before in the Tiers Livre (ch. 28) as Panurge begins to ponder the advantages and disadvantages of marriage. The husband Hans had married a much younger wife and was tortured by the fear of being cuckolded. One night he dreams that the devil offers him a bargain: he will give him a ring for his finger, and as long as he wears it, he will not be cuckolded. Hans accepts bargain and ring. Pleased and excited, he wakes up and finds that he has his finger in his wife's vagina.[27]

This gendered humor is based on the notion that women are not only driven to sex, but driven to be unfaithful to their husband. Another attribute of women is that they speak too much. In the context of the *question de marriage*, one interlocutor remembers that they all used to play together a *morale comoedie* at Montpellier. In addition to Rabelais himself, seven participating actors are named, who have all been identified as his fellow students of medicine.[28] What was this comedy?

To illustrate how much fun they had, Epistemon, remembering that he was present when the play was performed, gives a brief synopsis. A husband is married to a wife who is mute. By intervention of a physician and a surgeon, she is given the ability to talk. In fact, she soon talks so much that the husband revisits the same physician to ask for a remedy that would silence her. The physician replies that there are in his art medications for making women talk, but none for making them stop talking. The only remedy would be for him to lose his hearing. The husband indeed decides to go that route and by some magic potions ("par ne sçay quelz charmes") has himself be made deaf. Once his wife realizes that he is deaf and her talking is in vain, she gets enraged (*enragée*). When the physician asks to be paid, the husband says that he cannot understand what he is saying, since he is deaf. In his irritation the physician throws on the man's back some powder, which has the effect of making him mad (*fol* or *fou*). Mad husband and

25 I cannot give the full evidence for this statement here. But it should be noted that the view, for instance, of King Marc as a tragic character (as he loses Isolde to Tristan) is a romantic one. One might argue that (from a diachronic perspective) the switch from ridiculous cuckold to tragic victim goes through the theme of cuckoldry that is only imagined, as in Shakespeare's *Othello*.

26 Rabelais, *Oeuvres complètes*, p. 458.

27 Rabelais, *Oeuvres complètes*, pp. 442–443. Rabelais uses an euphemism: «et [Hans] trouva qu'il avoit le doigt en comment a nom? de sa femme.»

28 V.-L. Saulnier, "Médecins de Montpellier au temps de Rabelais", *Bibliothèque d'Humanisme et Renaissance* 19 (1957), p. 443.

enraged wife now become allies again and beat up physician and surgeon. Epistemon remembers that he had never before laughed as much.

This slapstick play, real or only imagined, is in the tradition of the declamations of the ancient satirist Libanius, who describes how a misogynist character called Dyskolos ('peevish') applies for a licence to kill himself because of a talkative wife; and perhaps also in the tradition of Pietro Aretino's play *Il Marescalco* (*The Stablemaster*), a tradition that, after Rabelais, was to lead to Ben Jonson's *Epicene, or The Silent Woman* as its finest example.[29] Although the humor in all such works relies on hallowed stereotypes of women, Rabelais's version seems to be the most 'medical' in what the physician does and does not do. He declares himself unable to do something about the wife's talkativeness. Is this a comic weakness of the art of medicine in the face of woman's nature or is it adherence to the physician's axiomatic and Hippocratic "Do no harm"? Perhaps it is both. One comic reversal consists in the physician's finally forgetting the maxim once payment becomes an issue: in an act of vindictiveness, he throws a powder at the husband that makes him mad. In a final reversal, *fou* and *enragée* together beat up physician and surgeon, whom they leave 'half dead' (*à demy mors*).

To call early modern medical humor Renaissance humor is not redundant verbiage. Like the academic medicine of the period, its medical humor harkens back to antiquity, with its prescriptions about the comportment of physicians (who should have *prudentia* and *gravitas*) and, most importantly, with its notions of hierarchy. These involve the physician's relationship to the other health professions and notions about gender and male-female relationships. Not surprisingly classical notions of sanity are linked to the classical ideals of temperance and balance, so that anyone off-balance, i.e. ruled by one of the physiological humors in excess, becomes ridiculous or in the old sense 'humorous'. Thus we saw that, from his vantage point of (neo-)classical humoral balance, a French physician has no compunction about calling an insane or melancholic laughable. This nexus with culture is the reason why medical humor that is in some way dated (and perhaps so much dated that one feels awkward to dredge it up) is 'thick' with meaning or most telling for the cultural historian.

29 The tradition is outlined in the prefatory material by the editor of B. Jonson, *Epicene, or The Silent Woman*, ed. by R. Dutton, Manchester / New York 2003.

DER *BONUS CHIRURGUS* UND DIE FEHLERVERMEIDUNG. ZUM BERUFSETHOS DER CHIRURGIE IN DER FRÜHEN NEUZEIT[1]

Klara Vanek

> Der Nutzen der Chirurgie ist sehr groß,
> aber ihre Ausübung ist unsicherer als ihre Theorie.[2]

Die Chirurgie erfuhr in der frühen Neuzeit sehr unterschiedliche Bewertungen. Angesichts zahlreicher Schilderungen blutiger Eingriffe mit verheerenden Folgen für die Patienten entsteht der Eindruck, als sei die Chirurgie zu dieser Zeit keine allzu vertrauenserweckende Praxis gewesen. Welch „Schaden, Jammer und Verderben des Leibes und des Lebens der Kranken“ von „unerfahrenen und groben Waghälsen“ tagtäglich angerichtet werde, könne jeder sehen, beklagte etwa Wilhelm Fabry von Hilden (1560–1634) und wünschte sich, dass die Obrigkeit dem Wüten dieser „ungeschickten und unerfahrenen groben Kerle“ in „dieser edlen und sehr notwendigen Kunst“ Einhalt gebiete.[3] Die Chirurgie war gefährlich, nicht nur an sich riskante Operationen, sondern auch kleinere Eingriffe konnten schnell lebensgefährlich werden, wenn sie unsachgemäß durchgeführt wurden. Dieser Einschätzung steht der in der frühneuzeitlichen Literatur gern und oft zitierte Topos von Celsus (7, 1) gegenüber, wonach innerhalb der Medizin die Chirurgie das Fach mit den sichersten Ergebnissen sei.[4] In welchem Zusammenhang

1 Dieser Aufsatz entstand im Rahmen des DFG/ANR-Projekts „Fallibilität und Fehlerkultur in der frühneuzeitlichen Medizin“. Mariacarla Gadebusch Bondio danke ich für ihre wertvollen Anregungen und Verbesserungsvorschläge und Manuel Förg für sein scharfes Auge.

2 Dieser Aphorismus geht auf den osmanischen Polyhistor Kâtib Çelebi (1609–1657) und seine bibliographische Enzyklopädie *Kashf al-zunūn* zurück, ich zitiere hier nach E. Savage-Smith, „The Practice of Surgery in Islamic Lands: Myth and Reality“, *Social History of Medicine* 13/2 (2000), S. 307-321, S. 307.

3 *Gründlicher Bericht vom heissen und kalten Brand welcher gangraena et sphacelus oder S. Antonii- und Martialis-Feuer genannt wird*, nach der 2. dt. Ausg. v. 1603 hg. v. E. Hintzsche, Bern / Stuttgart 1965, S. 144.

4 Celsus: *De medicina*, Buch 7, Abs. 1: „Ea non quidem medicamenta atque uictus rationem omittit, sed manu tamen plurimum praestat, estque eius effectus inter omnes medicinae partes euidentissimus.“ hg. v. F. Marx (Corpus Medicorum Latinorum; I), Leipzig / Berlin 1915, S. 301. In der deutschen Übertragung lautet die Stelle: „Freilich wendet auch dieser Teil der Medizin die Behandlung mit Arzneimitteln und Diät an, aber die Hauptbehandlung ist doch immer der chirurgische Eingriff, und von allen Teilen der Heilkunst hat die Chirurgie den evidentesten Erfolg aufzuweisen.“ Dt. Übersetzung und Kommentar von E. Scheller und W. Frieboes, 2. Aufl. Braunschweig 1906, S. 362.

stehen diese widersprüchlichen Äußerungen? Lassen sie sich überhaupt miteinander vereinbaren?

Fehler ließen sich in das Lehrgebäude der Chirurgie integrieren, indem sie als Verstöße gegen Vorschriften zur Ausübung der Kunstlehre gedeutet und damit auf diejenigen Personen zurückgeführt wurden, die die operativen Eingriffe tätigten. Dazu passt der Celsus-Topos gut, denn wegen der Verbindung von manuellem Eingriff und Ergebnis der Operation kann bewertet werden, ob der Eingriff richtig war oder nicht. Entscheidend ist, dass dieser Gedanke erstens *überhaupt* eine Verbindung zwischen dem Eingriff als solchem und seinem Ergebnis postuliert – etwa im Unterschied zur Pharmakologie, in der die Wirkung einer Medikamentengabe angesichts möglicher anderer einflussnehmender Faktoren unklar sei[5] – und damit die Chirurgie epistemologischen Überlegungen zugänglich macht. Zweitens folgt daraus, dass die Ausgestaltung und Qualität eines Eingriffs unter anderem wesentlich vom Chirurgen abhängt.

Die Rolle des Handelnden für das Gelingen einer Operation bildet den zentralen Aspekt des vorliegenden Aufsatzes.[6] Aus dieser Perspektive ist ein misslungener Eingriff auf den Operateur zurückzuführen, der gegen die Grundsätze der Kunstlehre – und zwar aus Gründen, die in seiner Person liegen – verstößt:

> Deshalb werden wir jenen Chirurgen als weniger vollkommen empfinden, der all diese Dinge und Einzelheiten nicht redlich und genau bedacht hat. Denn wer nicht schnell, geschickt, beherzt und entschlossen operiert, fügt den Kranken Schaden zu und zeigt sich als ein Unkundiger dieser Kunst. Wer weniger kunstgerecht und anständig handelt, der wird keinen Ruhm beim Volk erwerben, und den Kranken weder beliebt noch geschätzt sein.[7]

5 Celsus führt im Anschluss an die eben zitierte Stelle aus (7, 1–2): „Siquidem in morbis, cum multum fortuna conferat, eademque saepe salutaria, saepe uana sint, potest dubitari, secunda ualetudo medicinae an corporis an beneficio contigerit. [...] At in ea parte, quae manu curat, euidens omnem profectum, ut aliquid ab aliis adiuuetur, hinc tamen plurimum trahere." – „Da aber bei den Krankheiten das Glück eine so große Rolle spielt und dieselben Mittel bald heilen, bald wirkungslos sind, so kann man wirklich im Zweifel sein, ob die Herstellung der Gesundheit den angewandten Mitteln oder der Selbsthilfe des Körpers zuzuschreiben ist. [...] Bei dem chirurgischen Teil der Medizin ist aber offenbar der meiste Erfolg dem chirurgischen Eingriffe selbst zuzuschreiben, wenn er auch zum Teil von den anderen Teilen der Heilkunst unterstützt wird." ebd.

6 Andere Gesichtspunkte zum Themenkreis des wissenschaftlichen Status der Chirurgie im Verhältnis zur Medizin blende ich bewusst aus – man denke etwa an die vieldiskutierten Fragen der Zuständigkeiten und Kompetenzen zwischen Ärzten und Chirurgen; verwiesen sei allein auf Johannes Battista Silvaticus, der in seinen *Controversiae medicae numero centum* von 1601 unter der Kontroverse Nr. 94 die Frage „An manu faciendæ operationes ad medicum spectent nec ne" ausführlich erörterte.

7 „Minus itaque perfectum esse dicemus illum chirurgum, qui hæc omnia, & singula probè, & ad amussim non obseruauerit: cùm enim neque celeriter, neque eleganter, neque iucundè, neque promptè operatur, ægrotantibus damnum affert artisque propterea sese ignarum ostendit. Dum verò etiam minus concinnè, & indecorè agit, gratiam apud vulgus acquirit nullam, ægrotantibusque gratus non est, nec carus." J. B. Silvaticus, *Medicinam Practicam, In prima sede profitentis, Medicus*, Mediolani, Apud Hieronymum Bordonum. M. DC. XI, S. 161 (die Übersetzungen stammen, sofern nicht anders gekennzeichnet, von mir).

Die Ursache für einen Fehler ist nach Giovanni Battista Silvaticus (1550–1621) im Chirurgen zu suchen. Damit sind Fehler von Chirurgen und Vorstellungen über den *bonus chirurgus* eng miteinander verknüpft und gleichsam zwei Seiten der gleichen Medaille. Berufsethische Vorschriften, wie sich ein guter Chirurg zu verhalten habe, sollen das Einhalten der Regeln der Kunstlehre der Chirurgie sichern – und die Fehlervermeidung verbessern. Umgekehrt gehen misslungene Operationen auf die Verletzung dieser Regeln zurück. Freilich ist die Rede über den Fehler begehenden Chirurgen ohne die Folie des *bonus chirurgus* nicht denkbar, da seine Wesenszüge die Tugenden des guten Chirurgen *ex negativo* spiegeln. Die Kritik an den Fehlern der Chirurgen und die Bestimmung der Eigenschaften des *bonus chirurgus* bildeten in der frühen Neuzeit zwei komplementäre Diskurse, die eng miteinander verbunden sind.

So wie man über den guten und erfolgreichen Arzt nachdachte,[8] findet sich in der frühneuzeitlichen Literatur einiges über den guten Chirurgen. Doch anders als dem *optimus medicus*[9] hat sich die medizinhistorische Forschung dem *bonus chirurgus* bislang nur vereinzelt gewidmet.[10] Es zeigt sich jedoch, dass Mediziner und Chirurgen im 16. und 17. Jahrhundert trotz oder gerade wegen dieser gefährlichen Praxis und der Beispiele ihres Missbrauchs intensiv über die Gestalt von guter Chirurgie und ihres Berufsethos nachdachten.

8 Man denke an entsprechende Schriften wie Gabriele Zerbi: *Opus perutile de cautelis medicorum* (ca. 1495, ed. und dt. Übers. in Vorbereitung von Mariacarla Gadebusch Bondio und Kay Peter Jankrift), Giovanni Antonio Sicco: *De optimo medico* (1551), Alfonso de Miranda: *Diálogo del perfecto médico* (1562), Leonardo Botallo: *Tractatus de medici et aegri munere* (1565), Johannes Sporisch: *Idea medici* (1582), Enrique Jorge Enríquez: *Retrato del perfecto médico* (1595), Roderico de Castro: *Medicus politicus* (1614), Pietro Castelli: *Optimus medicus* (1617) oder auch an die frühneuzeitliche Rezeption von Galens *Quod optimus medicus sit quoque philosophus* etwa durch die Neuübersetzung von Erasmus von Rotterdam (1526).

9 Vgl. etwa Y. David-Peyre, *Le personnage du médecin et la relation médecin-malade dans la littérature ibérique. XVIe et XVIIe siècle*, Paris 1971; D. E. J. Linden, „Gabriele Zerbi's ‚De cautelis medicorum' and the Tradition of Medical Prudence", *Bulletin of the History of Medicine* 73/1 (1999), S. 19–37; D. Linden, „The Perfect Physician: 16th Century Perspectives from the Iberian Peninsula", *Sudhoffs Archiv* 84/2 (2000), S. 222–231; A. Wigger, *Vom ‚metasanos' zum ‚médico perfecto'. Zum literarischen Bild des Arztes im Spanien des 16. Jahrhunderts*, Berlin 2001; R. French, *Medicine Before Science. The Rational and Learned Doctor from the Middle Ages to the Enlightenment*, Cambridge 2003; I. J. Polianski, „Der ‚gute Arzt'. Ärztlicher Moralhaushalt und das Selbstverständnis der Medizin seit der Frühen Neuzeit", *Medizinhistorisches Journal* 46 (2011), S. 171–211; M. Gadebusch Bondio, „Vom Gewicht des Wortes. Der redegewandte Arzt als humanistisches Ideal", in: G. Maio (Hg.), *Macht und Ohnmacht des Wortes. Ethische Grundfragen einer personalen Medizin*, Göttingen 2012, S. 315–333; M. Gadebusch Bondio –„‚Medical Virtues'. Neue Fragen und alte Vorbilder", in: M. Gadebusch Bondio – A. Bettels (Hgg.), *Im Korsett der Tugenden. Moral und Geschlecht im kulturhistorischen Kontext*, Hildesheim / Zürich / New York 2013, S. 125–148, v.a. S. 137–142.

10 Über den *bonus chirurgus* schreibt beispielsweise V. Nutton, „Humanist surgery", in: A. Wear – R. French – I. M. Lonie (Hgg.), *The Medical Renaissance of the Sixteenth Century*, Cambridge et al. 1985, S. 75–99, S. 84f.

Ziel der folgenden Darstellung ist die Rekonstruktion dieses omnipräsenten Bildes des *bonus chirurgus* aus der Analyse von einschlägiger chirurgischer Fachliteratur heraus. Dazu greife ich auf weit verbreitete italienische und französische Lehrwerke und Programmschriften der Chirurgie vorwiegend aus dem 16. Jahrhundert zurück, sowie mit ihnen sich im Einklang befindliche kleinere Schriften. So soll gewährleistet werden, dass es sich bei den formulierten Ansichten um standardisierte, weitgehend unumstrittene und repräsentative Vorstellungen über diese Sache handelt. Es geht zudem darum, die vielseitigen Bezüge, Übernahmen und Aneignungen vorgängiger Literatur zum Thema freizulegen und damit letztlich aufzuweisen, wie topisch diese Gedanken in dieser Zeit waren.

Die Figur des guten Chirurgen wird im Folgenden systematisch entlang von Eigenschaftsgruppen dargestellt, die sich aus dem historischen Material ergeben. Die Notwendigkeit und Dringlichkeit dieses Idealbilds für die Chirurgie demonstrieren in jedem Abschnitt entsprechende Stellen über den schlechten Chirurgen. Die Spiegelbildlichkeit der Charakteristika der Figuren des guten und schlechten Chirurgen wird deutlich und offenbart, wie eng diese beiden Diskurse miteinander verknüpft waren. Am Schluss werfe ich noch einen Blick in die deutsche, dezidiert handwerkliche chirurgische Literatur. Damit soll das Bild, das in der gelehrten Chirurgie vom idealen Praktiker entworfen wurde, mit den Vorstellungen zu vervollständigen, die sich Handwerkschirurgen über den vollendeten Standesgenossen gemacht haben.

Wie stellte man sich also einen guten Chirurgen vor? Wie sollte ein Chirurg richtig handeln? Was musste er wissen? Welche Eigenschaften hatte er für seine Arbeit mitzubringen?

KÖRPERLICHE UND GEISTIGE VORAUSSETZUNGEN FÜR EINEN *IDONEUS CHIRURGUS*

Bei der Frage, wer für den chirurgischen Beruf geeignet war und wer nicht, ging es zunächst um eine Reihe von Voraussetzungen, die diese Person mitbringen musste. Nicht jeder sollte diese gefährlichen und gefürchteten Eingriffe vornehmen dürfen, wie die folgende Charakterisierung eines Chirurgen impliziert:

> Et partant que le Chirurgien Barbare, est celuy qui, comme Satyre, d'vne presomptueuse ignorance, masqué, de quelque apparence d'experience brule, taille, couppe & tranche à toute reste: plustost par vne nature cruelle & Barbare que de Chrestien [.][11]

Angesichts der Drastik, die Schilderungen von Operationen in der frühen Neuzeit nur zu häufig anhaftete, scheint es zunächst schwierig, sich den Operateur anders denn als groben Schlächter vorzustellen, als *chirurgien barbare*, wie ein gewisser Estienne Thevet, Chirurg von François de Bourbon, Fürst von Condé (1558–

11 E. Thevet, *Les errevrs et abvs ordinaires commis av fait de la Chirurgie. Diuisez en quatre liures*, A Poictiers, Par Iean Blanchet Imprimeur ordinaire du Roy, & de l'Vniuersité, 1603, S. 20^{v}.

1614), ihn 1603 in seinem Pamphlet über *Les erreurs et abus commis au fait de la chirurgie* nannte. Diesem furchteinflößenden *chirurgien barbare* stellte Thevet freilich den „vray & legitime Chirurgien" gegenüber. In puncto der Voraussetzungen für einen guten Chirurgen war man sich zu dieser Zeit weitgehend einig, wie der Blick in die chirurgische Fachliteratur zeigt. Im Proöm zum Standardwerk *Practica in arte chirurgica* (zuerst erschienen Rom 1514)[12] forderte etwa der päpstliche Chirurg Johannes de Vigo (1450–1525),[13] ein Chirurg solle jung sein („Chirurgus autem debet esse adolescens: aut saltem adolescentiæ propinquus").[14] Den geeigneten Chirurgen (*idoneus chirurgus*) beschrieb Vigo folgendermaßen:

> Darüber hinaus muss er mit fester Hand, die niemals zittert, mit der scharfsinnigen und klaren Kraft seiner Augen, im Herzen unerschütterlich und unerbittlich seine Eingriffe in den menschlichen Körper auf tapfere Weise ausführen. Er soll sich weder vom Schreien der Patienten dazu verleiten lassen, weniger zu tun, als notwendig ist, aber auch nicht mehr, als die Sache verlangt. Ja, vielmehr soll er wagemutig handeln, und zwar nicht anders, als wenn aus dem Wimmern des Anderen kein Gefühl bei ihm entstünde. Außerdem soll er mit der linken nicht anders als mit der rechten Hand gewandt sein. Dies alles nämlich gehört (wie Celsus im Buch 7 seiner Chirurgie sagt) zum geeigneten Chirurgen.[15]

In dieser Äußerung über die Qualitäten des guten Chirurgen bezog sich Vigo ausdrücklich auf Celsus. Von dessen Enzyklopädie, die im Mittelalter weitgehend unbekannt und erst 1426 von Guarino di Verona (1374–1460) in Bologna wieder-

12 Vigos *Practica* gab es in zwei Fassungen: in einer längeren, in der in neun Büchern die Sachen der Chirurgie *copiose dictae*, sowie in einer kürzeren, in der sie in fünf Büchern *compendiose dictae* wurden. Beide Fassungen, die oftmals zusammen erschienen, wurden in dieser Zeit breit rezipiert: E. J. Gurlt, *Geschichte der Chirurgie und ihrer Ausübung*, Bd. 1, Berlin 1898, S. 919 zählt von der *Practica in arte chirurgica copiosa* für das 16. Jahrhundert 14 Ausgaben und Übersetzungen in viele Sprachen: ins Französische (1525 u.ö.), Italienische (1540 u.ö.), Englische (1543 u.ö.), Spanische (1557 u.ö.), Portugiesische (1613) und auch ins Deutsche (von Johannes Scultetus d.J., Nürnberg 1677 und 1685).

13 Vigo wurde in Rapallo geboren, dort studierte er bei einem gewissen Meister Battista di Rapallo. Vigo praktizierte in Genua, um 1495 kam er in in Savona in die Dienste des Kardinals Giuliano della Rovere. Als Letzterer 1503 Papst Julius II. wurde, begleitete ihn Vigo nach Rom. Nach Julius' Ableben 1513 wurde er Leibchirurg von Julius' Neffen Sisto della Rovere, nach dessen Tod 1517 zog sich Vigo aus dem öffentlichen Leben zurück. Seine Lebensdaten sind umstritten. Vgl. E. Nicaise, „Introduction", in: P. Franco, *Chirurgie. Nouvelle édition avec une introduction historique, une biographie et l'histoire du Collège de Chirurgie*, Paris 1895, S. VII–CLXIV, S. XXXIII f.; Gurlt: *Geschichte der Chirurgie 1* (1898), S. 919–942; Art. „Da Vigo", *Dizionario Biografico degli Italiani*, Bd. 33, Rom 1987, C. H. Talbot, Art. „Vigo", *Dictionary of Scientific Biography*, Bd. 14, New York 2008, S. 27f.

14 *Practica D. Ioannis A Vigo Genvensis, Olim Ivlii II. Pont. Max. Chirvrgici Clarissimi*, Lvgduni, Apud Bartholomæum Honoratum. M. D. LXXXII, fol. *4^{v}.

15 „Insuper manu strenua, nec vnquam intremescenti, acri oculorum potentia, & clara, animo intrepidus, immisericors, suas operationes in corpore humano viriliter exercendo: ne clamore patientis minus facere, quàm necesse est, nec plus, quàm res desiderat: imò omnia audacter agat: non secus ac si nullus ex vagitibus alterius | affectus oriatur: & non minus sinistra, quàm dextra manu promptus esse debet: hac enim omnia (vt inquit Cel. lib. 7. suæ chirurgiæ) ad idoneum pertinent chirurgum." ebd., fol. *4^{v}–*5^{r}.

entdeckt worden war, überlebten nur die Abschnitte über die Medizin.[16] Im siebten Buch über die Chirurgie erörterte Celsus in den ersten Absätzen die Definition der Chirurgie als jene Medizin, in der man mit der Hand heile, die Stellung der Chirurgie als dritter Teil innerhalb der Medizin, die Augenscheinlichkeit der Wirkung gelungener chirurgischer Eingriffe sowie das Alter und die Geschichte der Chirurgie.[17] Anschließend kam er auf die Eigenschaften des Chirurgen bzw. des Arztes, der mit der Hand heilt, zu sprechen – und das sollte sich, wie man bei Vigo und vielen anderen gut sehen kann, für das Bild des Chirurgen für eine lange Zeit als prägend erweisen. Denn es war Celsus, der meinte, ein guter *chirurgus* sollte jung sein, von fester Hand, geschickt mit beiden Händen, mit guter Sehkraft ausgestattet und unerschrockenen Geistes.[18]

Diese Forderungen finden wir auch in der *Chirurgie fort utile* (1580) von Dominique Reulin wieder.[19] Nachdem dieser Arzt aus Bordeaux zu Beginn seines Kapitels „Des qualitez que le Chirurgien doit auoir, & du suiet de la Chirurgie" auf eine ganz ähnliche Weise die Ansprüche an einen guten Chirurgen beschrieben hatte,[20] fuhr er fort:

16 Freilich gehörte *De medicina* nach der sehr frühen *editio princeps* (Florenz 1478) zu den am häufigsten gedruckten medizinischen antiken Schriften der frühen Neuzeit.

17 Celsus, *De medicina* 7, 1–3.

18 „Esse autem chirurgus debet adulescens aut certe adulescentiae propior; manu strenua, stabili, nec umquam intremescente, eaque non | minus sinistra quam dextra promptus; acie oculorum acri claraque; animo intrepidus; misericors sic, ut sanari uelit eum, quem accepit, non ut clamore eius motus uel magis quam res desiderat properet, uel minus quam necesse est secet; sed perinde faciat omnia, ac si nullus ex uagitibus alterius adfectus oriatur." Celsus, *De medicina* 7, 4, ed. Marx (1915, CML 1), S. 301f.

19 Über Reulin wissen wir nur, dass er Arzt in Bordeaux war und abgesehen von seiner *Chirurgie fort utile* drei weitere – bemerkenswert verschiedenartige – Schriften verfasste, nämlich eine griechische Grammatik (*Methodicae totius Grammatices graecae descriptionis libri tres*, 1558), eine diätetische Schrift (*De recto cibariorum ordine usuque libri duo*, 1560) sowie eine polemische Entgegnung auf die *Erreurs populaires* von Laurent Joubert (*Contredicts aux erreurs populaires de L. Joubert*, 1580). Vgl. Art. „Reulin", in: L. M. Chadon – F. A. Delandine (Hgg.), *Nouveau dictionnaire historique*, Bd. 10, Lyon 1804, S. 443f.; Art. „Reulin", *Dictionnaire biographique universel et pittoresque*, Bd. 3, Paris 1834, S. 145; Gurlt, *Geschichte der Chirurgie 2* (1898), S. 844ff. Zu Reulins *Contredicts* vgl. auch J. Coste, *La littérature des ‚erreurs populaires'. Une ethnographie médicale à l'époque moderne*, Paris 2002, S. 38–41 und D. Brancher, „Jeux de la médiation dans les ‚erreurs populaires' de Laurent Joubert", in: A. Carlino – M. Jeanneret (Hgg.), *Vulgariser la médicine. Du style médical en France et en Italie (XVIe et XVIIe siècles)*, Genf 2009, S. 213–242, S. 216, 228.

20 „Qviconque voudra se dedier à bon escient à cest art de Chirurgie, & le bien apprendre, doit prealablement, selon Celse, estre institué & versé aux bonnes lettres: & avant le pouuoir deument exerçer est requis qu'il soit en aage viril, ou pres d'iceluy, ayant sa main vigoureuse & ferme, sans qu'elle bransle ou tremble, & qu'il ait sa senestre si agile, & prompte, s'il est possible, comme la dextre: que sa veüe soit claire & ague: qu'il ne soit timide, & ne s'estonne d'aucune operation qu'il luy conuienne entreprendre: & ne soit induit par les cris, pleurs, ou doleances de son patient, ou des assistans, à ne faire l'entiere incision, cauterisation, extirpation, ou autres œuures Chirurgicales requises, ains, sans en estre aucunement destourné, doit icelles dextrement executer & parfaire." *La Chirvrgie de Dominiqve Revlin medecin de Bordeavx: fort vtile & necessaire à tout homme exerçant cest art: comprise en cinq liures: le*

Secondement que le Chirurgien soit ingenieux, subtil, prudent, & de bon iugement, ayant le corps commode & bien proportionné: singulierement les mains bien fermes & non tremblantes, & les doigts | d'icelles gresles, & les yeux cler voyans.[21]

Zu den erwähnten körperlichen Voraussetzungen der guten Augen und der festen Hand kommen das angenehme Äußere hinzu sowie geistige Eigenschaften: Der *chirurgien* sollte einfallsreich, scharfsinnig, klug und von guter Urteilskraft sein. Reulin bezog sich hier explizit[22] auf Guy de Chauliac (ca. 1298–1368), eine Autorität, die in der frühneuzeitlichen Chirurgie viel gelesen und zitiert wurde. Tatsächlich zeigt der Vergleich mit Guys *Inventarium seu collectorium in parte cyrurgicali medicine*, genannt *Chirurgia magna* (1363), [23] wie eng sich Reulin in diesem Punkt an seine Quelle hielt. Im dortigen Anfangskapitel „Capitulum singulare in quo premittuntur quedam communia valde necessaria cuicumque volenti proficere in arte cyrurgie" heißt es doch – ich zitiere den Text der französischen Übersetzung des Anatomen und Chirurgen Laurent Joubert (1529–1583) von 1579:

Tiercement qu'il soit ingenieus, & de bon iugement & bonne memoire. C'est ce que disoit Haly rodoan au troisieme du Techni: Il faut que le Medecin ayt bonne souuenence, bon iugement bonne inuention, bonne veuë & sain entendement, & qu'il soyt bien formé: comme (suppleez) qu'il ayt les doigts greiles, les mains fermes & non tremblantes, les yeus clairs, & c.[24]

tout deduit par bon ordre, & facile methode, A Paris. De l'Imprimerie de Leon Cauellat, rue S. Iean de Latran: au Griphon d'argent, 1580, S. 12.

21 Ebd., S. 15f.

22 „Guy de Cauliac requiert en vn bon Chirurgien quatre choses principalement." ebd., S. 12.

23 Der früheste heute greifbare lateinische Druck erschien 1497 in Venedig, allerdings verzeichnet Edouard Nicaise als *editio princeps* eine verlorene venezianische Ausgabe von 1490. Der Text wurde im 16. Jahrhundert mehrmals nachgedruckt, darunter sind die berühmte humanistische venezianische Giuntine (1546) und eine kritische Ausgabe mit ausführlichem Kommentar von Laurent Joubert (1585). Außerdem gibt es schon im 14. und 15. Jahrhundert zahlreiche Übersetzungen ins Französische, aber auch ins Alemannische, Englische, Hebräische, Italienische, Niederfränkische, Okzitanische und Ripuanische. Diese vernakuläre Tradition wurde auch im Zeitalter des Buchdrucks weitergeführt, von den mindestens 24 französischen Ausgaben im 15. und 16. Jahrhundert sei etwa die Fassung von Jean Canappe (Lyon 1538) genannt sowie eine Neuübersetzung von Laurent Joubert aus dem Jahre 1579, die bis weit ins 17. Jahrhundert immer wieder aufgelegt wurde (Lyon 1579, 1580, 1592, Tournon 1598, 1609, 1611, Rouen 1615, Tournon 1619, Rouen 1632, 1641, 1649, Lyon 1659). Außerdem sind mindestens fünf italienische, zwei katalanische, fünf spanische, eine englische und vier niederländische frühneuzeitliche Übersetzungen bekannt. Zur komplizierten Überlieferungs- und Übersetzungsgeschichte von Guys *Chirurgia magna* vgl. E. Nicaise, „Introduction", in: Guy de Chauliac, *La grande chirvrgie de Gvy de Chavliac composée en l'an 1363, revue par E. Nicaise*, Paris 1890, S. ix–cxci, S. clxix; Gurlt, *Geschichte der Chirurgie 2* (1898), S. 78; S. Tittel, *Die ‚Anathomie' in der ‚Grande Chirurgie' des Gui de Chauliac. Wort- und sachgeschichtliche Untersuchungen und Edition*, Tübingen 2004, S. 27ff.

24 *La grande chirvrgie de M. Gvi de Chavliac, medecin tres-famevx de l'Vniversité de Mompelier, composee l'an de grace M. CCC. LXIII. Restitvee novvellement a sa dignité, Par M. Lavrens Iovbert. Voyez au prochain feuillet, ce que M. Iovbert ha faict (oultre sa nouuelle traduction) & fourny du sien, en recognoissant cest' œuure*, A Lyon, par Estienne Michel, M.

An dieser Stelle bezog sich Guy de Chauliac allerdings nicht auf Celsus (der ja im Mittelalter vergessen war), sondern auf *Haly Rodoan*, gemeint ist der Kommentar des arabischen Arztes Ali ibn Ridwan (ca. 988–1061/8) zu Galens *Tegni*.

Eine ausführliche Erörterung der nötigen Voraussetzungen für einen *optimus chirurgus* finden wir in der monumentalen Darstellung der Chirurgie des gelehrten venezianischen Chirurgen Giovanni Andrea Della Croce (1515–1575).[25] Diese im Jahre 1573 erschienenen *Chirurgiae libri septem* werden von einer längeren programmatischen *Praefatio in suam chirurgiam* eingeleitet, in der Della Croce unter anderem seine grundsätzlichen Ansichten über die Chirurgie umfassend in acht von insgesamt 18 Abschnitten auf etwa elf Folioseiten darstellte – und dabei aus der ganzen Vielfalt der inzwischen greifbaren griechischen, römischen und arabischen Autoritäten schöpfte.[26] Della Croce betonte beim *bonus chirurgus* die Bedeutung des sinnlichen Wahrnehmungsvermögens: Guter Seh- (*visus*), Takt- (*tactus*) und Hörsinn (*auditus*) helfen bei Diagnose und Therapie,[27] an anderer

D. LXXIX, S. 14 (das Zitat ist bei Joubert am Textrand durch Anführungsstriche hervorgehoben, die Umsetzung dieser Auszeichnung hier mittels Kursivierung). Der lateinische Text lautet folgendermaßen: „Tercio, quod sit ingeniosus ac boni iudicii et rememoracionis, et hoc dicebat Haly Rodoan in 3° Tegni: Oportet medicum esse bone rememoracionis, boni iudicii, bone solercie, ac bone visionis et sani intellectus cum bonitate forme, ut (supple) quod habeat digitos graciles, manus firmas non tremulas, oculos claros, et cetera." *Guigonis de Caulhiaco (Guy de Chauliac) Inventarium sive Chirurgia magna*, Bd. 1, hg. v. M. McVaugh, Leiden / New York / Köln 1997, S. 9.

25 Auch Dalla Croce oder Crucejus. Der gebürtige Venezianer erlernte das Handwerk des Barbiers bei seinem Vater Matteo Guiseppe und studierte zugleich die Lehren der antiken Medizin und Chirurgie. 1532 wurde er Mitglied im hochangesehenen *Collegio chirurgico di Venezia*, dem später auch Fabrici d'Aquapendente, Falloppia und Sassonia angehörten. 1538 bis 1546 bekleidete er einen Posten als Chirurg in Feltre, kehrte anschließend nach Venedig zurück, wo er unter anderem als Flottenarzt arbeitete. 1559 zog er sich aus gesundheitlichen Gründen von öffentlichen Ämtern zurück, auch um sich intensiv seiner anatomischen und chirurgischen Schriftstellerei zu widmen. 1575 verstarb er zusammen mit seiner ganzen Familie an der Pest. Zu Della Croce vgl. Gurlt, *Geschichte der Chirurgie 2* (1898), S. 335–361; Art. „Della Croce", *Dizionario Biografico degli Italiani*, Bd. 36, Rom 1988. Zum *Collegium chirurgorum* in Venedig vgl. auch R. Palmer, „Physicians and Surgeons in Sixteenth-Century Venice", *Medical History* 23 (1979), S. 451–460.

26 Die folgende Darstellung von Della Croces Ansichten basiert auf den Gedanken, die er in dieser *Praefatio* ausbreitete: *Chirvrgiae Ioannis Andreae A Crvce, Veneti medici Libri Septem, Quamplurimis instrumentorum imaginibus Arti Chirurgicæ opportunis suis locis exornati, Theoricam, Practicam, ac uerißimam Experientiam continentes. In quibus ea omnia, quæ optimo Chirurgo in curandis vulneribus conuenire videntur, ordine quodam amplissimo concerni possunt: Nvnc primvm in lvcem editi*, Venetiis, Apud Iordanum Zilettum, 1573, S. 1^r–6^r, eine italienische Übersetzung erschien 1574. Außerdem findet sich diese Übersetzung geringfügig verändert (zum Teil wurde die Reihenfolge umgestellt) in seinem *Chirurgiae universalis opus absolutissimum* wieder, das 1573 erschien und 1596 wieder aufgelegt, außerdem 1583 ins Italienische sowie 1607 ins Deutsche übersetzt wurde.

27 „Vnaqvaeqve actio Chirurgica præcipuè sumitur à membrorum affectorum similitudine & dissimilitudine, in unitate, forma, numero, quantitate, & situ: & horum omnium cognitio acquiritur *visv*, ut inflammationum, siue tumorum omnium præter naturam, solutionum continui, & cutaneorum affectuum. *Tactv*, ut in luxatis, aut fractis ossibus, scirrhosis, aut ædematosis dispositionibus, ac effectibus calidis & figidis. *Avditv*, ut in magnis ossium fracturis,

Stelle kommen noch der Geruchs- (*odoratus*) und Geschmackssinn (*gustus*) dazu.[28] Im weiteren Verlauf betonte Della Croce die schon genannten positiven Eigenschaften, er sprach über die geistigen Voraussetzungen wie scharfer Verstand (*acutum ingenium*), beste Urteilskraft (*optimum iudicium*) und gutes Erinnerungsvermögen (*tenax memoria*)[29] und hob auf das gepflegte Auftreten und gute Aussehen,[30] die Eleganz[31] und die Jugend des *bonus chirurgus* ab.[32]

RICHTIGES HANDELN UND TUGENDEN DES *OPTIMUS CHIRURGUS*

Zur grundsätzlichen Befähigung kommt bei einem guten Chirurgen das an Tugenden orientierte Verhalten und die richtige Einstellung zu seiner Arbeit und zum Patienten hinzu. Eine körperlich und geistig geeignete Person wird erst dann zu einem guten Chirurgen, wenn sie sich geschickt anstellt und moralische Grundsät-

nempe crepitu, & rumore; aut uocis raucedine, uel mentis alienatione." ebd., S. 3v (Hervorhebungen in der Vorlage).

28 „In optimo etiam Chirurgo omnium sensuum salus requiritur; *visvs* præsertim, vt primo ægrotantis faciem pernotet, & vt minima quæque in profundo, aut abscondito sinu videre possit; vt corruptionis initium, aut alterius morbi agnoscat, ac medicaminum, vel instrumentorum, bonitatem percipiat. *Avditvs*, in ossium fracturis, quæ strepere solent; aut in caluariæ terebratione, quæ magis auditu, quàm tactu tutò perficitur. auditui etiam subiecta sunt sternutamentum, tussis, hominis strepitus præternaturam loquentis dum mente non constat. *Gvstvs*, ob simplicium medicamentorum facultates, & quibus vescuntur, rerum temperaturas. *Odoratvs*, ob vlcerum, aut abscessuum digestiones, aut putredines, vel deiectionum, aut lotij, aut respirati acris qualitates, & medicaminum bonitatem. *Tactus*, ad durities, & lenitates percipiendas ad intemperiei qualitates, & vlcerum dispositiones dignoscendas, ac vomicarum maturationes perscrutandas." ebd., S. 6r (Hervorhebungen in der Vorlage).

29 „Speciales verò siue præcipuæ optimi Chirurgi conditiones in eius animi operationum promptitudine consistunt; ob id Prudens esse debet, & acuti ingenij, ut medicorum axiomata intelligat, ac ea indicationibus, & operationibus opportunis applicare sciat, nec non vt accidentia, quæ de recenti contingunt, aptè corrigat, atque propellat. Sit tenacis memoriæ ob vniuersalium theorematum reminiscentiam; & vt eorum, quæ apud peritos præceptores aliàs viderit, operando reminiscatur. Sit optimi iudicij, vt morborum facultates, qui primò ac per se actiones lædunt, & causas, quæ non per se & primò, sed per accidens easdem offendunt, ac symptomata, quę morbos tales esse demonstrant, & concomitantur, perscrutetur; hæc nanque præter naturam sunt omnia, & illi vim inferunt, ac eius ordinem peruertunt, summeque pręsagiendo circunspectus esse debet." ebd., S. 5v.

30 „nam medici gubernationem esse dicimus (ait Hippocrates) vt videat, quo bono corporis habitu, & colore præditus sit iuxta existentem in ipso naturam. vulgus enim existimat eos, qui non fatis benè dispositum corpus habent, nec sibi, nec cæteris benè prospicere posse." ebd.

31 „Ornatè, sed expeditè, induatur, vt liberè operetur, & operando ne deturpetur: grauis sit in vestimentorum longitudine, & indumentorum bonitate: anulos aliquot in digitis gerat: manus, faciem, pilos in barba & in capite, ac alias corporis partes quàm purissimas habeat: ungues digitos ne excedant, neque admodum breues sint, ne, dum vulnera probe ad decorè vnire tentauerit, infirmo maleficium inferat." ebd.

32 „Aetas sit juuentutis, aut iuuentuti propinqua, hoc est intra consistendi ætatem & virilem, quæ & sensibus, & robore viget, ob varias vtilitates, nempe labores ferendo, studendo, deambulando, & medelam opportunè præstando." ebd.

ze beherzigt. Entsprechend kritisierte der Züricher Barbiermeister Felix Würtz (1500/10–1590/6) in seiner *Practica der Wundarzney* die Mitleidslosigkeit so manch eines Arztes:

> Nach dem Hefften vnd Blutstellen ist das neheste / welches mit dem kleinen eysernen Instrumentlein / so vom suchen her das Sucherlein genennet / begangen wirdt. Mit demselbigen haben ihren viel ein solches suchen/ gruͤblen/ vnd stupffen in den Wunden / als ob sie etwas in selbigen verlohren hetten: vnd woͤllen vber eins wissen / wie weit die Wunden / wie tieff der Stich / welches Aederlein entzwey / welches Beinlein gebrochen oder noch gantz seye. Solches thund sie nicht nur einmal / als zu dem ersten Gebaͤnd / welches noch zuverzeihen were: sondern so offt sie die Wunden auffbinden / als offt muß solches geschehen.Vnd wann ihren drey oder mehr Artzet beysamen seind / so ist es nicht gnug / daß der eine mit dem Sucheysen seinen vnverstand | vnd vnbarmhertzigkeit beweyse: sonder nach dem ersten muß auch der ander / vnd nach diesem der dritte / sein verlohrnen pfenning in der Wunden suchen / vnd darinnen herumb stopffen / je einer groͤber vnnd ungestuͤmer als der ander. Wie meint aber einer / daß ein solcher armer verwundter dardurch gepeyniget vnd gemartert werde?[33]

Das mehrmalige Sondieren von Wunden sei eine überflüssige und unnütze, für den Patienten extrem qualvolle, aber leider gängige Art, um Wunden zu untersuchen: Dazu benutzen die Behandelnden eiserne Sonden, mit denen sie in die Wunden stechen, um die Tiefe und die Art der Verletzung zu ermitteln. Dem Patienten eine solche äußerst schmerzhafte Untersuchung gleich mehrmals zuzumuten, zeuge von besonderer *vnbarmhertzigkeit* der Ärzte, zumal sie aus medizinischer Sicht ohne größeren Nutzen sei. Würtz selbst war der Meinung, dass man Wunden nach dem Reinigen am besten den Selbstheilungskräften der Natur überlassen sollte. Mit der gängigen Methode des Sondierens von Wunden werde, implizierte Würtz, lediglich dem Geltungsstreben der Ärzte entsprochen. Dass dem Patienten – ohne medizinische Notwendigkeit – Schaden zugefügt werde (nämlich starke Schmerzen), kümmere sie nicht.

Dem Gebot der Schmerzvermeidung begegnen wir bei Della Croce: Im Abschnitt „De optimi Chirurgi generalibus conditionibus“ seines Vorworts bestimmte er die Art und Weise der manuellen Therapie, der *chirurgus* solle *cito*, *laete* und *tuto* operieren, und möglichst *sine dolore*.[34] Im folgenden Abschnitt „De optimi Chirurgi præcipuis conditionibus“ zitierte er den entsprechenden *locus classicus*:

33 *Practica Der Wundartzney/ Was für schädliche Mißbräuch bey der Wundartzney in gemeinem schwanckt vnd warumb die abzuschaffen seind. Item Wie man allerley Wunden/ sie seyen Geschossen/ Gehawen/ Gestochen/ Gefallen/ Geschlagen/ ohn einigen Mißbrauch/ wie auch die Beinbrüch/ Curieren solle. Deßgleichen Von allerley Zufällen der Wunden/ wie dieselbigen zuerkennen/ vnd ehe sie kommen/ wie man ihnen begegnen soll/ vnd so sie vorhanden/ wie die abzuschaffen. Sampt einem grundtlichen bericht Von den Salben/ Pflastern/ Oelen/ Blutstellungen/ sc. insonders von den Wundtränckern. Alles nach newer Form vnnd Art mit viel geschwinden Handgriffen/ Exempeln vnd Arcanen/ alles durch selbs eigene Erfahrung beschrieben/ deßgleichen zuvor in Truck niemals außgangen: durch Felix Wirtz/ Wundartzet zu Basel*, getruckt zu Basel [letzte Seite:] Durch Sebastian Henricpetri Anno Christi CIↃ IↃ XCVI, T. 1, cap. 6, S. li–lii.

34 Della Croce, *Chirurgiae libri septem* (1573), S. 5^{r}.

manu vtraque pro dextra, intremula, & sana vtatur: nam agens (ait Hippocrates) vti vtraque manu ad omne opus debet, & ambabus simul: siquidem ambæ similes sunt, id spectant, vt rectè, vt decorè, vt eleganter, vt celeriter, vt iucundè, vt promptè agat.[35]

Diese Stelle stammt aus der hippokratischen Schrift *De officina medici*, die in der lateinischen Übersetzung von Vidus Vidius (1509–1569) vorlag:[36] die *Chirurgia è Graeco in Latinam conversa* (Paris 1544).[37] Auf den gleichen Text bezogen sich auch andere frühneuzeitliche Aussagen über den *bonus chirurgus*, etwa vom Mailänder Arzt Giovanni Battista Silvaticus (auch: Selvatico, 1550–1621).[38] Die-

35 Ebd., S. 5^{v}. Die Stelle im *Corpus hippocraticum*, auf die sich Della Croce bezieht, lautet: „Τὰ ἔργα πάντα ἀσκέειν ἑκατέρῃσι δρῶντα καὶ ἀμφοτέρῃσιν ἅμα· ὅμοια γάρ εἰσιν ἀμφοτέρῃσι στοχαζόμενον ἀγαθῶς, καλῶς, ταχέως, ἀπόνως, εὐρύθμως, εὐπόρως.“ – „Qui operatur, eum operationes omnes exercere decet utrisque seorsim manibus et ambabus simul; ambae namque sunt similes, scopum intuentem recte, decore, cito, jucunde, concinne, prompte.“ Hippokrates, *De officina medici* 4, in: *Hippocratis de medici officina liber et Galeni in eum commentarius I*, in: *Medicorum graecorum opera quae exstant*, hg. v. C. G. Kühn, Bd. 18, Teil 2, Leipzig 1830, S. 629–718, S. 716. Es sei noch darauf hingewiesen, dass der Gedanke des sicheren, schnellen und beherzten chirurgischen Eingriffs schon in der Antike von mehreren Autoren topisch gebraucht, zuweilen auf Asklepiades von Bithynien (124–60 v.Chr.) zurückgeführt und auch bei Celsus (*De medicina* 3, 4, 1) zu finden ist.

36 Der gebürtige Florentiner Guido Guidi (latinisiert Vidus Vidius) lebte bis 1541 in Rom und wurde 1542 vom französischen König Franz I. als erster Professor für Medizin an das *Collège Royal* (später Collège de France) berufen. Dort wurde er unter anderem wegen der anatomischen Demonstrationen, die er in seine Vorlesung einführte, zu einem beliebten Universitätslehrer. 1548 kehrte er nach Italien zurück und wurde Leibarzt von Cosimo I. sowie Professor für Philosophie und Medizin in Pisa, wo er dann 1569 starb. Vgl. Nutton, *Humanist surgery* (1985), S. 87f. Weiterführend zu Vidius sind W. Brockbank, „The Man Who Was Vidius“, *Annals of the Royal College of Surgeons of England* 19/5 (1956), S. 269–295 und M. D. Grmek, „Contribution à la biographie de Vidius (Guido Guidi) permier lecteur royal de médecine: ses origines et sa vie avant la période parisienne“, *Revue d'histoire des sciences* 31/4 (1978), S. 289–299.

37 Die *De officina medici* hatte schon Galen ausführlich kommentiert, die griechische *editio princeps* erschien 1526 in Venedig. Vidius' *Chirurgia* leitete die breitere Rezeption der chirurgischen Schriften im Hippokratischen Korpus ein, im Einzelnen waren dies *De medici officina*, *De fracturis* und *De articulis* (diese drei hippokratischen Schriften zusammen mit Galens Kommentar), dann *De ulceribus*, *De fistulis* und *De capitis vulneribus*, außerdem das pseudogalenische *De fasciis* sowie die beiden Schriften *De laqueis* und *De machinamentis* des Oribasius.

Auch wenn diese Ausgabe wohl nicht nachgedruckt wurde, rezipierte man sie rege. Davon zeugt ein Eintrag über ein Exemplar in Girolamos Fabrizi d'Aquapendente Bibliothek (als Nr. 13 in seinem Katalog, dazu F. Zen Benetti, „La libreria di Girolamo Fabrici d'Acquapendente“, *Quaderni per la storia dell'università di Padova* 9/10 (1976/1977), S. 161–183, S. 173), Conrad Gesner übernahm einen Teil dieser Ausgabe (Vidius' Übersetzungen von (Ps.-)Galens *De fasciis liber* sowie Oribasius' *De laqueis* und *De machinamentis*) in seine chirurgische Anthologie von 1555. Außerdem verzeichnet Gurlt, *Geschichte der Chirurgie 2* (1898), S. 304 zwei französische Übersetzungen (Lyon 1555 und Paris 1634); und Nutton, *Humanist surgery* (1985), S. 87ff. berichtet allgemein über den Einfluss, den Vidius' *Chirurgia* in seiner Zeit ausübte.

38 Der gebürtige Mailänder studierte in Pavia und ließ sich in seiner Heimatstadt als praktischer Arzt nieder. Später wurde er dort Professor für Medizin. Silvaticus war ein produktiver Schriftsteller, wir wissen von Schriften über den Aderlass (1583), die Simulation von Krank-

ser zitierte in seinem *Medicus* von 1611 die Stelle[39] und erörterte anschließend die einzelnen Prinzipien des *celeriter*, *eleganter* und *iucunde* entlang von Galens Hippokrates-Kommentar. Im Grunde stellt das Kapitel zwölf („Chirurgus in operationibus manuum quomodo se gerere debeat") eine ausführliche Besprechung dieser Prinzipien dar. Dabei ging es dem Silvaticus – mit Bezug auf Galens zweiten Kommentar zu Hippokrates' *De officina medici*, Abs. 1[40] – auch darum, dass wer sich bei der manuellen Therapie auf diese Weise gemäß den Regeln der Kunst richtig verhalte, seinen Ruhm als Chirurg vergrößern könne.[41]

Und Reulin schrieb – wieder mit Guy – über dieses Thema:

> Finablement qu'il soit vertueux & bien morigeré, aux choses seures & manifestes hardy, aux douteuses & dangereuses tardif, & craintif, à ses patiens modeste & affable, discret & bien aduisé en la prediction des issues & succés des maladies, chaste, sobre, & pitoyable, se faisant payer selon le merite de son œuure, & la puissance du patient, sans exaction & auarice.[42]

Im Zusammenhang mit den Tugenden und dem richtigen Verhalten des Chirurgen wurde also üblicherweise zu Sittenstrenge, Keuschheit und Abstinenz aufgefordert, zudem zur Zurückhaltung bei Prognosen, vor allem im Hinblick auf mögliche Heilungsversprechen. Ein guter Chirurg solle in seiner Behandlung keine unnötigen Risiken eingehen und auch bei scheinbaren Routineeingriffen immer von Vorsicht geleitet sein. Schließlich ging es um die Arzt-Patient-Beziehung: Der Chirurg solle bescheiden, freundlich und mitfühlend auftreten sowie die Höhe seines Honorars von der finanziellen Situation des Patienten abhängig machen. Auch Della Croce forderte moralische Vorbildhaftigkeit, worunter er unter anderem die Kenntnisse der Moralphilosophie und die guten Sitten (*boni mores*) des Chirurgen fasste:

heiten (1595), Aneurysmata (1595), Theriak (1597) und populären Themen wie Einhörner und Wundersteine (1605), außerdem eine Schrift, in der er sich zu den gängigen medizinischen Streitpunkten positionierte (1601) sowie über die Geschichte des Mailänder *Collegium medicorum* (1607). Vgl. Gurlt, *Geschichte der Chirurgie 2* (1898), S. 541–544.

39 Silvaticus, *Medicus* (1611), S. 159.

40 *Hippocratis de medici officina liber et Galeni in eum commentarius II*, ed. Kühn 18/2 (1830), S. 719–815, S. 723.

41 „Quod clarè satis sermone de Chirurgo instituto, Galenus docuit 2. in lib. Hipp. de offic. Med. com. 1 elegantiam in actionibus suis manuum, illius gloriam augere apud vulgus, affirmans." Silvaticus, *Medicus* (1611), S. 159.

42 Reulin, *La chirurgie fort utile* (1580), S. 16. Die entsprechende Stelle bei Guy lautet: „Quatriemement i'ay dit, que faut qu'il soit bien morigeré. Soit hardi en choses seures, craintif ez dangiers, qu'il fuye les mauuaises cures ou practiques. Soit gratieus aus malades, bienueulhant a ses compagnons, sage en ces predictions. Soit chaste, sobre, pitoyable & misericordieus; non conuoyteus ni extortionnaires d'argent, ains qu'il reçoiue moderement salaire selon son trauail, les facultez du malade, la qualité de l'yssue ou euenement, & sa dignité." Guy de Chauliac, *La grande chirurgie*, trad. fr. L. Joubert (1579), S. 14. Die lateinische Fassung lautet: „Quarto dixi, oportet quod sit morigeratus; sit audax in securis, timidus in periculis, malas curas fugiat. Sit infirmis graciosus, sociis benivolus, cautus in pronosticando; sit castus, sobrius, pius, et misericors; non | cupidus neque extorsivus, sed secundum laborem suum et facultatem infirmi et qualitatem finis et dignitatem ipsius salaria recipiat moderate." Guy de Chauliac, *Chirurgia magna*, ed. M. McVaugh (1997), S. 9f.

> Er sei angefüllt mit den Vorschriften der Moralphilosophie, damit er im Stande ist, sich bei seinen eigenen Handlungen richtig zu verhalten. Er sei mit guten Sitten versehen: zu den Armseligen rechtschaffen, mit allen freundlich, aber nur mit sehr wenigsten tatsächlich vertraulich. Mit den Unkundigen sollte er nicht viel sprechen. Er sei ansprechbar, frohen Mutes, aber zugleich verschwiegen und keusch.[43]

Zum richtigen Handeln zählte auch der geschickte Umgang mit chirurgischen Instrumenten. Das finden wir bereits bei Vigo,[44] besonders ausführlich beschäftigte sich Della Croce damit. Er leitete diesen Abschnitt mit den Worten ein:

> Die Werkzeuge oder Instrumente aber, die für verschiedene Eingriffe benötigt werden, die beim guten Chirurgen im täglichen Gebrauch sind, muss der Chirurg immer griffbereit haben. Sie werden auf verschiedene Weise und aus unterschiedlichem Material hergestellt. Auch müssen sie auf solche Weise in die Nähe des Operateurs gelegt werden, dass sie dort, wo operiert wird, die Arbeit nicht stören, aber auch nicht so weit entfernt liegen, dass sie [vom Operateur] nicht gefasst werden können.[45]

Anschließend stellte Della Croce die einzelnen Instrumente vor, geordnet nach ihrer Funktion, *ad explorandum, coniungendum, incidendum, perforandum, aperiendum, extrahendum, imponendum, restaurandum, anatomizandum, cauterizandum.*[46] In einer späteren Fassung des Vorworts finden wir eine verlängerte Passage über den Umgang mit Instrumenten, der dort explizit zu den Voraussetzungen eines guten Chirurgen zählt: „Zu diesen vnd dergleichen nothwendigen Stuͤcken gehoͤrt auch/ daß er mit allerley noͤtigen instrumenten versehen sey/ vnnd dieselbige so viel muͤglich allenthalben bey sich trage“, so heißt es in der deutschen Übertragung durch den Frankfurter Stadtarzt Peter Uffenbach (um 1566–1635) aus dem Jahre 1607.[47] Auf etwas mehr als zwei ganzen Folioseiten werden Schermesser, Scheren, Pinzetten, Sonden, Nadeln und Skalpelle vorgestellt, ihre

43 „Philosophię moralis præceptis abundet, vt in propriis actionibus se rectè regere valeat. Bonis sit moribus præditus: miseris pius, cunctis amicus, sed quàm paucissimis familiaris intimus: cum imperitis non multa fabuletur: Sit affabilis, lætus: sed secretus, & castus.“ Della Croce, *Chirurgiae libri septem* (1573), S. 5ᵛ.

44 Vigo, *Practica* (1582), fol. *5ʳ.

45 „Organa autem, siue instrumenta ad uarias operationes requisita, quæ apud bonos Chirurgos in quotidianum vsum veniunt, quibus etiam munitus perpetuò esse debet Chirurgus, vario modo & ex diuersa materia formantur, & propè operatorem ea exponenda sunt, ne, ubi operari expedit, operam impediant, si longius distent, quàm ut possint capi:“ Della Croce, *Chirurgiae libri septem* (1573), S. 4ʳ.

46 Ebd., S. 4ʳ–4ᵛ. Die zentrale Rolle der operativen Instrumente in den chirurgischen Schriften von Della Croce bespricht ausführlich Gurlt, *Geschichte der Chirurgie 2* (1898), S. 335–361.

47 *Officina avrea. Das ist/ Güldene Werckstatt der Chirurgy oder WundtArtzney/ Von allen Gliedtmassen deß gantzen Menschlichen Leibs vnd derselbigen eusserlichen Gebrechen. Als/ den viel vnd mancherley vnnatürlichen Geschwülsten/ Wunden/ Geschwärn/ Frantzosen/ Beinbrüchen/ Verrenckungen/ vermischten vnnd vnvermischten Artzneyen vnd allen nohtwendigen Instrumenten gantz conterfätisch vorgestelt: Erstlich Von Ioanne Andrea de Crvce einem erfahrnen Wundtartzt zu Venedig beschrieben/ Nun mehr aber Allen Wundtartzten vnnd Liebhabern solcher Kunst/ die der frembden Sprachen vnerfahrn/ zum besten/ auß dem Italianischen/ als seinem Original in vnsere hoch Teutsche Sprach versetzt/ Durch Petrvm Vffenbachivm der Artzney D. vnd bestalten Medicum in Franckfort*. Getruckt zu Franckfort am Meyn bey Johann Saurn/ in Verlegung Jonæ Rhodii/ M. DC. VII., S. 11.

unterschiedlichen Anwendungsbereiche erklärt und anhand von Abbildungen verschiedene Variationen im Aussehen gezeigt.[48]

ERFAHRUNG UND WISSEN DES *CHIRURGUS PERITUS*

Als wesentlich für das Gelingen von Operationen galt die Erfahrung und das Wissen des Chirurgen. Sollte ein Chirurg keine Erfahrung gesammelt, dem Meister beim Operieren nicht assistiert, dessen Ausführungen nicht zugehört haben und es dennoch wagen zu praktizieren, würde er in seiner Unverfrorenheit viele Irrtümer begehen. Mit entsprechenden Versen warnte der französische Chirurg Ambroise Paré (1510–1590) den *brave chirurgien*:

> Celuy qui a bien leu, et pour cela pense estre
> Braue Chirurgien, sans auoir assisté
> Aux operations, et lecture du maistre,
> Se trompe tout contant, et n'est qu'vn effronté.[49]

Das Lernen von Anderen und die Erfahrung kam auch in der gelehrten Chirurgie zur Sprache, hatte sich doch auch Guy darüber geäußert.[50] Reulin paraphrasierte ihn folgendermaßen:

> Tiercement qu'il ait bonne experience de l'art, auant qu'il se mette à l'exercer, tant pour auoir veu, & bien obserué les operations des excellens Chirurgiens, que pour s'estre auec iceux souuent exercé, & accoustumé en icelle operations & curations.[51]

Erfahrung erwerbe ein Chirurg dadurch, dass er vorbildhafte *excellens Chirurgiens* beobachte sowie einzelne Eingriffe einübe. Auch Della Croce hob auf diesen Punkt ab, sollte doch ein *optimus chirurgus* sich in dieser Kunst häufig üben sowie Anderen, in dieser Kunst besser Bewanderten, beim Operieren zusehen (in

48 Ebd., S. 11–14.

49 Ambroise Paré, *Canons et reigles chirvrgiqves* (1575), in: *Œuvres complètes d'Ambroise Paré*, hg. v. J.-F. Malgaigne, Bd. 3, Paris 1841, Regel 33, S. 650.

50 „En segond lieu i'ay dit, qu'il faut qu'il soit expert, & ayt veu operer d'autres: iouxte le dire du sage Auenzoar, Il faut que tout medicin sache premierement, & que en apres il ayt l'vsage & l'experience. De mesme tesmognent Rasis au quatrieme liure a Almansor, & Halyabbas sur le testament d'Hippocras au premier de sa Theorique." Guy de Chauliac, *La grande chirurgie*, trad. fr. L. Joubert (1579), S. 14. „Secundo dixi, oportet quod sit expertus et viderit alios operari. Iuxta illus sapientis Avenzoaris: Oportet unumquemque medicum prius scire, deinde usum et experienciam habere. Et Rasis in 4° Almansoris, Haly Abbas in testamento Ypocratis primo Theorice, illud idem testantur." Guy de Chauliac, *Chirurgia magna*, ed. M. McVaugh (1997), S. 9.

51 Reulin, *La chirurgie fort utile* (1580), S. 16. Damit bezieht sich Reulin wieder auf seine Vorlage Guy de Chauliac, allerdings lässt er hier die von Guy genannten arabischen Autoritäten aus (Avenzoar, *Teisir*; Rhazes, *Almansor* 4,32; Haly Abbas, *Regalis dispositio* 1,1,2, Angaben nach M. McVaugh – M. S. Ogden, *Guigonis de Caulhiaco (Guy de Chauliac) Inventarium sive Chirurgia magna. Volume Two: Commentary*, Leiden / New York / Köln 1997, S. 21f.).

arte frequenter se exerceat, & cæteros artis peritiores operari sæpissimè uideat).[52] Allerdings sei – so Della Croce – immer darauf zu achten, dass ein junger Chirurg zuerst sorgfältig Bildung, die theoretischen Grundlagen des Faches und das notwendige Wissen für die chirurgische Tätigkeit erwerbe, bevor er praktisch tätig wird und beginnt, eigene Erfahrungen zu sammeln.[53] Denn ein Chirurg kann noch so erfahren, klug, einfühlsam und geschickt im Umgang mit den Instrumenten sein, er würde trotzdem Fehler begehen, wenn er die Grundlagen des Faches nicht oder falsch verstehe. Dies lässt sich mit einem eindrücklichen Fall veranschaulichen:

> Allein wenn sie [die Chirurgen] nach dem Aderlass das Blut in der Schüssel – wegen des eingeschlossenen aufgeblähten Geistes – erzittern sehen, nehmen sie an, dass mit dem Blut das Leben herausfließt. Deswegen zwingen sie den Patienten dazu, ihr Blut, bevor es schnell erkaltet, hinunterzuschlucken.[54]

Neben vielen anderen Unzulänglichkeiten und Fehlern der *vulgares chirurgi* kritisierte der humanistische Arzt Johannes Lange (1485–1565)[55] in seinen *Epistolae medicinales*[56] ihre falsche Auffassung, dass beim Aderlass jenes Blut, das in der Schüssel schaumig werde, mit dem *spiritus* vermischt sei und in diesem Fall offensichtlich das Leben selbst mit aus dem Körper fließe. Deshalb würden solche Chirurgen ihre Patienten dazu zwingen, ihr eigenes Blut zu trinken. Und das sei,

52 Della Croce, *Chirurgiae libri septem* (1573), S. 4^{v}.

53 „& quæ ab alijs facta viderit, ac ipse expertus fuerit, memoriæ mandet, ac diligenter obseruet: nam dictum est, artium omnium opera frequenti exercitio firmantur; & artis necessaria sæpè tractanda sunt, ut inferius ad unguem in singularium morborum curatione explicaturi sumus." ebd., S. 4^{r}.

54 „attamen cum secta vena sanguinem in lebete, ob flatulentum inclusum spiritum, contremiscere vident, vitam cum sanguine effusam suspicantur: quem ob id repente, antequam tepescat, patientem absorbere cogunt." Johannes Langius: *Epistolarvm medicinalivm volvmen tripartitvm, denvo recognitum, & dimidia sui parte auctum. Opus varia ac rara cum eruditione, tum rerum scitu dignissimarum explicatione refertum: vt eius lectio non solum Medicinæ, sed omnis etiam naturalis historiæ studiosis plurimum sit emolumenti allatura*, Francofvrdi Apud heredes Andreæ Wecheli, Claudium Marnium & Ioann. Aubrium, MDLXXXIX, ep. 8, S. 36.

55 Johannes Lange studierte zunächst in Leipzig, begab sich dann auf eine ausgedehnte *peregrinatio academica* nach Italien, wo unter anderem in Ferrara Niccolò Leoniceno (1428–1524) sowie in Rom Johannes Vigo kennenlernte und in Pisa in Medizin promovierte. Er stand anschließend bis zu seinem Lebensende im Dienste der Kurfürsten von der Pfalz, unternahm vor allem mit Friedrich II. viele Reisen und starb dann auch hochbetagt mit 80 Jahren in Heidelberg. Zu Lange vgl. E. Gurlt, Art. „Lange, Johannes", ADB 17, 1883, S. 637–638; Nutton, Caius & Lange (1984); Nutton: *Humanist surgery* (1985), S. 91–96.

56 Langes wichtige Hinterlassenschaft ist sein Briefwechsel mit vielen berühmten Ärzten seiner Zeit aus verschiedenen Ländern. Nach der Erstveröffentlichung von 83 Briefen im Jahre 1554 erschienen 1560 weitere 61 Stück. Posthum wurden erweiterte Sammlungen dieser *Epistolae medicinales* veröffentlicht und Conrad Gesner nahm eine Auswahl von elf Briefen unter dem Titel *Themata chirurgica* in seine chirurgische Anthologie aus dem Jahre 1555 auf (fol. 311^{r}–325^{r}). Zu den *Themata chirurgica* vgl. auch E. J. Gurlt, *Geschichte der Chirurgie und ihrer Ausübung*, Bd. 3, Berlin 1898, S. 33–37.

so stöhnte Lange, allein auf das „vermessene Unwissen der Chirurgen" (*audax chirurgorum ignorantia*) – hier der Säftelehre – zurückzuführen.[57]

Langes Kritik spiegelte sich in der Forderung an den *bonus chirurgus* wider, über solides Fachwissen zu verfügen. In seinen *De chirurgica institutione libri quinque* entwarf der Professor an der Medizinischen Fakultät in Paris, Jean Tagault (bis 1545),[58] ein regelrechtes Bildungsprogramm für Chirurgen auf.[59] Der *peritus ac rationalis chirurgus* sollte neben praktischen Kenntnisse (*peritia*), die für die Ausführung nötig sind, einen genauen Begriff (*exacta cognitio*) von der Chirurgie besitzen.[60] An die Seite des sachlichen Wissens über Chirurgie, das er systematisch nach Definitionen, Gegenstand, Ziel und die Frage der Reihenfolge des Lernens abhandelt, stellte Tagault das Wissen, das den Chirurgen in seinem operativen Handeln überhaupt erst in die Lage versetzte, richtige Entscheidungen über Behandlungsmethode, Prognose und Heilmittel zu treffen. So werde gewährleistet, „dass der Chirurg auf kundige, entschlossene und rechte Art jenes ausführen kann, was zur Kunstlehre, die er ausübt, gehört."[61]

Mit diesem ambitionierten Programm begann Tagault das erste Kapitel „Generalis et compendaria chirurgi institutio, facili, & artificiosa methodo tradita". Dieser Abschnitt ist deswegen bemerkenswert, weil Tagault ein Programm der wissenschaftlichen Chirurgie in einem knappen merksatzartigen Stil entwarf, der in der Renaissance für viele propädeutische Schriften typisch war. Am Ende dieses Kapitels kam Tagault nochmal eigens auf die Anforderungen an den *bonus chirurgus* zu sprechen: Unter die *conditiones requisitæ ad manuales operationes*

57 „O audax chirurgicorum ignorantia, qui nesciunt, aerem, vitalis & animalis spiritus fomentum, non modo per arterias cerebri, pulmonis & cordis cauernas, sed per occultam quoque inspirationem & poros, vniuersos corporis artus perreptare." Lange: *Epistolae medicinales*, ed. auct. (1589), ep. 8, S. 36.

58 Tagault kam in Buleux, einem Dorf in der Nähe von Amiens in der Picardie, auf die Welt, studierte in Paris Medizin, promovierte 1524 und wurde 1534 zum Dekan der Medizinischen Fakultät gewählt. Vgl. Gurlt, *Geschichte der Chirurgie 2* (1898), S. 624.

59 Die *De chirurgica institutione libri quique* erschienen meistens zusammen mit einem sechsten Buch *De materia chirurgica* von Jacques Houllier (bis 1562). Die Erstausgabe kam in Paris 1543 heraus, anschließend finden wir Editionen von 1544, 1547, 1549, 1560 und 1567. Außerdem druckte sie Conrad Gesner in seiner chirurgischen Anthologie 1555 mit ab und wir finden sie 1610 im *Thesaurus chirurgiae* von Peter Uffenbach. Tagaults Chirurgie erfuhr außerdem zahlreiche Übersetzungen, zunächst 1549 ins Französische (auch 1576, 1610, 1618, 1629, 1679), im Folgejahr ins Italienische (auch 1570, 1585), sowie 1557 ins Niederländische (auch 1621) und 1574 ins Deutsche (auch 1584 und 1618).

60 „In perito, ac rationali Chirurgo, duo potissimùm desyderantur.
1. Exacta cognitio eius partis tertiæ therapeutices medicinæ: quæ, quia manu medetur χειρουργικὴ Græcis nominatur.
2. Peritia, ac solers promptitudo, seu prompta quædam dexteritas exequendi ea omnia, quæ ad affectus Chirurgiæ subiectos attinent." Johannes Tagault, *De Chirurgica institutione libri quinque, iam denuò accuratius recogniti, ac à mendis plerisque uindicati*, Venetiis. Ex officina Erasmiana apud Vincentium Vaugris prope horologium Diui Marci. M. D. XLIIII, fol. β vi^{r}.

61 „Vt peritè, promptè, ac dextrè exequatur Chirurgus, quæ ad artem quam exercet, pertinent." ebd., fol. β vi^{v}.

probè exercendas zählte er neben Scharfsinn und Tugendhaftigkeit auch das Wissen und Bildung (*doctrina atque eruditio*) des Chirurgen.[62] Darunter fiel das theoretische Feld der *res naturales, non naturales* und *praeter naturam* sowie die zum eigentlichen Praktizieren gehörigen Haltungen und Kenntnisse über Medikamente und Lebensführung, über die der Chirurg allerdings im Zweifelsfall den Arzt konsultieren sollte.[63]

Wie Tagault in seiner *Ad lectorem praefatio* ausführlich darstellte, verstand er seine Chirurgie als eine modernisierte Fassung der *Chirurgia magna* von Guy de Chauliac, die er sprachlich und inhaltlich verbesserte und weiterführte. Eine besondere Stellung hatte dieses einleitende programmatische Kapitel inne, das eine in weiten Teilen starke Umarbeitung von Guys Einleitungskapitel („Capitulum singulare in quo premittuntur quedam communia valde necessaria cuicumque volenti proficere in arte cyrurgie") darstellt. Darin zeigte Tagault eine in der Renaissance verbreitete, aber nicht unumstrittene Haltung, zum einen die Autoritäten wiederzubeleben und an ihnen festzuhalten, zum anderen ihre Texte sprachlich zu modernisieren und ihre Inhalte zu aktualisieren.

Tagaults Umgang mit Guy rief bei seinen Zeitgenossen geteilte Reaktionen hervor, Reulin etwa schrieb im Vorwort zu seiner *Chirurgie fort utile*:

> Guy de Cauliac l'a [gemeint ist: *la chirurgie*] bien descrite, mesmement pour son temps, auquel les sciences & arts n'estoient si esclercis & fleurissans, comme sont au nostre, qui nous a produit de plus agus & subtils esprits & engins: qui à bon droit desirent Chirurgigraphes, & autres aucteurs consonans & conformes à leur dexterité. Si le docte Tagaut les eust voulu contenter en cela, comme il pouuoit bien faire, il eust, ce me semble, mieux fait, que d'auoir enrichy ledit Guy de bon langage, esclercy, & embelly.[64]

In seinem Abschnitt über die Kenntnisse des guten Chirurgen, in dem Reulin sich eng an Guy hielt,[65] führte er zunächst ausführlich auf zweieinhalb Seiten das Wissen der *theorique* über die (natürlichen, nicht-natürlichen und widernatürlichen) Krankheitsursachen aus, sowie anschließend wesentliche knapper die *pratique*.[66] Reulin betonte mit Guy die Relevanz von Bildung und theoretischem Wissen des *bonus chirurgus*, im Vergleich dazu wurden die positiven Eigenschaften und die Tugend des Chirurgen lediglich in Gemeinplätzen abgehandelt.

62 Ebd., fol. δ^r.
63 Ebd., fol. δ^r – δ^v.
64 Reulin, *La chirurgie fort utile* (1580), S. 3.
65 „Guy de Cauliac requiert en vn bon Chirurgien quatres choses principalement. Premierement qu'il soit bien lettré & versé non seulement en | la Theorique de l'art, mais aussi en la Pratique." ebd., S. 12f. Die entsprechende Stelle bei Guy lautet: „Il est donc requis en premier lieu, que le Chirurgien soit lettré, non seulement ez principes de la Chirurgie, mais aussi de la Medecine, tant en theorique que en pratique." Guy de Chauliac, *La grande chirurgie*, trad. fr. L. Joubert (1579), S. 13. „Requiritur ergo primo quod cyrurgicus sit litteratus, non tantum in principiis cyrurgie sed eciam phisice, tam in theorica quam practica." Guy de Chauliac, *Chirurgia magna*, ed. M. McVaugh (1997), S. 9.
66 „Touchant la pratique, le Chirurgien doit bien entendre, & estre versé aux maladies subiectes à son art, & pour la curation d'icelle, sçauoir ordonner diete & maniere de viure commode, medicamens, & autres remedes conuenables, & iceux appliquer: & generalement faire toutes autres choses requises pour l'exercice dudit art" Reulin, *La chirurgie fort utile* (1580), S. 15.

Eine ausführliche Beschäftigung mit dem Wissen der Chirurgie finden wir bei Della Croce, der im Abschnitt „De optimi Chirurgi præcipuis conditionibus“ im Anschluss an die Erläuterung der guten Eigenschaften zunächst beschrieb, mit welchen allgemeinen Bildungsgütern der *optimus chirurgus* ausgestattet sein sollte:

> Darüber hinaus sei er ein eifriger Student der humanistischen Wissenschaften, damit er die griechischen und lateinischen Schriftsteller verstehe. Er soll in der Logik beschlagen sein, um zu zeigen, dass er das Wahre vom Falschen unterscheiden kann und das Vermögen hat, sich vor [Spitzfindigkeiten von] Sophisten zu schützen.[67]

Grundlegend für das Gelingen eines Eingriffs seien außerdem die Umstände, die ein Chirurg bei seiner Arbeit beachten muss.[68] Ein *bonus chirurgus* sollte immer die Bedingungen des Kranken selbst, der Umstehenden und Helfenden bedenken und allgemeine Umstände wie Licht und Zeit berücksichtigen. Zentral war sein Wissen über die betroffenen Körperteile und Säfte, über die Beschaffenheit des Gewebes und über die Position des Kranken bei der Operation. Schließlich musste der Chirurg auch über Art und Weise der diätetischen Anweisungen und des Medikaments Bescheid wissen. Die Vorlage für diesen Abschnitt bildet wieder das hippokratische *De officina*, das Della Croce am Anfang des Kapitels – in Großbuchstaben – in lateinischer Übersetzung zitierte und anschließend kommentarartig ausführte.[69]

Schließlich ging Della Croce noch auf drei Hinsichten ein, die von einem erfahrenen Chirurgen (*peritus chirurgus*) bei seiner Arbeit notwendigerweise berücksichtigt werden müssen („à perito chirurgo in suis operationibus necessariò considerantur“):[70] die Anatomie, das Ziel der *unitas corporis* und die Beherrschung der geeigneten Heilmittel, Lebensführung und Instrumente. Die Anweisung zur Anatomie lautet, „der Chirurg sei also bei den Handhabungen der Anatomie, das heißt bei der richtigen Art der Leichenöffnung, sorgfältig und geübt.“[71] Die Nützlichkeit der Anatomie sei nicht unwichtiger als andere Kenntnisse („talis cognitio non minoris est utilitatis“):

> Da in den inneren wie in den äußeren Körperteilen Schmerzen und verschiedene Arten von Krankheiten entstehen, kann hingegen niemand glauben, der davon keine Kenntnis hat, die

67 „Sit præterea humanarum litterarum studiosus, vt Græcos & Latinos scriptores intelligat. Logicen calleat, vt demonstrando, verùm à falso discernat, & à sophistis valeat se tueri.“ Della Croce, *Chirurgiae libri septem* (1573), fol. 5^{v}.

68 Ebd., fol. 3^{v}–4^{r}.

69 Hippokrates, *De officina medici* 2. Der Wortlaut ist: „Τὰ δ᾽ ἐς χειρουργίαν κατ᾽ ἰητρεῖον.“ Und: „Ὁ ἀσθενέων, ὁ δρῶν, οἱ ὑπηρέται, τὰ ὄργανα, τὸ φῶς, ὅκου, ὅκως, ὁκόσα, οἷσιν, ὅκως, ὁκότε, τὸ σῶμα, τὰ ἄρμενα, ὁ χρόνος, ὁ τρόπος, ὁ τόπος.“ Die lateinische Übersetzung lautet: „Quae autem ad chirurgiam in medici officina spectant.“ Und: „Aegrotans, agens, ministri, machinamenta, lumen, ubi, quomodo, quot, quibus, quo pacto, quando, corpus, instrumenta, tempus, modus, locus.“ ed. Kühn 18/2 (1830), S. 664 und 667.

70 Della Croce, *Chirurgiae libri septem* (1573), fol. 3^{r}.

71 „Sit ergo Chirurgus in anatomicis administrationibus, id est corporum mortuorum recta sectione diligens & exercitatus.“ ebd.

> Heilmittel anwenden zu können. Also ist es notwendig, möglichst viele Körper von Toten aufzuschneiden und ihre Eingeweide sowie die äußeren Teile zu untersuchen.[72]

Mit der Anatomie kommt Della Croce auf ein Wissen zu sprechen, das die frühneuzeitliche Chirurgie wesentlich prägte. Forderungen nach besseren anatomischen Kenntnissen hatte freilich schon Guy de Chauliac erhoben, der ihnen das erste Hauptkapitel widmete und sie im Eingangskapitel unter die *res naturales* zählte, die zum Wissen des *bonus chirurgus* gehörten. Entsprechend paraphrasierte Reulin in seiner *Chirurgie fort utile*:

> Entre lesquelles causes, le Chirurgien doit specialement cognoistre les parties du corps, par l'Anatomie, sans l'intelligence de laquelle il ne peut deument exercer la Chirurgie.[73]

Abgesehen von solchen Autoritätsbezügen avancierte die Anatomie mit dem Beginn der systematischen anatomischen Sektionen in der frühen Neuzeit zur wahrscheinlich wichtigsten empirischen medizinischen Disziplin, man denke allein an die Entwicklungen an der Universität Padua, wo die Anatomie im Laufe des 16. Jahrhunderts die Chirurgie in ihrer Wichtigkeit als Fach überholte.[74] Sehr bald schon war das Bild des *bonus chirurgus* nicht mehr ohne fundierte Anatomiekenntnisse denkbar.

DER *WOL ERFAHRNE WUNDARTZT* IN DER HANDWERKLICHEN CHIRURGIE

Das Bild des Chirurgen, das sich aus diesen Zeugnissen der italienischen und französischen Chirurgie im 16. Jahrhundert zusammensetzt, ist ambitioniert: Der *bonus chirurgus* sollte exzellente physische und psychische Voraussetzungen mitbringen, von tadellosem Äußeren und tugendhaftem Wesen sein, professionell-

72 „At, cùm in interioribus, & exterioribus membris & dolores, & morborum uaria genera nascantur, nemo putet se ijs adhibere remedia posse quæ ignorat. Ergo mortuorum corpora quàm plurima secare oportet, eorumque viscera, ac partes externas scrutari;" ebd.

73 Reulin, *La chirurgie fort utile* (1580), S. 13. Guy hatte formuliert: „Et premierement faut qu'il entende les choses naturelles, principalement l'anatomie, car sans icelle il n'y ha rien de fait en Chirurgie, comme il apperra cy dessoubs." Guy de Chauliac, *La grande chirurgie*, trad. fr. L. Joubert (1579), S. 13. „Primo enim oportet quod ipse cognoscat res naturales, precipue anathomiam, nam sine ipsa factum est nichil in cyrurgia, ut inferius apparebit." Guy de Chauliac, *Chirurgia magna*, ed. M. McVaugh (1997), S. 9.

74 Erst mit Vesal, der den Lehrstuhl für Chirurgie innehatte, wurde die Anatomielehre an der Universität Padua institutionalisiert, auch Realdo Columbo und Falloppio lehrten beide Fächer. Erst 1584 wurde der Lehrstuhl dann offiziell zur Professur für Anatomie und Chirurgie umbenannt. Vgl. dazu: J. Facciolati, *Fasti Gymnasii Patavini ab anno MDXVII. quo restitutæ scholæ sunt ad MDCCLVI*, Patavii, Typis Seminarii, MDCCLVII. Apud Joanem Manfrè, S. 385–389. Vgl. außerdem J. J. Bylebyl, „The School of Padua: Humanistic Medicine in the Sixteenth Century", in: C. Webster (Hg.), *Health, Medicine and Mortality in the Sixteenth Century*, Cambridge / London / New York / Melbourne 1979, S. 335–370. Zur frühneuzeitlichen Anatomie im Allgemeinen vgl. etwa R. French, *Dissection and Vivisection in the European Renaissance*, Aldershot 1999.

freundliche Umgangsformen pflegen, bei großen Meistern gelernt haben und über einen breiten Erfahrungs- und Wissensschatz in der Chirurgie verfügen. Dieses notwendigerweise überzeichnete Idealbild musste mit der Realität zusammenprallen. Besonders krass klafften Anspruch und Wirklichkeit im Falle von Barbieren auseinander. Ein Beispiel für eine solche Kritik:

> Und in der Tat ist es daher so, dass nur wenige unserer Chirurgen auch nur ein bisschen mehr können als Haare schneiden, Bärte rasieren, ungeschickt zur Ader lassen, Schröpfköpfe anbringen, Köpfe waschen, den Dreck aus den Ohren holen und herumschwätzen. Keiner außer denen, die mit Bildung und in vernunftgeleiteter Weise mit der Kunstlehre [der Chirurgie] in Berührung gekommen sind, kann die Chirurgie wirklich verstehen und ausüben.[75]

Für Johannes Freitag (1581–1641), Professor für Medizin und fürstbischöflicher Leibarzt, war die Sache klar: Wegen der Untüchtigkeit (*inertia*) und des stumpfsinnigen Unverstands (*Chirurgorum barda inscitia*) konnten Chirurgen nicht heilen.[76] Es gebe nichts gewagteres als Unwissenheit (*ignorantia*), weswegen Chirurgen umso unerträglichere Fehler (*intolerabiliores errores*) begingen![77] So wie Johannes Freitag in seinen *Noctes medicae sive de abusu medicinae tractatus* von 1616 im Kapitel 13 *De chirurgis, horumque spissa ignorantia & imposturis* polemisierte, taten es Viele in dieser Zeit. Abgesehen davon, dass die Scharlatanerieschelte wohl einen tatsächlichen Missstand der Zeit widerspiegelte,[78] diente der Vorwurf der Scharlatanerie auch als rhetorische Waffe gegen Konkurrenten und zur Abgrenzung der eigenen beruflichen Kompetenzen: studierte Ärzte gegen die

75 „Verum itaque & vero verius est, paucos nostrorum chirurgorum paulo plus scire, quam capillos & barbas radere venas rustice secare, cucurbitulas affigere, capita lauere aurium sordes extergere, nugari, nullos, præterquam literis tinctos & arte rationaliter imbutos vere chirurgiam intelligere & exercere." Johannes Freitag: *Noctes medicæ Siue de abvsv medicinæ tractatvs qvo vniversvm medicastrorum examen Empiricorum modernorum vberrima annona, vromantes seu lotiophysici, agyrtæ, ophthalmici dentifrangibuli chirurgi, genethliaci, seplasiarioinstitores, myrolopæ, pseudochymici, vmbratici doctores Paracelsistarum sectæ, magomedicastri, sagæ & superstitiosam vulgò curam exercentes perstringuntur, de magia vetita & magorum suppliciis agitur, artis Paracelsicæ fundamenta luculenter traduntur, examinantur & euertuntur, scitu necessariæ & iucundæ omnibus omnium facultatum studiosis quæstiones mouentur*, Francofvrti, Ex Officina Typographica Iohannis Bringeri. Sumptibus Ioannis Berneri. M. DC. XVI, S. 55.

76 Ebd., S. 54.

77 „atqui cum ignorantia nihil sit audacius, intolerabiliores errores errant." ebd.

78 Dass sich diese Polemik wirklich speziell gegen eine ausgewiesene Gruppe richtete, illustriert eine weitere Stelle in diesem Kapitel 13 der *Noctes medicae*, an der Johannes Freitag ausdrücklich die gelehrten Chirurgen („iis, qui rationalis chirurgiae praecepta medica [...] acceperunt") von der Kritik ausnimmt: „Hic aduertendum, me non loqui de iis, qui rationalis chirurgiæ præcepta medica (est enim chirurgia antiquissima medicinæ pars cæterarumque fons & origo quæ externis corporis affectibus, | medetur) rationali methodo in academiis primo acceperunt, eique doctis præeuntibus & manu ducentibus magistris encheriam & operationis manualis solertiam & artificia coniunxerunt, quorum rari in Germania nostra visuntur, sed de plerisque istis & vulgaribus sycophantis qui cum nihil penitus in sua professione intelligant artemque suam exercentes fortunæ temeritati quorsum res vergat, committere cogantur, nihilominus adeo frontem perfricuerunt, vt se supra Galenum ipsum sapere arroganter deierarent & si in viuis esset, impudenter obstrigillarent." ebd., S. 53f.

nicht-akademischen heilkundig Tätigen, die handwerklichen Chirurgen gegen die ungelernten Heiler – man denke an das Eingangszitat von Wilhelm Fabry über die *groben Kerle*, die chirurgisch tätig waren. Man denunzierte ihre Fehler, die auf Unwissen, oder ihre unwirksamen oder lebensgefährlichen Kuren, die auf die Geldgier und betrügerische Absicht zurückgingen.[79]

Die handwerkliche Chirurgie brachte in diesem Spannungsfeld zur akademischen Medizin in der frühen Neuzeit eigene, umfassende chirurgische Literatur hervor, in der sie auch über die Frage nach dem idealen Praktiker nachdachte. Der Straßburger Chirurg und Feldarzt Hans von Gersdorf (1450/60–1529)[80] bestimmte 1517 in seinem *Feldbuch der Wundarztney* den Unterschied zwischen akademischen Ärzten und Chirurgen folgendermaßen:

> das ist ein handtwürcker/ oder wundartzet. | In dem entscheidet von dem artzt/ dz der phisicus oder leibartzt kein handwürckung thůt. Darumb ist des chirurgici ampt/ mit der handt zů würcken an des menschen leib wo der offen ist/ gehawen oder zercbrohen/ den wider zůsamen fügen/ oder gantz zemachen als es vor ist gewesen noch müglichen dingen.[81]

Nur dem Chirurgen – nicht nicht dem *medicus* („phisicus oder leibartzt") – seien manuellen Eingriffe erlaubt. Um seine Arbeit gut zu erledigen, führt Gersdorf an dieser Stelle des kurzen Kapitels *Von der ordenung vnd schicklicheit des Chirurgici/ wie sich der halten sol in alle weg handtwürckunge der wundartzney*[82] weiter aus, müsse der

> [...] Chirurgicus ein gůte vernunfft hab vnd ein gůte verstaͤntnüß. Nit zůschnell in seiner würckung/ sonder allzeit wolbedocht/ was schaden im oder dem krancken erwachsen moͤcht durch seine vngeschicklicheit.[83]

Gersdorf gebietet demjenigen *wundartzt*, der noch keine „volkümenliche verstaͤntnüß" erworben hat, sich nicht zu schämen, sondern bei den Erfahrenen zu lernen: „so schaͤme er sich nit/ nem ein erfarenen alten scherer/ oder der mer verstaͤntnüß hab dann er zů jm".[84] Und schließlich fordert er noch anatomische Kenntnisse:

79 Scharlataneriepolemik gab es viel und lange, so auch noch Ende des 17. Jahrhunderts, man denke etwa an den satirisch gewendeten *Medicus machiavellus*, vgl. dazu: K. Vanek, „Der ‚Machiavellus medicus' und die gelehrte Scharlatanerie", in: T. Asmussen – H. Rößler (Hgg.), *Scharlatan! Eine Figur der Relegation in der frühneuzeitlichen Gelehrtenkultur*, Frankfurt a. M. 2013, S. 309–333.

80 Über Gersdorff (auch Schyl Hans genannt) ist wenig bekannt. Er scheint lange als Kriegschirurg gearbeitet und in Straßburg im Spital viele Amputationen durchgeführt zu haben. Vgl. E. Wickersheimer, Art. „Gersdorff", *NDB* 6, 1964, S. 322–323. Ausführlich zu Gersdorf jetzt: M. Panse, *Hans von Gersdorffs ‚Feldbuch der Wundarznei'. Produktion, Präsentation und Rezeption von Wissen*, Wiesbaden 2012.

81 *Feldtbůch der wundtartzney. Mit Keyserlicher freyheit getruckt zů Straßburg durch Joannem Schott* [Ende Vorrede:] Anno domini M CCCCC Xvij, Tract. 2, Kap. 1, S. XIX^{r}–XIX^{v}.

82 Ebd., Tract. 2, Kap. 1, S. XIX^{r}–XIX^{v}.

83 Ebd., S. XIX^{v}.

84 Ebd.

> Sol mer ein fleissig vffsehen haben vff alle glider wie die geschickt seyen in den gleychen vnd in dem geåder so er sye schniden/ etzen/ cauterisieren. i. brennen mitt ysenen oder guldin instrumenten wil. domit kein schad dem glid doruß erwachßen mőg.[85]

Mit seiner Forderung nach Anatomiekenntnissen folgte Gersdorf, wie andere Autoren seiner Zeit auch, Guy de Chauliac. Ein profunderes Verständnis der Bedeutung anatomischer Sektion und der daraus resultierenden Kenntnisse für die chirurgische Arbeit demonstrierte dagegen Wilhelm Fabry von Hilden,[86] der in seiner Zeit als Stadtchirurg von Bern eine Schrift *Von der Fürtrefflichkeit und Nutz der Anatomy* (1624) verfasst hatte. Dort kritisierte Hildanus beispielsweise die fehlenden Anatomiekenntnisse der *Oculisten*, denn „es ist keiner würdig, solch edles Gliedt anzugreiffen, er habe dann eine grundliche Erkandnuß desselben." Überhaupt gingen viele tödliche Fehler von Chirurgen auf ihre mangelnden Anatomiekenntnisse zurück:

> Den Stein, die Brüch vnd andere Gewechs zu schneiden, erfordert auch die Erkandnuß der Anatomy, wo es anders recht sol zugehen. Bey meiner Zeit, als ein fremder, vermessener vnd der Anatomy vnerfahrner Schnittartzet gen Genff kompt, vnd daselbst einer jungen Dochter ein Gewechs am Halse außzuschneiden sich vnderstehet, vnd auff die *venas jugulares* nicht Achtung gibt, ist sie vnder seinen Händen vnd in derselben Stund gestorben. Also ist auch ein Graf von Waldeck drauff gangen vnd in derselben Stund, als ein stoltzer vnd vnverzagter Bruchschneider ihm ein Gewechs in der Dicke des Schenkels solte außschneiden, verscheiden, darumb daß der Schnittartzet wegen seiner Vnerfahrenheit in der Anatomy auff den großen *ramum* oder Zweigen der *venae cavae*, das ist der Blutader, so auß der Leber zu dem Schenkel hinab gehet, nicht Achtung gab.[87]

Hildanus gelang es, die geschilderten Fehler auf konkrete fehlende Kenntnisse in der Anatomie des tätigen Chirurgen zurückzuführen und auf diese Weise anschaulich die Notwendigkeit und den Nutzen dieser Kenntnisse auch für die nichtstudierten Chirurgen zu vermitteln.

85 Ebd.

86 Wilhelm Fabry wurde 1560 in Hilden im Bergischen Land geboren und ging in Neuss bei einem Bader in die Lehre, wurde Geselle bei Cosma Slot in Düsseldorf und ging 1585 auf Wanderschaft. Anschließend ließ er sich in der Schweiz nieder, zunächst in Genf, wo er zusammen mit Jean Griffon praktizierte sowie Marie Colinet, eine berühmte Hebamme und Wundärztin, heiratete. Nach seinem Aufenthalt in Lausanne wurde er 1602 zum Stadtchirurg von Payerne/Peterlingen bestallt, 1615 zum Stadtchirurgen von Bern , wo er 1634 starb. Unterbrochen wurde seine Tätigkeit als Stadtchirurg immer wieder von zum Teil ausgedehnten Reisen, in deren Abwesenheit er von Marie Colinet vertreten wurde. Abgesehen von vielen medizinischen Einzel- und einzelnen religiösen Erbauungsschriften verfasste Hildanus eine große Anzahl von *observationes*, die in sechs Zenturien im Laufe seines Lebens und posthum erschienen. Vgl. C. P. Leporin, *Das Leben Des Vortrefflichen Gvilielmi Fabricii von Hilden*, Quedlinburg / Aschersleben 1722; Gurlt, *Geschichte der Chirurgie 3* (1898), S. 107–147; E. Jones, „The Life and Works of Guilhelmus Fabricius Hildanus (1560–1634)", *Medical History* 4 (1960), S. 112–134, S. 196–209, S. 112–120; W. Wennig, „Wilhelm Fabrys Lebenslauf", in: W. Wennig (Hg.), *Fabrystudien IV*, Hilden 1975, S. 9–19; M. Stolberg, Art. „Fabricius, Wilhelm", *DMB* 2007, S. 469–471

87 Wilhelm Fabry, *Von der Fürtrefflichkeit und Nutz der Anatomy*, 2., erw. Aufl. nach dem in der Stadtbibliothek von Bern befindlichen Manuskript hg v. F. de Quervain u. Hans Bloesch, Leipzig 1936, S. 23 (Hervorhebungen in Vorlage).

Vor allem die Anhänger von Paracelsus unter den Handwerkschirurgen neigten dazu, die Rolle der Erfahrung des Chirurgen über alles andere zu stellen. Ein Exponent dieser paracelsistischen Auffassung war Felix Würtz,[88] aus dessen *Practica der Wundarztney* oben bereits die Kritik an der Unbarmherzigkeit der Ärzte zitiert wurde.[89] Würtz verlieh seiner Geringschätzung der Büchergelehrsamkeit in der Vorrede deutlich Ausdruck:

> Solches nun beyzubringen / wirdt mir zweiffels ohn ein jeder wol erfahrner Wundartzt leichtlich zugeben vnd bekennen: Daß ja die Wundartzney nicht ohn grosse muͤhe vnnd arbeit erlernet werde. Dann sie lest sich mit nichten / wie ihren viel vermeinen / daheimen auff den Kussen oder mit lesen der Buͤchern / so daruon geschrieben / ergreiffen.

Um ein *wol erfahrner Wundartzt* zu werden benötige man statt Bücher „Lange zeit / vnd ernsthaffte uͤbung / wirdt darzu auch erfordert / so man in dieser Kunst etwas rechtgeschaffens außzurichten begeret." Nur durch Erfahrung, Reisen („wanderschafften vnd reisen hin vnd wider") und gute Vorbilder erwerbe ein Chirurg sein Können. Dem Felix Würtz war sein (gleichnamiger) Vater der Lehrer:

> Er hat mich auch hiemit aller seiner Curen vnd Heylungen/ wie vnd welcher gestalt er die vollbracht/ vnnd was er darbey auß der Erfahrung gelernet/ nicht allein muͤndlich vnderrichtet vnd gelehrt/ sonder auch augenscheinlich gezeiget/ vnd an die Hand gegeben/ so viel dessen immer muͤglich gewesen. Nach solchem/ hat er mich/ der Erfahrung nachzuziehen/ von sich gelassen: mit vnderrichtung darneben/ wessen ich mich in der frembde verhalten/ wie vnd was gestalt ich aller sachen warnemmen/ vnd alles fleissig mercken solte.[90]

Die individuelle Erfahrung galt dem Würtz als wesentliches Element der Kompetenz eines Chirurgen. Vermittelt wurde Erfahrung auf verschiedene Weise, durch den *mündlichen underricht* und das *augenscheinliche zeigen*. Nach der Lehre ging

88 Felix Würtz (auch: Wirz oder Wirtz) wurde zu Beginn des 16. Jahrhunderts in Bern oder Zürich geboren, nach Lehre und Wanderschaft ließ er sich als Bader in Zürich wieder, war Mitglied der Schererzunft „Zum schwarzen Graben" und genoss einen derart guten Ruf, dass er für sich eine Ausnahme von dem üblichen Verbot der Anwendung innerer Medizin für nicht-studierte Heilende in Zürich erwirken konnte. 1559 ging er nach Straßburg. Die Autorschaft der *Practica der Wundarztney* ist nicht sicher, entweder sie stammt aus der Feder von Felix Würtz und wurde später von seinem gleichnamigen Sohn herausgegeben und/oder weitergeschrieben, oder aber sie geht ganz auf Felix Würtz den Jüngeren zurück, über den wir nur wissen, dass er Bader war, in Basel wirkte und dort 1586 das Bürgerrecht erworben und 1587 bis 1596 dort zünftig war. Vgl. Art. „Würtz, Felix", *Zedler* 59, 1749, Sp. 1237; Hermann Frölich, Art. „Würtz, Felix", *ADB* 44, 1898, S. 352–354; Gurlt, *Geschichte der Chirurgie 3* (1898), S. 238–263; Alice Steinbrecher, Art. „Würzt (Wirtz, Wirz), Felix", *Enzyklopädie Medizingeschichte* 2005, S. 1503.

89 Auch wenn Würtz in seinem Text weitgehend ohne Bezüge auf Autoritäten auskam, so ließ er sich doch zu einem Lob des Paracelsus hinreißen: „Daher dann auch an ettlichen Orten/ die ich wol weiß/ an Eydstat verbotten worden/ die Buͤcher Theophrasti Paracelsi (welchem doch die beruͤmbtesten Wundaͤrtzten weichen muͤssen) zulesen. Aber/ meins schlechten beduncken/ wirdt damit gantz thoͤrlichen gehandelt." Würtz, *Practica der Wundartzney* (1596), S. xc.

90 Ebd. (ohne Paginierung, fol. a vi^r).

der Geselle auf Wanderschaft, um dort Erfahrungen zu sammeln.[91] Würtz berichtete, wie ihn der Vater dazu anhielt, sich auf seiner Reise in seinem Verhalten der Fremde anzupassen und alles gut zu merken. Er sei „ganz trewlich vnd Vaͤtterlich vermahnt" worden, sich vom *allgemeinen Brauch* zu distanzieren, gemeint ist die gängige Art, die Chirurgie zu praktizieren. Instrument gegen diese schlechte Praxis waren dem Würtz die eigene Erfahrung, seine Wahrnehmung und eine systematische kritische Überprüfung der gängigen Praktiken. Folgerichtig endet die Vorrede mit den Worten:

> Als ich nun dieser vnd dergleichen sachen wargenommen/ vnnd gesehen hette/ was in gemein im Brauch oder nit im brauch were: hab ich die Erfahrung/ deren ich nachgezogen/ dargegen gehalten/ vnd eins gegen dem andern nach seinen gruͤnden vnd vrsachen Examinirt vnd erwegen/ vnd auß solchem baldt befunden/ warinn der jrrthumb vnnd fehler begangen werde/ derohalben das rechte fundament od' grund der Wundartzney gesucht/ dahin ich auch endtlich gelanget bin: also dz ich vor allen Mißbraͤuchen/ so viel deren heut diß tags in der Wundartzney im schwanck gehen/ mich selber huͤten/ vnd andere warnen kan.[92]

Würtz entwarf also ein Programm der radikalen Prüfung der gängigen Chirurgie, eine von „vielen schaͤdlichen Mißbraͤuchen vnd greifflichen Irrthumben"[93] massiv gestörte Praxis. Instrument der Kritik und der Verbesserung war dem Würtz die Erfahrung, mit der das „rechte fundament od' grund der Wundarztney" gelegt werden könne.

FAZIT

Die Schilderungen der zuweilen schrecklichen *errores*, die Unsicherheit der chirurgischen Praxis und die unbeständigen Kompetenzen der Chirurgen verdeutlichen, als wie drängend die Probleme in der Chirurgie empfunden wurden, die gängige Missstände sollten abgebaut und der Beruf des Chirurgen professionalisiert werden. Einige der italienischen und französischen Lehrbücher und Programmschriften der Chirurgie von Vigo, Della Croce und Tagault entwarfen im 16. Jahrhundert ein Bild des in Hinsicht auf die moralischen Qualitäten, intellektuellen Fähigkeiten, manuelle Geschicklichkeit und Haltung gegenüber dem Patienten idealen Chirurgen, der um die angemessenen Handlungsweisen weiß, sich extensive medizinische und chirurgische Kenntnisse aneignet und über einen reichen Erfahrungsschatz verfügt. Entsprechend ging es bei der Reflexion all dieser Eigenschaften letztlich um die Festlegung eines chirurgischen Berufsethos: Wissensstandards, Kontrolle des äußeren Erscheinungsbilds und Regulierung von

91 Zur handwerklichen chirurgischen Ausbildung im frühneuzeitlichen Zürich vgl. exemplarisch den Lehrweg von Würtzens Zeitgenossen Jacob Ruf, konzise nachzulesen in H. Steinke, „Vom Schererlehrling zum Chirurgenmeister", in: H. E. Keller (Hg.), *Mit der Arbeit seiner Hände. Leben und Werk des Zürcher Stadtchirurgen und Theatermachers Jakob Ruf (1505–1558)* (Jakob Ruf. Leben, Werk und Studien; 1), Zürich 2008, S. 63–73.

92 Würtz, *Practica der Wundartzney* (1596), fol. a ii^{r}.

93 Dieser Ausdruck findet sich häufig in der ganzen *Practica*, in der Vorrede beispielsweise auf fol. a v^{v}.

Verhalten – dem guten Chirurgen sollte es sehr wohl möglich sein, Fehler weitgehend zu vermeiden.

War die Medizin in der frühen Neuzeit in erster Linie eine von akademischer Büchergelehrsamkeit geprägte universitäre Disziplin, besaß die Chirurgie – auch in ihrer akademischen Ausprägung – einen hohen praktischen Anteil. Die im Vergleich zur Medizin stärkere Handlungsorientierung spiegelt sich in den Vorstellungen über den idealen Chirurgen anschaulich wider, man denke an die Rolle des praktischen Wissens sowie an den Stellenwert, der etwa den manuellen Fertigkeiten, der Jugend und der Beherztheit des Chirurgen beim Operieren zugesprochen wurde. Der Umfang und die Inhalte des Wissens des *bonus chirurgus* wurden freilich unterschiedlich gewichtet: Die Bandbreite reicht von der weitreichenden Forderung nach humanistischer Gelehrsamkeit als Voraussetzung für die Lektüre und Aneignung der antiken Schriften in Griechisch und Latein (Della Croce) bis hin zur Beschränkung des Wissens auf das, was zur Anwendung nötig ist (Würtz).

In den hier zur Sprache gekommenen Programmschriften und Lehrbüchern der Chirurgie, die über den *bonus chirurgus* und seinen Berufsethos nachdachten, orientierte man sich an den autoritativen Schriften der antiken medizinischen Literatur Hippokrates, Celsus und Galen sowie an den gängigen Topoi. Bemerkenswert ist die intensive Rezeption des Chirurgen Guy de Chauliac aus dem 14. Jahrhundert. Andere bekannte, ebenfalls in der frühen Neuzeit edierte Autoren wie Guglielmo da Saliceto oder Henri de Mondeville fanden in dieser Sache keine Erwähnung, obwohl sie sich ebenfalls über den *bonus chirurgus* geäußert haben.[94] Guys Attraktivität lag abgesehen von der guten Editionslage und Zugänglichkeit durch die vielen volkssprachlichen Übersetzungen wohl auch daran, dass er im präliminatorischen Kapitel ein prägnantes und gut fassbares Konzept des guten Chirurgen entworfen hatte, dessen vier Grundelemente er konzise fassen konnte:

> Für den Chirurgen sind vier Bedingungen notwendig: erstens, dass er belesen ist, zweitens, dass er erfahren ist, drittens, dass er einfallsreich ist und viertens, dass er von guten Sitten erfüllt ist.[95]

An der lebendigen Guy de Chauliac-Rezeption lässt sich die wichtige Rolle der mittelalterlichen Schriften als Mittler antiken und arabischen Gedankenguts veranschaulichen. Guy besaß zudem schon im 14. und 15. Jahrhundert eine eigene volkssprachliche Überlieferung. Überhaupt spielten vernakuläre Übersetzungen aus dem Lateinischen oder aus anderen Volkssprachen in der Chirurgie eine große Rolle. So konnte etwa Vivian Nutton am Büchermarkt in Lyon angesichts der

94 Zu Guglielmo vgl. etwa J. Agrimi – C. Crisciani, „The Science and Practice of Medicine in the Thirteenth Century according to Guglielmo da Saliceto, Italian Surgeon", in: L. García-Ballester et al. (Hgg.), *Practical Medicine from Salerno to the Black Death*, Cambridge 1994, S. 60–87, S. 75ff. oder zu Mondeville: D. Jacquart, „Medical Practice in Paris in the First Half of the Fourteenth Century", in: L. García-Ballester et al. (Hgg.), *Practical Medicine from Salerno to the Black Death*, Cambridge 1994, S. 186–206, S. 191ff.

95 „Condiciones que requiruntur in cyrurgico sunt quatuor: prima quod sit litteratus, secunda quod sit expertus, tercia quod sit ingeniosus, quarta ut sit morigeratus." Guy de Chauliac, *Chirurgia magna*, ed. M. McVaugh (1997), S. 9.

vielen französischen Fassungen chirurgischer Bücher aufweisen, dass wir es in der Chirurgie mit einem weniger gebildeten Publikum zu tun haben, das oftmals über wenig Lateinkenntnisse verfügte.[96] Doch sogar ein dem gelehrten Bildungsgut so feindlich gesinnter Praktiker wie Würtz kannte Guy. Daraus lässt sich schließen, dass profunde Kenntnisse und ein gelehrter Umgang mit der Chirurgie nicht nur für die universitär gebildeten Ärzte-Chirurgen gefordert wurden. Vielmehr muss angesichts vieler Übersetzungen von einer breiteren Leserschaft der gelehrten chirurgischen Traktate ausgegangen werden, die einen eigenen Absatzmarkt für entsprechende volkssprachliche Übertragungen bildete.

Und so ist es wohl kein Zufall, dass ausgerechnet eine der umfassendsten und gelehrtesten Erörterungen des *bonus chirurgus* im Vorwort zur Chirurgie von Giovanni Andrea Della Croce nach einer italienischen Übersetzung 1583 im Jahre 1607 ins Deutsche übertragen worden war. Allerdings zeigt ein Blick in den deutschen Text, dass der Übersetzer Peter Uffenbach auf die vielen Quellen- und Autoritätsangaben, die noch den Rand des lateinischen Textes (und der italienischen Übersetzung) säumten, bis auf vereinzelte Hinweise auf Aristoteles, Hippokrates und Galen verzichtete und seine Fassung auf diese Weise von dem gelehrten „Ballast“ befreite. Es liegt nahe zu vermuten, dass er auf diese Weise den Lesegewohnheiten einer weniger gebildeten deutschsprachigen Leserschaft entgegen kommen wollte.

Neben der Übersetzung und Aufbereitung von akademischer chirurgischer Literatur für ein weniger gebildetes Publikum diffundierten die gelehrten Inhalte auch in die handwerklichen Chirurgien. Das zeigt sich an den vielen gängigen Topoi, die etwa Gersdorf in seiner Chirurgie von Guy de Chauliac übernommen hatte. Auch den Handwerkschirurgen ging es mit der Figur des *wol erfahrnen Wundartztes* um die Erneuerung und Sicherung ihrer Kunst. Und so argumentierte Jacob Ruf am Ende der Vorrede zu seiner *Augenheilkunde* von 1545, wie gefährlich chirurgische Eingriffe am Auge sind, wenn sie von unfähigen Praktikern durchgeführt werden:

> Da nun die Ausübung und Handhabung dieser Kunst nicht nur von höchster Subtilität, sondern auch insofern sehr gefährlich ist, als sie bisher in den Händen Unerfahrener lag und daher mit grösstem Risiko verbunden war, so müssen wir uns nun zu Recht mit allem Nachdruck und Kraftaufwand darum bemühen, diese Kunst den Händen der unerfahrenen und unredlichen Meister zu entwinden und aus Sorge um das öffentliche Wohl wieder in ihre ursprüngliche Würde und Reinheit einzusetzen. [...][97]

96 Nutton, *Humanist surgery* (1985), insb. S. 83.

97 „Cum ergo huius artis professio et tractatio non modo maximae subtilitatis, sed periculosa quoque admodum existat ex eo, quod imperitorum tractata manibus plurimum hactenus periculi dederit, merito nunc omnibus nervis, viribus et opera in hoc incumbendum [...], ut hanc imperitorum horum et improborum magistrorum manibus ereptam pristinae dignitati et puritati publicae necessitatis cura tacti restituamus.“ Jakob Ruf, *Practica in arte ophthalmica copiosa* [ca. 1545], hg. aus der Handschrift Wien, JB 6.452 mit Einleitung, dt. Übersetzung und Kommentar v. H. Steinke u. C. Müller, in: Jakob Ruf, *Werke 1545–1549. Kritische Gesamtausgabe*, Teil 2 (=Jakob Ruf. Leben, Werk und Studien dritter Band, hg. v. Hildegard Elisabeth Keller), Zürich 2008, S. 465–599, S. 492f.

THE DOCTOR AND THE MAGISTRATE. A LAWYER'S VIEW OF MEDICAL ETHICS

Vivian Nutton

Scholars today are familiar with what Michael McVaugh has termed the medicalisation of late medieval society, the penetration of medical ideas and institutions into the civic life of Western Europe from the thirteenth century onwards.[1] This was a process that developed at a different pace in different regions: Italy, Aragon and S. France appear to medicalise sooner than N. France or most of Germany; wealthy merchant cities before country towns, and the British Isles later than almost everywhere else. This is not a new insight. Studies abound of the development of medical (and surgical) professionalisation in the Middle Ages and Renaissance, buttressed by the legally established universities and colleges, and the role of civic authorities in the fight against plague has been illuminated in many excellent books and papers. Nor has legal medicine been neglected, particularly in its civil law manifestations – England, with its very different system of common law, has stood outside these discussions – and we have an excellent guide in Esther Fischer-Homberger's *Medizin vor Gericht*, particularly for developments from the seventeenth century onwards.[2] But in all this, the perspective has been that of the medical profession, and, more recently, that of the patient, and little attention has been paid to the new player in the game, the legally trained magistrate, and what he might think or might require in order to do his duty. Recent books have explored in detail the involvement of magistrates in the creation and administration of health boards as well as the ways in which their norms and values corresponded or conflicted with those of the medical profession or of society in general, but there has been much less interest in what legal advice was given to magistrates on matters medical.[3]

1 M. R. McVaugh, *Medicine Before the Plague. Practitioners and their Patients in the Crown of Aragon, 1285–1345*, Cambridge 1993, p. 3.

2 E. Fischer-Homberger, *Medizin vor Gericht. Gerichtsmedizin von der Renaissance bis zur Aufklärung*, Bern u. a. 1983.

3 Two fine recent studies typify this lacuna: J. Coste, *Représentations et comportements en temps d'épidémie dans la littérature imprimée de peste (1490–1725). Contribution à l'histoire culturelle de la peste en France à l'époque moderne*, Paris 2007, esp. pp. 415–453; S. K. Cohn, *Cultures of Plague. Medical Thinking at the End of the Renaissance*, Oxford 2010. The importance of legal sources, particularly as regards plague, was first established by M. Ascheri, *I giuristi e le epidemie di peste (secoli XIV–XVI)*, Siena 1997. He was followed by A. Pastore, "Governare la città appestata", in: A. Prosperi (ed.), *Piacere nel testo. Saggi e*

Of course, some doctors were well aware that, particularly in time of plague, it was the magistrate who exercised authority and who therefore needed the advice of the doctor if he was to intervene effectively. The German Johann Ewich, for instance, wrote a plague tract for the magistrates of Bremen in 1531, which was republished at Neustadt an der Haardt in 1582 as *De officio fidelis et prudentis magistratus tempore pestilentiae rempublicam a contagio preservandi liberandique*. A German version appeared at Bremen in 1565, and was republished at Muhlhausen in 1583, 1584 and 1597 under a longer and even more precise title: *Pestilentzordenunge. Nützer und notwendiger Unterricht von dem Ampt der Obrigkeit in Pestilentzzeiten, wie durch ihren Fleis die Pestilentz verhütet, und da dieselbe eingerissen gedempfft werden könnte*.[4] It enjoyed the rarity of an English translation, by John Stockwood, in 1583, and was still being republished in Germany as late as 1656.[5] Other doctors had more specifically forensic concerns in mind. The famous collection of rescripts and decisions published by Paolo Zacchia between 1621 and 1635 was aimed at legal faculties and magistrates at least as much as at doctors, and reflected his own experience in giving advice on matters medical before the legal tribunals of the Pope.[6] Fischer-Homberger provides an impressive list of similar writers from the late sixteenth century onwards: Giovanni Filippo Ingrassia in 1578, Giovanni Battista Codronchi in 1597, Fortunatus Fidelis in 1602, and Rodrigo de Castro in his *Medicus politicus* of 1614.[7]

Zacchia's collection is typical in its listing of the areas in which a magistrate ought to be aware of medical opinion: determining the causes of and responsibility for death, judging the legal capacity of testators and litigants; questions regarding marriage and, particularly, legitimacy; and, to a much lesser extent, public health.[8] In time of plague, this might involve the magistrate in deciding who was or was not a suitable practitioner to receive a civic contract, and, particularly in the sixteenth and seventeenth century, in imposing any necessary public health measures to prevent or defeat the epidemic. As we know from many cities, this

studi per Alberto Biondi, Rome 2001, pp. 423–444, and *Le regole dei corpi. Medicina e disciplina nell'Italia moderna*, Bologna 2007, esp. pp. 33–59.

4 I have been unable to locate a copy of the 1531 edition. I have consulted the German version, first published at Bremen in 1565, in the edition of 1597: *Pestilentzordenunge. Nützer und notwendiger Unterricht von dem Ampt der Obrigkeit in Pestilentzzeiten, wie durch ihren Fleis die Pestilentz verhütet, und da dieselbe eingerissen gedempfft werden könne*, Mühlhausen 1597. Later editions appeared at Magdeburg 1608 and, in Latin, at Bremen 1656.

5 J. Ewich, *Of the duetie of a faithfull and wise magistrate in preserving and delivering of the common wealth from infection, in the time of plague or pestilence*, London 1583.

6 P. Zacchia, *Quaestiones medico*-legales [...], Leipzig 1630. For a brief survey of Zacchia's work, see J. Duffin, "Questioning Medicine in Seventeenth-Century Rome. The *Consultations* of Paolo Zacchia", *Canadian Bulletin of Medical History* 28 (2011), pp. 149–170.

7 G. F. Ingrassia, *Methodus dandi relationes*, Catania 1938; G. B. Codronchi, *Methodus testificandi*, Frankfurt 1597; F. Fidelis, *De relationibus medicorum*, Palermo 1602; R. a Castro, *Medicus politicus*, Hamburg 1614.

8 The frontispiece to the 1679 Leipzig reprint of Fidelis' *De relationibus medicorum* (Fischer-Homberger, *Medizin*, p. 45) depicts his main concerns: virginity, hereditary diseases, birth, monsters, wounding, torture and poisoning. Plague does not figure.

was an action that was fraught with difficulties, and where, as Carlo Cipolla insisted, the costs, whatever the decision, might be astronomically high.[9] Failure to act in time, as in the plague of Venice of 1576, might lead to innumerable deaths; conversely, the introduction of anti-plague measures when the threat was slight might be disastrously expensive. The magistrate was faced with an unenviable decision, for which he needed as much help as possible. Doctors were willing to assist, but there was also a suspicion that, in all this, they might be serving their own purposes. To that end some lawyers composed their own treatises for fellow lawyers, both interpreting the opinions of doctors and setting out their own legal criteria for action.

The rest of this paper looks at two such treatises, one almost unknown, by Vincenzo Carrari, the other much more widely read and distributed, by Francesco di Santo Nazario, better known as Francesco Ripa, a Pavia-trained lawyer, who taught at the university of Avignon. His *Tractatus de peste* was first published at Lyons in 1522, and went through 14 printings in the sixteenth century, including an extended version at Lyons in 1538.[10] It was written during an epidemic of plague, when the prudent lawyer had fled Avignon to the small, and much healthier, country town of Maussane, in the hills of Provence.[11] Like a typical medical author of the time with his three-fold emphasis on causes, symptoms and remedies, Ripa divides his *iuridica remedia et salutifera consilia* into three sections: *Preludia* (in which he includes causes), *Privilegia* (i.e. contracts, wills and courts) and *Remedia* (further subdivided into preservative measures, those *ad conservandam ubertatem*, and curative measures). For the purposes of the present paper, the first and third are the most important.

Plague, the author admits, is a *quaestio physica*. It is not for lawyers to decide on its causes, which can be multifarious: bad air, putrid water, dirt and rubbish; imagination and fear; having had sex with a prostitute, over-exertion, over-eating, especially after a dearth, and the activity of demons.[12] Some of these causes he will treat later when discussing the appropriate remedies a magistrate might apply, but his aim in his first section is to stress the upheaval in society that plague

9 C. M. Cipolla, *Cristofano and the Plague*, London 1973; id., *Public Health and the Medical Profession in the Renaissance*, Cambridge 1976. For the plague of Venice, see R. J. Palmer, "Girolamo Mercuriale and the Plague of Venice", in: A. Arcangeli – V. Nutton (eds.), *Girolamo Mercuriale. Medicina e cultura nell'Europa del Cinquecento*, Florence 2008, pp. 51–66.

10 F. de Ripa, *Libri de peste*, Avignon 1522. I have cited it from a later edition, *Tractatus de peste [...] cui novissime accesserunt singularium materiarum summaria cum repertorio*, Lyons 1538. Biographical and bibliographical details are given by Ascheri, *I giuristi*, pp. 12–23. This tract thus predates Giovanni Previdelli, *Tractatus legalis de peste. In quo continetur quid de iure fieri debeat, et possit tam circa ea quae salubritatem civitatum respiciunt quam circa ultimas voluntates, iudicia et ceteros actus inter vivos, tempore quo peste affligimur*, Bologna 1524, which, however, says almost nothing about doctors. On this author, see also Ascheri, *I giuristi*, pp. 23–26; Cohn, *Cultures of Plague*, pp. 240–241.

11 Ripa, *De peste*, f. 1v.

12 Ibid., f. 2r. Similarly Previdelli, *Tractatus*, f. 31v, states: *morbum pestilentiae medicis puto relinquendum*, before giving a brief account of its causes.

brings. Witnesses fail to turn up, engagements are broken off, contracts cannot be fulfilled, children are baptised in private houses because it is too dangerous to go to church, peasants take their corn to be ground at a different mill, clients die before they can pay their lawyers, and teachers of law on a salaried contract move to more salubrious surroundings elsewhere, or demand compensation for working in a plague-ridden town.[13] Peasants have their animals seized, or kill them themselves in desperation.[14] Plague orders bring their own consequences.[15] Those who break them are to be punished severely, even with death by hanging, when they can then be handed over for a public dissection, after a sung mass and appropriate funeral rights, "as I have often seen at Pavia", says Ripa. He adds a caution: this should not be done if the body already smells, and preferably not in summer. All these are questions that are likely to come before a lawyer or a magistrate, who should be aware of medical and legal opinion, and particularly where there are disputes within the professional groupings.

As a magistrate or his adviser, the lawyer must also be involved in putting into practice the plague precautions, ensuring that there is sufficient money in the town's funds, appointing a suitable treasurer, and defining the financial contributions and reimbursements of the citizens.[16] He should know beforehand what public notices of plague are required, as well as how to produce plague passes. These should be checked carefully to see if any have been passed on to a third party or bear suspicions signs of alteration. It was the magistrate's job to enforce quarantine and house-confinement, taking care that men and women should not be placed together, for, so it was believed, plague was a source of innumerable carnal sins: indeed, women after the death of their husbands were often seduced into second marriages with those who were beneath them in status or wealth.[17] Finally, it was the magistrate's duty to set up a hospital in a remote and healthy place ("for a change of location is the best medicine"), and to oversee the necessary doctors in the town.[18]

The legal basis for this was the decisions in the late-antique Code of Justinian on the status and number of civic physicians, suitably modified to fit the sixteenth century.[19] Ripa argued that the Code did not insist on a physician at all, let alone a graduate physician, for the term *medicus* could include a surgeon, or even a vet. The great Dr Bartolo had indeed insisted that because the law specified that only a *medicus* could attend upon nuns at a time when graduate physicians were few or non-existent, this term must also have covered non-graduates such as surgeons,

13 Ibid., ff. 2r–12v. The question of contracts and court cases occupies Previdelli throughout his treatise, esp. ff. 4v–14r (wills), 14r–20v (courts) and 10v–27r (contracts), although he is neither as full nor as eloquent as Ripa.

14 Ripa, *De peste*, ff. 19r–v.

15 Ibid., ff. 21r–19v. For the anatomy, f. 18r.

16 Ibid., ff. 22v–26r, 29r–v.

17 Ibid., f. 30r.

18 Ibid., ff. 30r–31v, 32r–35r. Previdelli is briefer, ff. 28v–31r (hospitals, taxes and doles), 33r–34v (quarantine).

19 K.-H. Below, *Der Arzt im römischen Recht*, München 1953.

and even slaves, who could in Antiquity become doctors. But barber-surgeons, who were known in antiquity, must have been definitely excluded by the restriction to *medici*.[20] Nonetheless, the law should still pay appropriate regard to the dignity of the doctorate.

But who should serve as a plague doctor? The ancient Roman lawyers had emphasised that the choice of a civic physician should be made on the grounds of the experience and the morals of suitable candidates, and Ripa concurred. Even if a candidate was young and an orphan, that should not be enough to place him first, for "the mere shadow of an experienced doctor" was worth more than the eloquence of youth, too quick to rush to judgment and too ambitious to succeed. The *imperitia* of the young might be fatal to the state.[21]

Paolo Zacchia, a century later, took a slightly different line, perhaps only too well aware of the ravages of the plagues of the 1570s and after. His preference was for an experienced practitioner, and, failing that, for bringing someone out of retirement. But if that were not possible, a recent graduate would do, even if unlicensed, or even a medical student. If the worst came to the worst, surgeons, barbers, pharmacists and the like might be press-ganged to serve, provided they had completed at least one year of training.[22] In plague, the queen of all diseases, one must make do with what one can.

Questions relating to the contract of a plague doctor also vexed Ripa. Authorities differed over whether a doctor could continue acting as a *medico condotto*, and receiving payment, once his contract had lapsed; most thought not, unless the city had actually failed to take the opportunity, if it were offered, to choose a replacement.[23] What should be the starting point for any payment was another problem. Ripa allowed payment to be made to a foreigner if he happened to be delayed while on his journey, but if he arrived on a Sunday or a feast day, he could not claim any extra payment for that day: Christ the true physician cured for nothing on the Sabbath, and doctors should do likewise.[24] Besides, doctors and surgeons were notoriously slow in treating the sick in plague, unless they were given an increased salary, and hence many citizens were likely to die unnecessarily from their delays. Better perhaps to pay more for a successful cure than simply for treatment. The inhabitants of Auray paid a gold coin for a success, but only a silver florin for a failure, with good effect, for the town rapidly escaped the plague and most sufferers were cured, a consequence, says Ripa, of the doctors' insatiable greed which drove them to greater efforts to cure.[25] He himself accepts that,

20 Ripa, *De peste*, f. 32v. For *dignitas*, f. 29v. Previdelli, *Tractatus*, says almost nothing about the doctor, except, f. 31r, that someone who pretends to the insignia of a doctor should be severely punished.

21 Ripa, *De peste*, f. 32r.

22 Zacchia, *Quaestiones*, lib. VI.1.6, pp. 456–457 in the edition of Lyons 1673–1674. He discussed the problem of the *medico condotto* at greatest length in a *consilium* delivered between 1656 and 1659, in this edition, pp. 108–112, and for substitutes and replacements, p. 112.

23 Ripa, *De peste*, f. 34r.

24 Ibid., f. 34v.

25 Ibid., f. 35r.

unless specific provision has been made to the contrary, the public doctor must always be paid for his services. This he deserves far more than lawyers, since he brings an assured benefit. But, in return, the privilege of the *condotta* should compel him to do more than the arrogant outsider: he should work harder, and gladly treat the poor for free. A public doctor who treated the poor worse than the rich should be sacked and expelled from the community forthwith. Likewise any doctor who deliberately made matters worse or who demanded money inappropriately should be punished. Nor could he refuse to offer treatment in a desperate case, for, so the lawyer thinks, his ministrations would hardly worsen the situation, and the patient's death would hardly be considered his fault. Beside, as every doctor knew, patients do not always obey their doctors: and as a result, *peccant graviter*.[26]

The personal morality of the doctor, whether or not he has a contract, also exercises Ripa. Basing himself on his Roman texts, he stresses the need for the doctor to act opportunely, to understand the individual nature of his patient, and to be flexible enough to deal with new conditions when they arise. He should exercise diligence in overseeing apothecaries in order to ensure that his remedies are properly made up, and he should avoid spending time with the rich or taking on more cases than he can properly manage. Gentleness, sobriety and *pudicitia*, a chaste self-control, all help to distinguish the good doctor from the bad, as do his religious beliefs.[27] Ripa devotes five vigorous paragraphs to warning the people of Avignon against Jewish doctors, for one of the marks of the good doctor was his willingness to advise his patients to trust in God, something impossible for a non-Christian. Nonetheless, he admits, there might be times when no Christian doctor was available and hence it was permissible then to employ a Jew. And better a Jew than an evil and perfidious Christian, by which he may mean a Protestant or, just possibly, one of the surviving heretics of the Languedoc.[28] Ripa himself insists on the importance of a proper religious attitude on the part of patients also, spending many sections on the role of penitence and confession in time of plague before concluding that a *meditatio mortis*, thinking about death, is the best philosophy against plague.[29]

Throughout his book, Ripa displays a certain degree of scepticism about doctors. He supports them, but he is well aware of their failings, and of public suspicion of their activities. He raises the question of the possible nefarious involvement of the doctor if his male patient were to die and then the doctor were to marry the widow within a year. Such an action would certainly give rise to suspicion, but unless the magistrate could find evidence of a previous attachment and if their

26 Ripa, *De peste*, ff. 33r–v. For disobedient patients, ibid., f. 32v.

27 Ibid., f. 32v.

28 Ibid., f. 32v. For the possibility that Ripa might be thinking of Lutherans, cf. Pastore, *Le regole dei corpi*, p. 58.

29 Ibid., ff. 35r–39r, entirely appropriate given his and others' belief that plague might have a psychological cause. Previdelli, *Tractatus*, ff. 34r–v, also ends with a discussion of sin and repentance. At f. 4r, he demands the removal of brothel-keepers, who may corrupt "*simplices puellas et alias mulieres*".

fellow citizens judged them both to be of good character, the matter should be allowed to rest there.[30] Such reliance on public opinion can be traced in other legal rulings, particularly in the case of children born after the death of their possible father, where public opinion on the moral behaviour of the mother and her possible lover or second husband is given precedence in disputed cases over the dubious evidence of the facial similarity of the child to the new man in her life. Imagination in pregnancy, as every medieval scholar knew, could influence the child already in the womb, and hence confuse the question of paternity. One wonders how much more accurate was village gossip.[31]

Carrari, writing some fifty years after Ripa, dedicates his book to the papal governor of Bologna in a plea for financial support for his brothers, who want to become lawyers like him. He had been appointed governor of Tolentino, further south in the Papal States, and his book reflects some of his experiences. Although plague figures prominently, it is not his only theme. His title is broad *De medico et illius erga aegros officio*[32] (*On the doctor and his duty to the sick*), and his treatment substantial, far more detailed than the appellation *opusculum* warrants. He relies heavily on Ripa, Previdelli, and two other authors, one famous, the other much less so. Some of his comments about the status of doctors depend on the *Tractatus de nobilitate* of the Frenchman André Tiraqueau, an international best-seller, others on the *De probitate et improbitate, scientia et ignorantia, felicitate et infelicitate medicorum* by his fellow citizen of Ravenna, Hieronymus Rubeus.[33]

His aim is to provide a lawyer with guidance on all matters concerned with doctors. So for instance, a great part of Book III is taken up with discussion of the *condotta*. It should be voted on in a full council, by a majority decision, such is the importance of the post. It cannot be filled by a substitute in time of plague, although such substitutions are common.[34] Like Ripa, he frowns upon doctors who spend their time with the rich rather than the poor, and agrees that such doctors can be forced to deal with cases of plague or other new diseases. He agonises over the question of the taking of fees, suggesting that a doctor should receive 100 gold pieces for a cure, the same as a successful lawyer, but only from the wealthy and those who are in good health. [35] A doctor can legitimately treat a patient against his will, and claim his reward. Nonetheless, even if the law allows this, a salaried doctor might well be forced to pay it back by a judge, bowing to public opinion.[36] Enchanters, birth-women and magicians are in no way doctors, and he inveighs against the use of Jewish doctors. Bartolo's argument over the identity of

30 Ripa, *De peste*, f. 33v.

31 Zacchia, *Quaestiones*, lib. I.1.1–7, pp. 428–433.

32 V. Carrari, *De medico et illius erga aegros officio opusculum*, Ravenna 1581. He describes his career and his hopes for his brothers on p. 4.

33 I have used the following edition: A. Tiraqueau, *De nobilitate et iure primogenitorum*, Paris 1549. I have so far been unable to locate a copy of Rubeus' book, which, if it was ever published, seems to have had a very local circulation.

34 Carrari, *De medico*, pp. 112–113.

35 Ibid., pp.118–119, 122–123, 150 (a lawyer's fee).

36 Ibid., p. 121.

the *medicus* allowed to enter the doors of a nunnery he dismisses briskly, insisting on the privileges and status that only the *doctoratus* brings. Indeed, he argues that the only true doctor is one who has been examined further and whose name figures on a list of approved doctors (*sc.* in a local *Collegium).*[37]

Many of his recommendations for the ideal doctor agree with Ripa's. He should be resourceful, able to give a good account of himself, and no gossip, although Carrari is well aware that elderly doctors are inclined to be lazy, and an ignorant old doctor is hardly preferable to someone younger and with less experience, however rash he might appear.[38] One must balance the young man's desire for fame against his ability to bear better the "laborious exercise of healing". Better, perhaps, if the senior man would take a junior around with him to give him the necessary training.[39] Expertise and good morals are what count in civic appointments.

Carrari's greatest fear of the doctor is of his sexuality. He worries about his tendency to adultery, going well beyond the obvious statement that if a doctor has poisoned his rival, any marriage with the widow would be invalid. Marriage with the widow or even a daughter of someone dying in the plague is likely always to raise suspicions.[40] Indeed, it is best when treating beautiful women not to examine their breasts, abdomen or delicate white arms, in order to avoid any possible suggestion of adultery. Lust, he says, is a form of drunkenness, to be condemned at all times.[41] Whether this provision applied to ladies who were less than beautiful, Carrari leaves unanswered.

These two treatises, by Francesco Ripa and Vincenzo Carrari, offer different perspectives on the duties of a doctor as seen from the point of view of a lawyer who, whether in court or as an administrator, had to be acquainted with medicine and its practitioners. Although lawyers, lay and ecclesiastical, had long been concerned with such questions, and church councils (and others) had long legislated for what they believed at least some doctors should or should not do, Mario Ascheri may well be right in putting Ripa's treatise at the beginning of a new trend. Plague focussed the mind, even of lawyers, and many of the citations in Carrari, Zacchia and other similar writers relate to legal decisions in times of plague. Carrari ranges much more widely than the problems of plague, although one may wonder how much he owed to his fellow-citizen, Hieronymus Rubeus. All these writers base themselves on the decisions of the ancient Roman jurists – and, indeed, on classical literary sources in general – in their attempts to determine the role and function of doctors. They offer a different perspective from those of the doctors themselves, even of those, like Zacchia, concerned with legal matters, and one that is more critical and more practical than the encomia on med-

37 Carrari, *De medico*, pp. 164–165,168, 128, 116–117, 135–136.
38 Ibid., pp.186–187, 191–192.
39 Ibid., p. 192.
40 Ibid., pp. 95, 120.
41 Ibid., pp. 120–121, 198.

icine delivered by Erasmus and many others.[42] They also serve as a reminder that, increasingly, medicine was no longer a simple matter between doctor and patient, but one in which the city, or the state, and its officials had an interest and a responsibility. We are still a long way from the *medizinische Polizei* of the eighteenth century, but that should not be a reason for neglecting these legal sources.

42 J. van Beverwyck, *Epistolicae quaestiones, cum doctorum responsis. Accedit ejusdem, nec non Erasmi, Cardani, Melanchthonis, Medicinae encomium*, Rotterdam 1644.

"SPEAKS TRUE, WHO SPEAKS SHADOWS."* TRUTH AND LIES AT THE SICK-BED

Mariacarla Gadebusch Bondio

In the dialogue between the doctor and the terminally ill patient, a lie might be regarded as tactful consideration. For Karl Jaspers (1883-1969) "the well-known example of permissible, even required lying […], is the lie on the part of the doctor to the critically endangered or hopelessly ill patient."[1] He introduces his thoughts on the legitimacy of lying in the doctor-patient relationship with the statement that for "people on the whole", the "unconditional search for truth" is dangerous. His weighty volume on truth appeared in 1947, the year of the Nurnberg doctors' trials and the Geneva Declaration. By raising the question about the "possible meaning of truth here", Jaspers challenges the common arguments for and against doctors' lies. According to Jaspers, the "truth possible here" would require "not speaking the truth" and would generally remain unquestioned.[2]

The concept of truth and truthfulness in medicine is blurred. In addition, modalities of the passing on or withholding of information in dialogue between the doctor and the patient are culturally, historically and subjectively induced.[3] A range of emotional and cognitive factors accompany the two-way communication between patient and doctor: knowledge and ignorance, responsibility, trust, decision-making power, decision-making ability and dependency, hope, hopelessness, fear, doubt etc., all influence the decision to reveal something to a greater or lesser extent, to conceal or to present it differently.[4]

Concepts of truth and lies are fundamental when dealing with knowledge, lack of knowledge or conjecture in this context. The medico-ethical and philosophical consequences of this type of thinking are obvious. In pre-modern medicine, just as in countries like Japan or Italy today, the doctor's responsibility for

* The title is taken from Paul Celan. P. Celan, *Von Schwelle zu Schwelle* (1955), edited by J. Wertheimer, adapted by H. Schmull, in cooperation with C. Braun u. M. Heilmann, Frankfurt a. M. 2003.

1 K. Jaspers, *Von der Wahrheit*, München / Zürich 1997 (1. Aufl. 1947), p. 557.

2 Ibid.

3 The international medical and medico-ethical specialsed press over the past 20 years have documented the continuing relevence of this topic with hunders of articles. Accordingly searches via PubMed (U.S. National Institutes of Health, *Free digital archive of biomedical and life sciences journal literature*) for the keywords *lying* and *deception* result in 3,456 entries; with the search words *telling the truth* 652 entries appear. http://www.ncbi.nlm.nih.gov/pubmed [21.10.2013].

4 P. Langkafel – C. Lüdke, *Breaking Bad News. Das Überbringen schlechter Nachrichten in der Medizin*, Heidelberg 2008.

honest, accurate disclosure of a hopeless prognosis is far from self-evident.[5] The option of the mild lie produces, however, a sphere for reflection in which in early modernity philosophical and theological (both Catholic and Protestant) positions were already being discussed.

In medicine, sick-bed truth becomes both an issue in view of its consequences for the sick, and in terms of the moral attitude of the doctor. The following questions arise: when and how should the patient be told the truth? Is a doctor morally obliged always to tell the patient the truth, even when it causes stress? And what if the patient does not want to know the truth?

The fundamental questions which are more rarely discussed are, for example, what does "sick-bed truth" mean? Can a doctor present himself as a messenger of truth at all? Are we not dealing in most cases with probability based upon experience which contains ignorance?

Extensive articles on the topic of truth can be found (*truth telling*) in modern medico-ethical encyclopaedias, lexicons and standard German-language works of reference on bioethics and on medical ethics, at the centre of which is patient autonomy.[6] The possibility of the non-transference of "truth" is, as a rule, examined in connection with the so-called "right to know", and seen as an exception. The term "lie" (or deception, lat. *deceptio*) cannot be found anywhere in these works. In historical and philosophical dictionaries, on the other hand, the lemma "lie" is dealt with extensively.[7] In English language publications such as, for example, the *Encyclopedia of Bioethics*, questions such as "To tell or not to tell?" and "Why tell a lie?" are the starting point for a relatively detailed article on the topic of information disclosure.[8] The impression is given of a culturally influenced difference in the emphasis of withholding information as a real medical lever. The number and origin of medical and nursing publications in international journals shows that in some industrialised nations the mild lie is even regarded as a task of medicine.[9]

5 Y. Uchitomi – S. Yamawaki, "Truth-Telling Practice in Cancer Care in Japan", *Annals of the New York Academy of Sciences* 809 (1997), pp. 290–299; A. Surbone – C. Ritossa – A. G. Spagnolo, "Evolution of Truth-telling Attitudes and Practices in Italy", *Oncology Hematology* 52 (2004), pp. 165–172.

6 J. van de Loo, "Wahrheit am Krankenbett", in: W. Korff – L. Beck – P. Mikat (eds.), *Lexikon der Bioethik*, vol. 3, Gütersloh 1998, pp. 745–746; K. H. Brown, "Information Disclosure. I: Attitudes Toward Truth-Telling", in: *Encyclopedia of Bioethics*, vol. 3, New York et al. 1995 (Revised Edition), pp. 1221–1225; A. Jameton, "Information Disclosure. II: Ethical Issues", *ibid.*, pp. 1225–1232.

7 See G. Bien, "Lüge" s.v. in: J. Ritter – K. Gründer (eds.), *Historisches Wörterbuch der Philosophie*, vol. 5, Basel / Stuttgart 1980, pp. 533–544; K. Hörmann, "Lüge" s.v. in: id. (ed.), *Lexikon der christlichen Moral*, Innsbruck et al. 1976, col. 1003–1012; in the *Lexicon of Bioethics* the lemma "lie" is missing, this is also not discussed in the article on truth at the sick-bed, see van de Loo, Truth at the Sick-bed.

8 Brown, Information Disclosure I; A. Jameton, Information Disclosure II.

9 Uchitomi – Yamawaki, Truth-Telling Practice; Surbone – Ritossa – Spagnolo, Evolution of Truth-Telling.

Research on the history of medical ethics indicates an increasing discussion of the problematic nature of truth and lies in the early modern period.[10] What induced Renaissance doctors to take an interest in this subject?

Some sections of Hippocratic and Galenic writings may have inspired them to this. In ancient medicine, the patient's wellbeing is at the top of the medical scale of values, and as the highest principle regulates the flow of information. The Hippocratic passage in which deception (ἀπάτη) is described as a potential means of healing is well known.[11] It deals with a patient with an ear complaint. The doctor simulates the extraction of a foreign body (a small ball of wool) which he then throws into the fire. The patient believes he has been healed and feels better. Galen is sceptical of patient deception for therapeutic purposes – by means of the placebo effect. However he, too, advocates an individually tailored transfer of information.[12] People who are neither timid nor shy should be told the truth about their illness by a doctor who should conceal nothing; however in the case of patients who are anxious and prejudiced, or even foolish, information should be given which improves their disposition – without actually lying. These statements are in accordance with the Galenic medical ideal. The 'proper' doctor, *medicus verus*, is a friend of truth (*veritas*) and of moderation (*temperantia*).[13] However, the debate about the subject matter dealt with here by the two great physicians seems to be restricted to these few text extracts.

10 K. Bergdolt, *Das Gewissen der Medizin. Ärztliche Moral von der Antike bis heute*, München 2004, pp. 145–155: "Der Streit um Lüge und Betrug in der frühneuzeitlichen Medizin". See also: W. Schleiner, *Medical Ethics in the Renaissance*, Washington 1995, pp. 5–48: "Mentiamur sane. Lying for Health in Renaissance Medical Ethics".

11 See Hippokrates, *Epidemics* (vol. 7), VI, 5.7, ed. and tr. by W. D. Smith, Cambridge (Mass.) 1994, pp. 243: "If the ear aches, wrap wool around your fingers, pour on warm oil, then put the wool in the palm of the hand and put it over the ear so that something will seem to him to come out. Then throw it in the fire. A deception (ἀπάτη)." Galen doubts the authenticity of these Hippocratic passages. Galen, *Hippocratis Epidem. VI et Galeni in illum commentarius* V, sectio V, cap. 13, in: id., *Opera omnia*, vol. XVII, 2A, ed. by C. G. Kühn, Hildesheim 2001 (3. reprint of the edition Leipzig 1821), pp. 266–269: "Sed neque ob mitigandum dolorem, ut dixi, haec vox, dolus, seu deceptio adscribi potuit: adversatur enim illis verbis, ut aliquid ipsi exire videatur, eo, qui ita scripsit, indicante, decipiendorum aegrotantium causa ad hanc manuariam operam medicos accedere. Satius igitur fuerit, haec verba nequaquam esse Hippocratis extimare."

12 Galen, *Hippocratis Epidem. VI et Galeni in illum commentarius* II, Kühn, vol. XVII, 1 B, pp. 994–1001; Hippokrates, *Epidemics*, VI, 3.24, p. 223: "Arrangements for the sick person and inquiry about the disease: what is explained, what kind of things, how it must be accepted; the reasoning; what relates to the patient, what relates to those who are present, and the people elsewhere."

13 Galen, *Quod optimus medicus sit quoque philosophus*, Kühn, vol. I, p. 59: "σωφροσύνης γοῦν φίλος, ὥσπερ γε καὶ ἀληθείας, ὅ γ' ἀληθὴς ἰατρὸς ἐξεύρηται"; "Ex quo efficitur, ut, si quis verus medicus est, idem sit ut veritatis, sic etiam temperantiae amicus." Also of Hippocratic and Galenic origin is the ideal of the *medicus gratiosus*, who, with measure, self-control and tact, can win over the patient.

THE PRINCIPLE OF HOPE

As early as the decades around 1500, the dialogue between doctor and patient in medical texts which deal with professional ethos and medical conduct becomes the subject of normative endeavours. Medical texts which address the so-called *cautelae* (prudence/precautions) are full of advice for a balanced medical discussion. One of the earliest texts of this genre is the *Opus perutile de cautelis medicorum* (1495) by the professor of medicine, anatomist and papal physician Gabriele Zerbi (1445-1505). He regarded the doctor's approach to truth as a moral sphere for reflection.[14] A doctor, according to Zerbi, should not be a liar or somebody who denies the truth;[15] he should "never lie" where knowledge should be provided. "Rather a doctor should be truthful (*verax*) from the aspect of those things which belong to the speculative intellect. For truthful talk (*sermo verus*) is better in all things."[16]

When Zerbi gauges a doctor's attitude toward his patients, and above all to those who are suffering, he stresses that a doctor should never give up his promise to heal, and even in desperate situation should confirm their hopes.[17]

> And a doctor should always promise the hope of recovery by speaking pleasantly to the patient and encouraging cheerfulness and joy and nourishing his hopes. For this reason John of Damascus says in his aphorisms: 'It is necessary that you always promise the sick health, and you must never discourage them from hope, even if you yourself no longer have any. For the respective condition of the body is always inseparably linked to the state of mind'. And he adds: 'You should never cease to give hope to the sick'. And Cassiodor says: 'natural treatment consists of providing joy for the sick; strive to give the patient pleasure and he will recover.'[18]

14 Gabriele Zerbi, *Opus perutile de cautelis medicorum* […], Venetiis 1495, a3v–b2r: "Capitulum tertium. De modo se habendi medici secundum dispositiones tam animae quam corporis ex tempore acquisitas". See also: R. K. French, "The Medical Ethics of Gabriele Zerbi", in: A. Wear – J. Geyer-Kordesch – R. French (eds.), *Doctors and Ethics. The Earlier Historical Setting of Medical Ethics*, Amsterdam / Atlanta 1993, pp. 72–97; D. E. Linden, "Gabriele Zerbi's De cautelis medicorum and the Tradition of Medical Prudence", *Bulletin of the History of Medicine* 73 (1999), n. 1, pp. 19–37; Gabriele Zerbi, *Gerontocomia. On the Care of the Aged, and Maximianus, Elegies on Old Age and Love*, tr. by L. R. Lind, Philadelphia 1988, pp. 10–16; F. W. Bandtlow, *Die Schrift des Gabriel de Zerbis: De cautelis medicorum*, Diss. Med., Leipzig 1925.

15 Zerbi, *Opus perutile*, a4r: "Non mendax: ut negator veritatis: ne alterius mentem fallat."

16 Zerbi, *Opus perutile*, a4v: "Ex parte autem eorum quae intellectus speculativi sunt expedit medico veracem esse. Nam melior est sermo verus omnibus rebus ut ait Galienus primo de complexionibus et Aristoteles primo ethico."

17 Zerbi, *Opus perutile*, b2r–b4r: "Capitulum quartum. De modo se habendi medici erga patientes et maxime erga egrotantes".

18 Zerbi, *Opus perutile*, b3r: "Erit continuo medicus promittens spem salutis: immo et patientis animum mellitis suasionibus in laeticiam et gaudium alliciens: et eius spem nutriens. Unde Damascenus in Afforismis: Oportet te infirmis semper salutem promittere: numquam illos a spe eponere: et si ipse desperes. Complexio enim corporis affectioni animi semper inhaeret: et subdit: infirmos in eorum spe animare non desinas. Et Cassiodorus: naturalis cura est aegris dare laetitiam: nam fac invalidum gaudere: et sanatus erit." See footnote 21.

In order to help the critically ill to hold on to hope, the doctor should hide his doubts. In this case we are dealing with an appropriate, even necessary lie:

> And returning to the patient again, the doctor should promise him certain health and he should not fear using lies, as these are beneficial lies. And he should promise him health and assure him that all can abound in this. Doctors make promises, tradesmen practice their trade.[19]

Zerbi refers to Aristotle and Galen when he talks of the doctor's love of truth in an intellectual sphere.[20] In daily practice, however, it is the writings of Cassiodorus (485–580) and Damascenus (Johannes Mesué, approx. 777–857) which he quotes and uses.[21] Both had stressed that a doctor should brighten a patient's mood with persistent promises of health. Even in hopeless cases they advocated, as did Zerbi, a consistent, even therapeutic encouragement of hope in the patient. All authors who hold this position are convinced that the physical condition is dependent upon the mental condition, and that giving hope is one of the integral duties of a doctor.

Forty years after Zerbi, Clemente Clementini, Pope Leo X's physician, drafted the profile of the *medicus peritus*[22] in the foreword to his work *Lucubrationes* (1535). A practiced doctor should be gentle and kind (*benignus et clemens*) towards patients.[23] To the medical virtues, at the head of which stands *prudentia* (skill/prudence), is added the search for truth and goodness in all things.[24] It is of benefit to doctors if they are able to talk about subjects which give timely pleasure

19 Zerbi, *Opus perutile*, b4r: "Et ad infirmum denuo reversus firmam ei promittat salutem: et non vereatur etiam mendaciis uti: sunt enim hec officiosa mendacia: et salutem ei promittat: pollicitus enim dives quilibet esse potest iuxta illud. Promittunt medici: tractant fabrilia fabri."

20 Zerbi, *Opus perutile*, a4v: "Aristoteles primo ethicorum" see Aristotle *Nicomachean Ethics* 1096 a14–17 and "Galienus primo de complexionibus" is the medieval title for *De temperamentibus*, see G. Fichtner, *Corpus Galenicum. Bibliographie der galenischen und pseudogalenischen Werke*, Tübingen 2011 (extended and improved edition), entry 9, p. 15.

21 Cassiodorus, *Varia*, IX, 6, 2: "naturalis siquidem cura est aegris dare laetitiam: nam fac invalidum gaudere, sanatus est". http://www.intratext.com/IXT/LAT0253/_P9N.HTM [18.11.10]. Damascenus, *Amphorismi* [sic] *Iohannis damasceni*, Bologna 1489, Aiir: "Oportet autem te infirmo salutem promittere semper nec unquam illum a spe deponere et si ipse desperes."

22 Clementini, *Lucubrationes*, Basel 1535, a3v–a5r.

23 Clementini, *Lucubrationes*, a3v.

24 Clementini, *Lucubrationes*, a4r–a4v: "Itaque viri literati et maxime philosophi et medici plerunque sunt regulae morum et sapientes, et in rebus agendis primum consulunt illa quatuor genera virtutum, quae sapientes et felices homines faciunt, et duce prudentia inquirunt et prospiciunt veritatem vel bonitatem rei gerendae, et omnem diligentiam adhibent ne quicquam praeter rectum et laudabile agant, ob fortitudinem vero fiunt magnanimi et costantes, et nil nisi turpia timent, et adversam fortunam aequo animo tolerant, sed propter temperantiam nihil poenitendum appetunt, vitia cavent, et sub iugo rationis omnem cupiditatem et libidinem [a4v] domant, iustitiam colunt, et iniurias propulsant. Et quia fundamentum iustitiae est fides, medici debent esse valde fidi, et aegrorum saluti integerrime consulere, et diligere eos sicut vellent ab aliis diligi."

to their listeners. "Pleasant words" console the sick and nurture hope of recovery; they can more easily support those things that do a patient good.[25]

Through the cautious use of words, the doctor wins respect and trust. For Clementini, one further reason for being careful with statements about illness, particularly with prognoses, which the doctor should adhere to is the fact that the outcome of an illness – like that of a war – is always unsure.[26] The figurative comparison of the disease process with war is particularly significant here. According to the Hippocratic viewpoint, medicine is both a difficult and complex art, as the doctor must be ready to act at the right, fleeting moment (*kairos*), must respond and make decisions quickly; at the same time he must not only cooperate with the patient, but also with his family.[27] The allegory of war provides the Hippocratic characterisation of this basic, radical situation with clarity.

The metaphor of war will enjoy continuing success in the history of medicine, and persuade both doctors and patients to view illness as an enemy and foreign substance in the body.[28] In actual fact Clementini's comparison refers rather to unforeseeable aspects which cannot be planned for, and thus to the special status which people experience both in war and when sick.

The imperial physician to three rulers[29], Julius Alexandrinus von Neustein (1506–1590), also made use of the metaphor of war in his dialogue *De medicina et medico* (1557).[30] In certain cases, in the battle against illness, it is expedient for the doctor to lie (*licere mentiri*). Just as in war cunning strategies are necessary in order to achieve victory, so should a doctor use all the means at his disposal in order to achieve his highest aim, the patient's recovery. In brief: for the patient, or rather for the benefit of his health, we will do everything we can to tell beneficial lies – even if we occasionally have to lie to this end; we have said this as both for

25 Clementini, *Lucubrationes*, a4v: "[...] et blandis verbis consolantur aegrum, et spem salutis augent, et facilius persuadent, quae prosint infirmis."

26 Clementini, *Lucubrationes*, a5r: "Prognostica autem vivanda et dissuaenda aliis, qui maxima curiositate cupiunt scire finem aegritudinis, quondam eventus morborum est incertus, et sicut bellorum et aliarum rerum, et maxime quia medici non possunt scire solertiam astantium, neque obedientam infirmorum. Plurimae enim aedritudines ab inizio sunt salubres, quae postea ex malo redimine fiunt incurabiles vel mortales."

27 Hippocrates, *Aphorisms*, I, 1, in: *Hippocrates*, vol. 4 (The Loeb Classical Library; 150) tr. by W.H.S. Jones., London / Cambridge (Mass.) 1967, p. 99: "Life is short, the Art long, opportunity fleeting, experiment treacherous, judgment difficult. The physician must be ready, not only to do his duty himself, but also to secure the cooperation oft he patient, oft he attendants and the externals."

28 See S. Sontag, Susan, *Illness as Metaphor,* New York 1978; L. J. Rather, "On the Source and Development of Metaphorical Language in the History of Western Medicine", *Bulletin of the History of Medicine*, Suppl.n.s. 6 (1982), pp. 135–153; M. Vegetti, "Metafora politica e immagine del corpo negli scritti Ippocratici", in: F. Lasserre – P. Mudry (eds.), *Formes de pensée dans la Collection Hippocratique*, Genf 1983, pp. 459–460.

29 This concerns Ferdinand II, Maximilian II and Rudolf II.

30 J. Alexandrinus, *De medicina et medico*, Zürich 1557; see J. Ruhräh, "Julius Alexandrinus 1506–1590", *American Journal of Diseases of Children* 44 (1932), n. 4, pp. 846–848; J. Hirn, *Erzherzog Ferdinand II. von Tirol*, vol. 1, Innsbruck 1885, p. 362; J. v. Aschbach, *Geschichte der Wiener Universität*, vol. 3, Wien 1888, pp. 343–347.

army commanders and leaders of state there was no shame attached to lying to either the army or the people in the cause of their health and benefit. On the other hand, however, if a patient tells a lie to us as doctors, we will be on our guard against it as if it were a highly dangerous evil.[31] When discussing practicable strategies for gaining the goodwill of a patient (*benevolentia aegri captanda*), Alexandrinus mentions the effect of pleasant dietetic and other prescriptions and recommends that a doctor should always guarantee the patient hope and total assurance: "A physician should be graceful when entering a sickroom and genial during his stay in it, always promising hope and assurance."[32] Military terms characterise Alexandrinus' considerations. He talks of battle (*pugna*) against and of victory (*victoria*) over illness, whilst the sick person in the "war camp" (*in castris*) follows the physician's advice.[33]

For the less-known author of the text *De optimo medico* (1551), Giovanni Antonio Sicco, the common fight of doctor and patient is also the basic underlying condition for the rehabilitation of health. The disclosure of information must therefore be considered very carefully. Following Galen's *Commentary on Epidemics* (VI.2, 44), Sicco distinguishes between two types of patient. If the patient appears sensible and not completely despondent he should be told the truth; on the other hand in the case of the less reasonable, more anxious patient he recommends "keeping nothing back that might help to encourage and to cheer up the patient's depressed mood."[34] Once the doctor has raised the patient's hopes and gained his trust in this way, the patient will then follow the doctor's advice and fight with him. Only if these conditions are met is there any chance of gaining victory over the illness.[35] However, a doctor should not resort to serious lies. Such an approach harmonises with the ideal of the *medicus optimus* propagated by Sicco who for him should be *verecundus* (respectful, modest, referential), and who should al-

31 Alexandrinus, *De medicina*, p. 334: "Breviter in aegroti, immo salutis potius illius gratiam, facere, tentemus omnia, ut etiam si mentiendum nobis aliquando hac de causa fuerit, mentiamur sane, quod diximus, quando neque exercituum ducibus, neque principibus civitatum, turpe unquam fuit mentiri in civitatum, aut exercituum suorum salutem atque usum. Contra autem ut mendaciis ad nos utatur aeger, cavebimus diligenter, tanquam perniciosissimum malum."

32 Alexandrinus, *De medicina*, p. 337: "[…] et accessio ad aegrum, ac sessio venusta, et hilaris, bonae semper spei plena at fidutiam [sic] promittens."

33 Alexandrinus, *De medicina*, p. 341.

34 G. A. Sicco, *De optimo medico*, Venedig 1551, p. 10v: "Ergo si aegrum prudentem et non parvi animi esse viderit, verum ei praedicet, nihil dissimulans: imprudenti vero et timido nihil reticebit eorum, quae iacentem animum possunt excitare, et demissum erigere."

35 Sicco, *De optimo medico*, pp. 10v–11r: "Adiunget praeterea, artem tribus constare: Medico, Aegroto, et Morbo: aegrotantem vero oportere una cum medico morbo adversari, atque obsistere: nam si solum finat aeger medicum certare cum morbo, aut a medico desciscens cum morbo ineat societatem, nullum medius fidius spei locum superesse: solus nanque medicus cum sit, parvo negotio a duobus superabitur. Contra vero, si a morbo aeger defecerit, et medico pro se pugnanti fuerit auxilio, plurimum de victoria sperandum esse: quoniam adversus unum morbum a duobus pugnatur. Hac aut alia simili oratione aegri obedientiam comparare necesse est: cui etiam vocis magnitudinem et sonum congruere oportet."

ways be able to distinguish between truth and deception.[36] Should there be any danger that the disclosure of truth might harm a patient, then a doctor should tactfully protect him from it. On the other hand the members of his family need not be spared the truth (*familiares nihil celabit*);[37] they should be informed of the actual condition of the sick person. The prudent and careful dosage of truth and lies at the sickbed must, according to Sicco be adapted to the specific conditions of each individual.

THE PATH TO THE *MEDICUS PIUS*

The ideal of the *medicus optimus* which has characterised Western medical culture since the second century A.D. was already being supplemented by the model of the *medicus pius*, the devout, virtuous, god-fearing Christian doctor, in Late Antiquity, and increasingly so in the Middle Ages.[38] In the second half of the 16th century, following the Council of Trent (1545–1563), several physicians favoured increasingily stricter views with regard to the question of truth. Their statements continue to relate typically to the classical medical authors of Antiquity (Hippocrates and Galen, complemented by Plato and Aristotle), but are sometimes overshadowed by the Gospel, the sayings of the Church fathers or by papal decrees and regulations, as we will see with Codronchius.

The physician Leonardo Botallo (1519–1588), who was born in Turin and worked in France, wrote a short text in 1565 on the behaviour of doctor and patient, *De medici et de aegri munere*.

> […] the wise doctor, possessing integrity and being experienced in the art of medicine, does not lust for transient fame, but desires rather secure recognition; he does not sow cunning lies, but endeavours with all his strength to be truthful and to stand by his words as well as his deeds. Consequently patients and those that care for them will give him the trust he deserves.[39]

The physician described by Botallo is careful in his use of language as it is "the most excellent way of expressing the innermost workings of the heart and the mind." It is therefore appropriate to control or to unleash the tongue as is fitting.[40]

36 Sicco, *De optimo medico*, p. 5r, p. 6v.

37 Sicco, *De optimo medico*, p. 10v.

38 See K. Deichgräber, *Medicus gratiosus. Untersuchungen zu einem griechischen Arztbild*, Mainz 1970.

39 L. Botallo, *Tractatus de medici et aegri munere*, in: id., *Opera Omnia*, Lyon 1660, pp.. 19–20: "Caeterum Medicus prudens et vitae integer artisque peritus, qui non in popularem auram inhiat, sed ut statam sibi laudem acquirat, non modo astuta mendacia non proseminat, sed omnibus viribus, dictis juxta ac factis, verum attingere curat. Huic igitur merito fidem adhibent patientes, assistentesque." See also: Leonardo Botallo, *I doveri del medico e del malato*, ed. by L. Carerj – A. Bogetti Fassone, Turin 1981, p. 78.

40 Botallo, *Tractatus*, p. 24: "Restant sermones, ex quibus potissime cordis et mentis intima exponuntur: quare non exigua prudentia est, linguam loco coercere, et, dum licet solvere. Non igitur sit haec garrula, vel ventosa, vel subdola, non maledica: nam sicuti cordis hilaritatem,

A doctor should be serious in discussion, but also show an appropriate sense of humour. Choice of words, tone and volume of voice, and also facial expression should all be used consciously by a doctor as they can arouse not only hope and cheerfulness in the patient, but also desperation and sadness. According to Botallo, everyone should "avoid being deceitful and talking ill of others". The man who expresses himself in an honest, open, flexible and polite manner appears "good, prudent and kind".[41] Apart from this, nothing can betray in speech what the soul alone cannot express better than either truthfulness or dishonesty. "Untruth has a short life. [...] the doctor with integrity will always remain faithful to the truth in both his life and his conscience; [...] he will be honest with everyone."[42] Botallo advises this doctor always to be prepared, to give hope through "compassionate and comforting words", without, however, concealing the true prognosis. If a patient insists, then he should be given the information he demands.[43] As far as the patient is concerned, he is obliged "to tell his doctor truthfully about past and present things" and to keep nothing secret.[44] Batallo documents with numerous examples just how damaging not telling a doctor the truth can be.

Whilst Zerbi, Clementini and Sicco differentiate between two contexts of a doctor's work in which either the love of truth or the patient's hopes are leading criteria, for Botallo, this differentiation does not appear to be of importance. In his view a doctor should never lie.

Battista Codronchius (1547–1628), a physician and philosopher from Imola, provides the earliest example of this tradition of Christian medical ethics in his *De christiana ac tuta medendi ratione* published in 1591, which had followers right

risus, moestitiam suspiria explicant; ita linguae protervia ac procacitas, dolus ac maledicentia animi petulantiam scurrilitatemque, fraudem et saevitiem, attestantur." Botallo, *I doveri*, p. 82.

41 Botallo, *Tractatus*, pp. 24–25: "Dolosam ac maledicam quisque hominum cavet bonus juxta ac malus. Probabile igitur ac pene necessarium argumentum esse videtur, si ex procaci, mendosa, atque maledica lingua improbum hominem esse concludamus: vel probum, prudentem, atque humanum, cuius oratio pura, docilis, comisque fuerit." Botallo, *I doveri*, p. 83.

42 Botallo, *Tractatus*, pp. 25–26: "Porro nil aliud sermo est, quam vera vel ficta significatio eorum, quae animus ipse per se significare non potest. Ast fictio exiqui tempori est. Ferum interdum fingere humanitatem spectamus, et ferociam humanum: Ast utrunque ocissime ad consueta reducit habitus. Caeterum cui malus est animus, vix huic bona manus est, quam durate coercet, ac tantum formidinae poenae, at cui animus bonus, vis mala manus erit. Sed quando ab audacia humanitas, a mendacio veritas, et, ut paucis absolvam, ab improbi tate probitas differat, res ipse edocet. Improbus namque secum ipse non modo audaciam, mendacium, vel improbitatem alienam, sed suam propriam accusat ac damnat, quaecunque bona laudans. [...] Nam Medicus vitae et animi purus, veritatem, undecunque venerit, amplectitur, nulla doli, nullaque improbae cupidinis labe persusus, honestum obsequium omnibus facere studens [...]." Botallo, *I doveri*, p. 83.

43 Botallo, *Tractatus*, p. 27–28: "Nam pium est (presagio non omisso) quos mors vel immedicabile corporis malum divexat, interea dum adhuc ipse patientis animus integer est, invisere, solari, spe fovere, et affectum (quantum conceditur) remediis mulcere. [...] reticere vero ex quibus haec parentur, tum quod patientes alias possunt citra medici consensum eisdem abuti praesidiis [...]." Botallo, *I doveri*, p. 84 and p. 87.

44 Botallo, *Tractatus*, p. 47; Botallo, *I doveri*, p. 115.

into the 19th century.[45] On the question as to whether a doctor should lie in certain situations, Codronchius is uncompromising. The Christian doctor is duty bound to persuade patients to confess their sins. If a doctor neglects to do this at the beginning of his treatment, then he is himself committing a cardinal sin.[46] As, according to Codronchius, the origin of an illness lies in the sins committed, he regards the comprehensive and merciless confrontation of all patients (sinners) with their fate as justifiable.[47] This should happen at any time and independently of the severity of the illness; as a result on the one hand the sick would not worry, and on the other provisions would have been taken should there be an unexpected deterioration in the patient's condition.[48] Should there be serious concerns about the recovery of a sick person, it is more advantageous for his mental and financial situation if he is informed of his impending death in a dignified manner.[49] If a patient's demise is imminent, then a doctor must persuade him to make confession and to write his will – even if he refuses to accept his life-threatening situation.[50] Codronchius regards Christian piety as the prudent and gentle way to inform a patient of his expected death.[51] The logical consequence is that Codronchius must

45 See Girolamo Bardi (1603–1667), *Medicus politicus catholicus*, Genua 1643, Thomas Browne (1663–1704) *Religio medici*, London 1643, Worthington Hooker (1806–1867), *Physician and Patient; or a Practical View of the Mutual Duties, Relations and Interests of the Medical Profession and Community*, London 1849. In addition to his deontological text (*De Christiana ac tuta medendi ratione*, Ferrara 1591), dedicated to the well-know physician Gerolamo Mercuriale, Codronchius also wrote two forensic treatises (*De morbis veneficis ac veneficiis libri quatuor* und *Methodus testificandi*, both published in 1595 in Venice).

46 B. Codronchius, *De Christiana ac tuta medendi ratione libri duo*, Ferrara 1591, p. 50: "Medicus itaque, qui initio curationis non suadet, neque hortatur infirmum ad peccatorum confessionem mortaliter proculdubio peccat, propter praecepta transgressionem, et sit periurus propter constitutionem."

47 Codronchius, *De Christiana*, pp. 47–59: 47: "Aegritudines saepe numero ab animi peccatis originem trahere sacrae literae, ac Doctores sancti clare ostendunt […]."

48 Codronchius, *De Christiana*, p. 51 and p. 52: "Itaque nisi moneat aegrotum a principio, et quotidie longius differat, cum urgente morbo manifestum periculum apparverit, hoc sequetur incommodi, quod aegrotus tanto terrore corripi poterit ex repentina, et praeter spem admonitione, itemque; morbi gravitate, ut inde mors sequatur, quod non accidisset, si initio de Confessione esset admonitus […]."

49 Codronchius, *De Christiana*, pp. 57–58: "Quod si forte dubitaret Medicus, an aegrotus periculose, et dubia spe vitae affectus, animam, rem ve familiarem composuerit huiusmodi finem vitae humaniter denunciare debet, et aeternae initium proponere, ut supra dictum est; in dubio enim unusquisque debet grave damnum proximi vitare, si potest; si vero infirmus confessus fuerit, ac testamentum condiderit, mortemque sibi imminere intelligat, vel se ad eam subeundam pie et religiose paret, eo munere Medicus levatur, et cuius odiosae sane denuntiationis eum taedebat, ab ea liberatur, nam notum illud est cum causa tollatur, eius effectum quoque aboleri."

50 Codronchius, *De Christiana*, p. 57: "[…] vel si aeger morbum letalem, vel se moriturum esse non percipiat, nisi det operam per se, aut alium, ut faciat utrunque […] mortemque non denunciat propinquam, si minus alia ratione potuit inducere ad confessionem, et testamentum, capitale delictum amittit."

51 Codronchius, *De Christiana*, p. 58: "Quaquam Christianae pietati valde consentaneum videtur, et aegrotanti utilius, prudenti quadam lenitate, per se, aut per alium, mortem vicinam

oppose Galen and Damascenus, for as a Christian physician he sees the psychological preparation for death of the person concerned as a doctor's most meaningful task. The medical approach favoured by Galen and Damascenus of giving hope, even in situations even when there is none, has no justification or sense for Codronchius in view of the imminent departure from physical life.[52]

THE MEDICUS POLITICUS

At the beginning of the 17th century there was a tendency to regard communication between doctor and patient less as an intimate and familiar matter, and more as the potential "public downside" of information brokering. The results of the spreading or withholding of information on the part of the patient or the doctor can be of either therapeutic, moral and religious, or a legal and forensic nature. The increasing sensitivity for the social dimensions of the medical profession is the main focus in the work of Roderigo de Castro.[53] In his text of the same name, the Jewish Portuguese physician (1546-1627) coins the phrase *medicus politicus*. Along with other *marrani* who left Spain and Portugal under pressure from the Inquisition and due to the worsening living conditions, de Castro went to Antwerp and Amsterdam in about 1580 and settled (in around 1596) in Hamburg.[54] Here he lived as a respected physician, keeping his Jewish faith hidden to begin with. Only in 1612, after he had achieved a high reputation both as a doctor and a citizen, did he publically profess his religious convictions.[55]

insinuare; credibile est enim hominem christianum cognita morte diligentius, ac ferventius se ad eam non modo moderate, sed hilariter ferendam comparaturum esse; quam si de ea nihil cogitaret, aut a nemine quidquam audiret, ad quod propositum quidam Religiosus vir dicere consuevit, *qui se quotidie recordatur moriturum, contemnit praesentia, et ad futura festinat* [emphasis by Codronchius] […]."

52 Codronchius, *De Christiana*, pp. 58–59.

53 Rodrigo de Castro was born in Lisbon and studied medicine and philosophy in Salamanca. In Hamburg in 1596 he battled against the plague and wrote his *Tractatus brevis de natura et causis pestis* […] (Hamburg 1596). As a result, an exception was made for him as a *marrano* and he was allowed to purchase a house in the Old Town. Benedict de Castro (born in Hamurg in around, died on 31st January 1684 ebd.), one of Rodrigo's sons, was like his father much in demand as a doctor at the princely courts of Europe. His many patients included, for example, Christine of Sweden. See H. Kellenbenz, *Sephardim an der unteren Elbe. Ihre wirtschaftliche und politische Bedeutung vom Ende des 16. bis zum Beginn des 18. Jahrhunderts*, Wiesbaden 1958, pp. 323–331.

54 J. Arrizabalaga, "Medical Ideals in the Sephardic Diaspora. Rodrigo de Castro's Portrait of the Perfect Physicians in Early Seventeenth-Century Hamburg", *Medical History Supplement* 29 (2009), pp. 107–124: 112.

55 Professed Jews were not given the right of abode in Hamburg until February 1612. In the list of the Jewish community in Hamburg (of 1612), the names of Rodrigo de Castro, his second wife and his children can be found. The Jewish community at this time consisted of 125 adults, amongst them two doctors. In around 1617, the hostility of the Lutherans towards the Jews of Portuguese origin increased in Hanburg; accordingly the Senate of Hamburg adopted restrictive property legislation which prohibited the Jews from owning houses. The Senate,

Castro cleverly dedicated his work to two senators of the Hanseatic city of Hamburg.[56] In view of the social and religious context, as well as of the life history of the man who, like many others who shared his fate, had to hold his ground amongst the many different beliefs and cultures of the time, it is not surprising that the complex themes of deception (*simulatio*) and the withholding of information are given such a prominent place in de Castro's work.[57] In different contexts, for example in relation to prognosis (Lib. III, chap. 7)[58] or in the chapter "How far and with what one should oblige patients" (Lib. III, chap. 8), de Castro advises a doctor not be too strict or to strive fanatically for the truth, but rather to act humanely and approachably.[59] The Hippocratic Galenic ideal of the *medicus gratiosus* who knows how to win over a patient with moderation, self-control and tact left its mark on de Castro.[60]

When de Castro deals with the promise of healing (Lib. III, chap. 9), he also pursues the question which had been the subject of controversial debate since Antiquity, namely whether a doctor may tell a lie for the benefit of an improvement in health.[61] De Castro refers both to well-known and other passages in the Hippocratic *Epidemics*, as well as to Galen's commentaries (VI, 4,8; VI, 5,13) in which

however, spared Rodrigo de Castro due to his many years of service. See Kellenbenz, *Sephardim*, p. 327; further detail in: J. Arrizabalaga, *Medical Ideals*, pp. 113–114.

56 R. de Castro, *Medicus-Politicus* [...], Hamburg 1614, p. A2r: "Amplissimis, clarissimis, sapientissimis Viris, Dn. Vincentio Mollero Jul. Peritissimo, et Dn. Hieronymo Vogelero, florentissimae Reipublicae Hamburgensis consulibus vigilantissimis. Rodericus a Castro Philosophus ac Doctor medicus."

57 Siehe M. Gadebusch Bondio, "Die Muse der Krankheit. Francisco Delicado, die Syphilis und die heilende Lozana", in: M. Pfister – K. Bergdolt (eds.), *The Renaissance and the Dialogue between Science, Art and Literature*, Wiesbaden 2011, pp. 136-160.

58 De Castro, *Medicus-Politicus*, p. 135: "In prognostico nisi certissima et infallibilia salutis aut mortis indicia adsint, sit medicus ambiguus: in promissionibus moderatus, sanitatis tamen potius semper spem praebeat, quam certam mortem praenunciet. Si enim a medico destitutus infirmus postea (quod saepe sit) casu vel natura restituatur, magnam incurrit infamiam. Et vero si sanitatis spem praebuerit, et mors sequatur, ignominia tanta non est, quia potuerunt incidere multa, errores, excessus, ac novus morbus, et facilior est a sanitate ad mortem commutatio, quam a morte ad salutem, quae naturae cursu est impossibilis."

59 De Castro, *Medicus-Politicus*, p. 138: "Nam ut sunt aliqui justitiae ac veritatis perfervidi zelatores, qui per summam injuriam summo utuntur jure, et ex nimio zelo nonnunquam impetu potius quodam quam judicio feruntur, ad reprehendenda, et castiganda vitia, et in ea re modum excedunt: ita perfecti alioqui in arte medica viri in circumstantiis quibusdam curationis saepe deficiunt [...]."

60 See de Castro, *Medicus-Politicus*, p. 141; see Deichgräber, *Medicus gratiosus*, pp. 13–52; Winfred Schleiner sees in Geronimo Bardi's (1603–1667) *Medicus politico catholicus* a critical reaction to de Castro's perception of a physician: I. Bardi, *Medicus politico catholicus seu de medicinae sacrae tum conoscendae ideae*, Genua 1643: Schleiner, *Medical Ethics*, pp. 94–97.

61 De Castro, *Medicus-Politicus*, p. 142: "Dictum fuit supra, fausta omnia languenti esse renuncianda, idcirco quaestio discutienda venit, dissensionis plena, et omnino controversa, liceat ne, medico aegrotum decipere salutis causa: idque ex mente Hippocratis, Galeni, et reliquorum philosophorum."

therapeutic deception is justified.[62] The previously discussed variable handling of medical details adjusted to the patients' individual frame of mind and strength or weakness of character date back to Galen.[63] Anxious patients should consequently be spared the truth about the severity of their health, although in these cases a doctor must always provide the family with exact information.

The range of sources which de Castro uses in his remarks is impressive: as well as the Old Testament, he refers to Plato (*Politeia*, III), Aristotle (*Nicomachean Ethics*, IV, 7), Celsus (*De medicina*, Lib. 3.6.5),[64] the *Aphorisms* of Damascenus and Aelianus' *De varia historia* (Lib. 12), from which de Castro takes a quotation from Pythagoras.[65] De Castro sees the platonic idea of the lie[66] in line with the platonic positions held by Hippocrates and Galen. In his *Politeia*, Plato states that "a lie is useless to the gods, and useful only as a medicine to men." The means of deception, or the pharmakon, should, however, only be available to those who govern the state ("for the sake of the enemy or the citizens, for the benefit of the city"). Those with no knowledge – here patients are also explicitly referred to – may not be allowed to make use of these means and may not lie.[67] De Castro justifies the right of a doctor to use deception with the anxiety of the majority of patients:

> [...] as it is in the nature of sickness itself to be anxious and mistrustful; the sick do not only pay close heed to words and the conclusions they draw from them, but also to the gestures and the facial expression of the doctor, fearing threats they interpret everything possible from

62 See Galen, *Hippocratis Epidem. VI et Galeni in illum commentarius* IV, chap. 8, Kühn, vol. XVII, 2–A, pp. 134–143; Galen, *Hippocratis Epidem. VI et Galeni in illum commentarius* V, chap. 13, ibid., pp. 266–269.

63 See Galen, *Hippocratis Epidem. VI et Galeni in illum commentarius* II, chap. 47, Kühn, Bd. XVII, 1–B, pp. 994–1001: p. 996.

64 De Castro, *Medicus-Politicus*, p. 142: "[...] prudentis ergo medici fuerit, quae aegro metum allatura putarit, aut animi perturbationem, ea simulatione tegere: quia ut scribit Celsus *aegros securos agere convenit, ut corpore tantum, non etiam animo laborent* [emphasis by de Castro]: ideo si quae sunt, quae exasperatura eorum animos sint, optimum est, eadem aegrotantium notitiae subtrahere; quam obrem Damascenus salutem aegro perpetuo promittendam, etsi de salute desperemus, praecepit."

65 De Castro, *Medicus-Politicus*, p. 143: "Sed enim Aelianus in libro *de varia historia* refert, Phytagoram dicere solitum, duo haec praeclara data esse hominibus a Deo, *vera dicere, et beneficia in alios conferre* [emphasis by de Castro]."

66 Plato, *The Rebublic*, (tr. By B. Jowett), Oxford 1908, 389b–c: "Again, truth should be highly valued, if, as we were saying, a lie is useless to the gods, and useful only as a medicine to men, then the use of such medicines should be restricted to physicians; private individuals have no business with them. [...] Then if any one at all ist o have the privilege of lying, the rulers oft he State should be the persons; and they, in their dealings either with enemies or with their own citizens, may be allowed to lie fort he public good. But nobody else should meddle with anything oft he kind."

67 Platon, *The Rebublic*, 389c–d: "[...] and although the rulers have this privilege, for a private man to lie to them in return is to be deemed a more heinous fault than for the patient or the pupil of a gymnasium not to speak the truth about his own bodily illnesses to the physicians or to the trainer, or for a sailor not to tell the captain what is happening about the ship and the rest of the crew, and how things are going with himself or his fellow sailors."

> the doctor's face; thus it becomes typical for the observant doctor to conceal through deception all those things that he anticipates as a threat, and which might cause the patient anxiety and confuse his mind.[68]

De Castro makes a careful distinction between that form of deception which withholds or conceals the truth (*simulatio, qua veritas tacendo subtrahitur, aut quovis velamine circumtegitur*), and that in which falsehood instead of truth is told (*qua falsum pro vero exprimitur*).[69] The former does not represent any wrongful act, rather it is virtuous (*virtus reputanda*).[70] As an example de Castro quotes an episode from the life of David. In order to save himself from the violence of King Achish, David pretended to be insane.[71] This trick saved his life.

In order to promote a patient's health, a doctor may be artful or cunning (*artificiose*) and thus deceive, or pretend to, accordingly.[72] With this view de Castro distances himself explicitly from Aristotle, whom he attempts to refute with skilful argument and the development of a typology of lying. For the Ancient philosopher, all variations of the untruth were without exception both bad and reprehensible. An honest person should never in any way lie about things known to him.[73] As *sententia validissima* de Castro adds here a traditional Pythagorean aphorism of Claudius Aelianus (170–c.222) in which it is said that the gods have given mankind two wonderful abilities: "to speak Truth, and to do Good [to others]".[74]

68 De Castro, *Medicus-Politicus*, p. 142: "[…] quia aegri sua propter natura suspiciosi cum sint, et formidolosi, accuratissime non solum verba, et ratiocinationes, sed gestus et nutus medicorum observant, a cunctis, quae vel ex vultu medici colligunt, sibi metuentes; prudentis ergo medici fuerit, quae aegro metum allatura putarit, aut animi perturbationem, ea simulatione tegere […]."

69 De Castro, *Medicus-Politicus*, p. 142

70 De Castro, *Medicus-Politicus*, p. 142: "Prima non modo inculpabilis, quinimo suo loco et tempore digna laude virtusque reputanda censetur […]."

71 De Castro, *Medicus-Politicus*, p. 142: "[…] qua ratione David, ut evaderet manus regis Laehis [Achisch], habitum mutavit, et insanum se finxit." See the Old Testament, *Samuel*, 21, 13–16.

72 De Castro, *Medicus-Politicus*, p. 142: "Nec vero simulare solum ac fingere, sed interdum mendacio uti medicum oportere, plerique censent, ut salutem aeger artificiose consequatur."

73 De Castro, *Medicus-Politicus*, p. 143: "Pugnat ex altera parte Aristoteles, qui *quarto Ethic.* omne genus mendacii, qualecunque fuerit, vituperans memorabilem illam pronunciavit sententiam, mendacium per se improbum est ac vituperabile: verum autem probum ac laudabile. Et *primo elench.: sapientis, inquit, est non mentiri, de quibus novit, et mentientes alios manifestare* [emphasis by de Castro]." Aristotle, *Nicomachean Ethics*, tr. by Ch. Rowe, Oxford 2002, 1127a: "In itself falsehood is a bad thing, and tob e censured, while truth is fine and something tob e praised." Aristotle, *On sophistical Refutations*, tr. by E.S. Forsters, London / Cambridge (Mass.) 1955, 165a: "[…] it is the task of a man who has knowledge of a particular subject himself to refrain from fallacious arguments about the subjects of his knowledge and to be able to expose him who uses them."

74 De Castro, *Medicus-Politicus*, p. 143: "Sed enim Aelianus in libro *de varia historia* refert, Phytagoram dicere solitum, duo haec praeclara data esse hominibus a Deo, *vera dicere, et beneficia in alios conferre* [emphasis by de Castro]". Claudius Aelianus, *His Various History*, tr. by T. Stanley, London 1665, Book XII, chap. LIX (Of Truth and Beneficence): "Pythagoras said that these two most excellent things are given by the Gods to Men; to speak Truth,

The Pythagorean praise of speaking the truth follows the discussion as to whether lying – if a lie is intrinsically bad (*mendacium per se est malum*), unnatural (*contra naturam*), or even an act which perverts God-given order (*actus per se inordinatus*) – can indeed be justified in certain situations.[75] For de Castro there are two constellations of this type which permit lying: 1. It is permissible to conceal the truth at the right time and in the right situation; this is not inappropriate behaviour, but rather deserves admiration. 2. Contrary to the damaging lie (*mendacium nocivum*) which has negative consequences for the majority, and which is also useless and reprehensible, the so-called lie out of kindness (*mendacium officiosum*) can generate a useful meaning (*sensus*) for those who hear it.[76] In this case it is necessary to be aware of the meaning and intention of the lie so that its usefulness becomes apparent. Then the lie is be used as a medicine. De Castro compares the medicinal use of a lie with that of the hellebore (*helleborus*) – just as the effective herb should always be used to the advantage of the patient (as it can also be deadly), "one should not lie if it is not to the great advantage of one's neighbours."[77] Twice as much damage is done if deception is used outside of an emergency situation by either doing or saying something in order to deceive somebody.[78] De Castro finally agrees with the Ancient authors: "The ancients considered the lie to be good if based upon a certain stratagem, above all if something is implemented against enemies and bandits."[79]

The discussion between Odysseus and Neoptolemos in Sophocles' *Philoctetes*, which de Castro does not explicitly mention here, conveys precisely this attitude. The physician Johann Heinrich Meibom (1590–1655) from Helmstadt recognised this in his learned commentary on the Hippocratic oath.[80] At the point at which Meibom declares the lie to be a legitimate means for a physician to attain

and to do Good [to others:] He added, that each of these resembled the actions of the Gods" [http://penelope.uchicago.edu/aelian/varhist12.xhtml (09.09.11)].

75 De Castro, *Medicus-Politicus*, p. 143.

76 De Castro, *Medicus-Politicus*, p. 143–144: "*Primum* est veritatem in tempore et loco tacere, non tantum sine vitio, sed etiam cum laude licere [144]. *Secundum* plurimum interesse inter mendacium nocivum, et mendacium officiosum: quippe illud semper est inutile et vituperandum; hoc etsi falsum, sensum perutilem tamen auditoribus generat; spectandus igitur semper est animus, et sensus: consilium etiam, propositum, et voluta intuenda, ne quid quis generit, sed quo voto egerit, inquirendum."

77 De Castro, *Medicus-Politicus*, p. 144: "[…] ex quo fit, ut prudenter quidam assimilaverint mendacium helleboro, quod si absque summi discriminis necessitate accipiatur, maximi sit exitii: si vero praesente exitiali morbo sumptum fuerit, sit salubre. Ita insuper mendacio utendum, uti medicamento et condimento, hoc est, nunquam magnopere mentiendum aut fine magna proximi utilitate."

78 De Castro, *Medicus-Politicus*, p. 144: "*Tertio* praemittendum, duplicem esse dolum; malum, nimirum qui est machinatio quaedam alterius decipiendi causa, cum aliud agitur, aliud simulatur, et comprehendit omnem calliditatem ac fallaciam, ad circumveniendum, fallendum, decipiendumve alterum adibitam […]." Here de Castro refers to the Roman lawyers Domitius Ulpianus (170–223) and Marcus Antistius Labeones (1st century AD).

79 De Castro, *Medicus-Politicus*, p. 144: "Bonum vero dolum veteres dixerunt solertiam quandam in rebus agendis, maxime si adversus hostem latronemque quis machinatur."

80 J. H. Meibom, *Hippokratis Magni Orkos, sive iusjurandum*, Lyon 1643, pp. 212–214.

his highest goal – the promotion of the health and wellbeing of the patient – he quotes the central statements in the dialogue between the crafty Odysseus and the young, upright Neoptolemos who asks: "Do you not always regard it as shameful when someone lies?" Odysseus replies: "Not if lying brings us salvation."[81]

Back to de Castro: for the benefit of a patient's recovery a doctor may conceal and promise much, as sometimes there is more chance of success through a pleasant lie and a particular skilfulness than with truthful talk.[82] In view of the arguments put forward, de Castro comes to the conclusion that Aristotle and Pythagoras also understood this sort of lie to be useless and associated with injuring people:[83] for Aristotle – de Castro says – every type of lie, even the pleasing lie, is reprehensible as they endanger the purity of truth. In order to reinforce his own position, de Castro cites several examples from the Old Testament: Abraham's white lie when, in order to save his own life during the famine in Egypt, he instructed his wife to tell people she was his sister instead of his wife (Moses 1, 12); the episode of the guileful Hebrew midwives (Moses 2, 1)[84] and the harlot Rahab in Jericho, who hid two scouts in her house and saved both their lives and hers by telling a white lie (Joshua 2); "[...] all these are in truth examples of the hidden meaning of a higher and more divine view."[85] But dictums against lying are also taken from the Bible.[86] Finally de Castro expresses the Galenic division of pa-

81 Sophocles, *Philoctetes*, pp. 108–110. The topic remains significant in the works of German physicians such as Johann Heinrich Meibom (1590–1655) (Commentary on the Hippocratic Oath: *Hippokratis Magni Orkos, sive iusjurandum*, 1643) and Johannes Bohn (1640–1718) (*De officio medici duplici*, 1704). Meibom refers to Hippocrates, Galen, Clemente Alessandrino, and sees the promotion of health and a patient's well-being as a doctor's highest goal. To these ends a doctor may use lies as a means to an ends: Meibom, *Hippokratis Magni Orkos*, pp. 212–14; J. Bohn, *De officio medici duplici clinici nimirum ac forensis* [...], Leipzig 1704; followers of a radical Christian point of view, which sees a doctor as always obliged to tell the truth, continued to cause a stir into the middle of the 19th century: W. Hooker, *Physician and Patient; or a Practical View of the Mutual Duties, Relations and Interests of the Medical Profession and Community*, London 1849, pp. 215–281.

82 De Castro, *Medicus-Politicus*, p. 144: "[...] interdum medico fallere, et veritatem obtegere, ut quod salutis aegri causa facere instituit, et veritatem non potest, dolo bono et arte quadam moliatur."

83 De Castro, *Medicus-Politicus*, p. 144: "Aristoteles, vero et Pythagoras de eo mendacio intelligendi videntur, quod aut inutiliter profertur, aut cum noxam alterius."

84 The King of the Egyptians wanted to prevent the people of Israel from becoming too large and powerful. He ordered the Hebrew midwives to kill all boys at birth. Out of fear of God they did not do this, and let the children live. When the pharaoh asked them why they had not obeyed, they answered: "Because the Hebrew women are not as the Egyptian women; for they are vigorous and give birth before the midwife can get to them" 2 Moses 1, here in: *The Bible. According to Martin Luther's translation* (bible text in the revised version of 1984), edited by the Evangelical Church in Germany, Stuttgart 2001, p. 58.

85 De Castro, *Medicus-Politicus*, p. 145: "Verum haec exempla divinioris altiorisque sunt contemplationis ac secretioris sensus."

86 At this point the following were instanced against lying: De Castro, *Medicus-Politicus*, p. 145: "[...] *non loquantur labia mea iniquitatem, nec lingua mea meditabitur mendacium* [emphasis by de Castro]", see Job, 27 and Psalm V; De Castro, *Medicus-Politicus*, p. 145: "*odisti, inquit, omnes, qui operantur iniquitatem, et perdes omnes qui loquuntur mendacium*

tients into two groups to which the prudent physician (*medicus prudens*) should adapt his statements. De Castro sets this medial ideal of a careful man (*vir prudens*) against the *histrio* (charlatan, mountebank, actor) who strives for fame and riches and is prepared to exceed the limits of a sense of shame, to lie brazenly or to promise the impossible.[87] With praise for the *medicus prudens* who never exaggerates, and who is extremely cautious in his prognoses, who neither flatters with excessive embellishment nor boasts by ostentatiously exaggerating the condition", de Castro increases the importance of moderation when dealing with patients.[88]

The detail with which de Castro explores the question appears to find a continuation in the medical forensic context. Two elements which were absent both with de Castro and with those authors presented appear in the deliberations of the Roman physician Paolo Zacchia (1584–1659): the patients will and the function of the doctor.[89] In the seven volumes of his *Quaestiones medico-legales*, which appeared between 1621 and 1651, the physician of Pope Innocent X and Alexander VII examines the mistakes which could be and were made through the withholding of advice.[90] Zacchia analyses and explains whether a doctor must announce an impending death (§ 13)[91] and whether he should ask a family member to encourage the sick person to make confession (§ 14).[92] On each question Zacchia discusses the opinions of physicians and canonists in order finally to clarify his own position.[93]

[emphasis by de Castro]", see Salomon, Sayings (XII, 12, 13, 17); De Castro, *Medicus-Politicus*, p. 145: "[…] *verbum mendacii longe fac a me* [emphasis by de Castro]".

87 De Castro, *Medicus-Politicus*, p. 145.

88 De Castro, *Medicus-Politicus*, p. 145–146: "Medicus tamen prudens et gravis salutem ubique non polliceatur, nec nisi illud addiderit, sanitatem quidem affuturam, Deo auxiliante, aegro vero omnia recte agente, et medici praeceptis obtemperante, ac servatis servandis, denique in prognostico magna cautione semper opus est, ne aut nimium blandiendo mitiorem, quam revera sit, morbum jactantes, eo graviore reddito, in ignominiae labem incurramus: aut nimium severe agendo, inanem metum aegro incutiamus."

89 P. Zacchia, *Quaestionum medico-legalium*, Tomus secundus, Lib. VI, Tit. I ("De medicorum Erroribus a Lege Punibilibus"), Quaestio IV ("De erroribus omissionis ad consilia spectantibus"), Frankfurt a. M. 1688, pp. 490–493.

90 More than 10 editions confirm the success of Zacchia's work, which was last printed in 1774, 115 years after Zacchia's death. See Z. Traunfellner, "Paolo Zacchia – Vater der Gerichtlichen Medizin, 400 Jahre nach seiner Geburt", *Zeitschrift für Rechtsmedizin* 94 (1985), pp. 159–163, G. Rossi – A. Pastore (eds.), *Paolo Zacchia. Alle origini della medicina legale 1584–1659*, Milano 2008.

91 Zacchia, *Quaestionum medico-legalium*, § 13, p. 492: "Insurgit […] alia dubitatio, num scilicet in morbo praecipiti, et periculi pleno, teneatur Medicus ultra confessionem, etiam ad Viatici assumptionem aegrum hortari."

92 Zacchia, *Questionum medico-legalium*, § 14, p. 492: "[…] dubitatur, an Medicus teneatur etiam mortem infirmo nunciare."

93 Zacchia refers here amongst others to Baptista Codronchius, *De Christiana* (Lib. 1, Cap. 17), Scipione Mercuri, *Degli errori popolari*, Venezia 1603 (Lib. 2, Cap. 25; Lib. 3, Cap. 4) and the canonist Ioannes Alphonsus de Fonseca, *Medicorum incipientium Medicina, seu medicinae christianae speculum*, Alcalá de Henares 1598.

A doctor – according to Zacchia – is not duty bound to make a patient's approaching death known to him, unless the patient should ask insistently about it and wishes to ensure his health or save his soul (*ob suae animae salutem*). It is advisable for a doctor always to inform the priest, the family and those close to the sick person about the actual situation, and to ask them to encourage him to make confession. As a doctor is responsible for bodily health, the announcement of death should be left to the pastor or the confessor. Otherwise the patient's disappointment, despair and anger might be directed at him, which, incidentally, could lead to a quicker death. As Galen (*Epid. Comm.* in VI, 4.8)[94], Zacchia also takes the view, referring to the Christian doctor (*medicus christianus*), that a doctor may never promise a dying person in a critical condition the health that he wants, but that at the same time he should never disclose to the patient that he will die (unless he is dealing with an emergency situation!).[95]

The positions held by de Castro with his ideal of the *medicus politicus*, and Zacchia with the *medicus christianus*, are based upon a clear hierarchy of medical values and aims, and are embedded in Hippocratic and Galenic medicine. The patient's wellbeing takes priority; the truth is secondary, although the family should be informed of it in order to protect a doctor from possible accusations.

CONCLUSION

Pre-modern doctors, such as Clemente Clementini or Julius Alexandrinus and Roderigo de Castro, were aware of the difficulty of predicting the outcome of an illness. This uncertainty, according to Karl Jaspers, places medical information in perspective. The "patient-doctor relationship" presupposes that both are capable

94 Zacchia, *Questionum medico-legalium*, § 14, p. 492: "Licet ergo Christianus Medicus non debeat (quod Gal. volebat *comment. 4. in sextum Epid. text. 8* [emphasis by Zacchia]) certam incolumitatem aegro polliceri, quando adest aliquod vitae periculum, ne spe corporeae salutis, a salutis aeternae desiderio distrahatur, nunquam tamen debet certam mortem enunciare, (nisi aliquid majus urgeat) sed hoc Parocho, confessariis, religiosis praestandum relinquere; cui sententiae videtur adhaesisse."

95 Zacchia, *Questionum medico-legalium*, § 14, p. 492: "Dico igitur, non videri ad Medicum pertinere, mortem aliquo modo aegro nunciare, nisi forte, ab ipso aegro, ut fit, instanter ob suae animae salutem, de hoc interrogetur; aut si nulla alia via sit, quam magnum scandalum evitari post aegri mortem posset, licet sufficeret etiam eo casu per alium hoc aegro denunciare. Satis ergo se ab omni culpa immunem Medicus reddet, si Parochum, Sacerdotes, Propinquos, assidentes, amicus ejus rei admonuerit. Et ratio est, quia Medicus corporeae saluti praepositus, dummodo satisfaciat debito de suadendo confessionem, quod ipse aeger scit ad Medicum pertinere, si mortem quoque ab eo sibi denunciari videat, a quo salutem expectat, absque dubio insolito timore ac terrore afficietur, forte etiam ira, et excandescentia in ipsum Medicum commovebitur, et mortem accelerabit, scio que infirmos nonnullos Medicis haec nunciantibus, et testamenti confectionem suadentibus iratos, et animos despondentes respondisse, hoc ad Medicum non pertinere; alios omne in posterum remedium recusasse, et alia inde mala ac scandala evenisse."

of understanding and realising the meaning of the possible truth here.[96] Three questions result from this premise. Firstly, Jaspers considers whether a doctor understands "how relative all knowledge is" and that therefore no prognosis can ever be absolutely certain.[97] Here the position adopted by some early modern doctors can be recognised, as well, however, as a conventional view in medical ethics held in the German Democratic Republic. Furthermore, Jaspers poses the question as to whether a patient's psychological situation allows such knowledge to be "comprehended methodically without falling into false conclusiveness.[98] The Galenic differentiation of the patient's mood, which leads to the variation of the truthfulness of the statement, is not far from this observation.[99] Finally, according to Jaspers the question that has to be addressed prior to medical information is whether the patient "is consciously able to discover and to accept his fate, as in every situation he can also maintain this possibility and can therefore have hope as long as he lives."[100] Such an open-minded and strong person has a right to the truth. At this point Jaspers again turns his attention to the physician. Only those who have an "unfailing sense" of these issues, and who regard themselves as fellow sufferers and not as an authority "have the right to speak the truth."[101] Open and honest discussion, the so-called *parrhesia* which in ancient times could only be practised by certain citizens, can, in view of these considerations, be regarded as a special, medical entitlement, an entitlement which in itself is not given, but for which a deep human understanding is required.[102]

96 Jaspers, *Wahrheit*, p. 558.

97 One topic for discussion in the GDR was the "pleaseant lie": the idea that a doctor may not claim for himself the right to make statements about the prognisis and the resultant life expectancy of a patient, and that he should therefore speak palliatively with him, was no exception. In the case of an unfavourable prognosis "to leave a patient in the dark with inappropriate formulations and (incomplete) presentations" was regarded as appropriate procedure. H. G. Berndt, "Gedanken zum Inhalt der Vorträge des Kolloquiums 'Ethik und Medizin im Sozialismus'", in: H. Hüller (ed.), *Ethik und Medizin im Sozialismus*, Greifswald 1974, pp. 1–6; see H. Bettin – M. Gadebusch Bondio, "DDR-Medizin – Eine eigene Ethik?", in: H. Bettin – M. Gadebusch Bondio (eds.), *Medizinische Ethik in der DDR – Erfahrungswert oder Altlast?*, Berlin 2010, pp. 7–19 and also H. Bettin – M. Gadebusch Bondio, "Greifswalder Ansätze zur Ethik in der Medizin – ein Rückblick in die jüngere Vergangenheit", *Journal für Anästhesie und Intensivbehandlung* 2 (2009), pp. 38–42.

98 Jaspers, *Wahrheit*, p. 559.

99 Ibid.

100 Ibid.

101 Ibid.

102 Galen of Pergamon discussed the *Parrhesia* in his work on mistakes and the methods used to avoid them: Galien, *L'âme et ses passions; les passions et les erreurs de l'âme; les facultés de l'âme suivent les tempéraments du corps*, ed. by V. Barras, Paris 1995. Galen, *De cognoscendi curandisque animi morbis*, Kühn, vol. V, book 1, chap. 5; Galen, *De cuiuslibet animi peccatorum dignotione atque medela libellus*, Kühn, vol. V, book 1, pp. 58–103; see also: M. Foucault, *Hermeneutik des Subjekts. Vorlesungen am Collège de France* (1981/82), Frankfurt a. M. 2009; T. Ricklin, "Parrhesia", in: I. Atucha et al. (eds.), *Parcours lexicographiques dans les cultures médiévales*, Louvain-La-Neuve 2011, pp. 507–516.

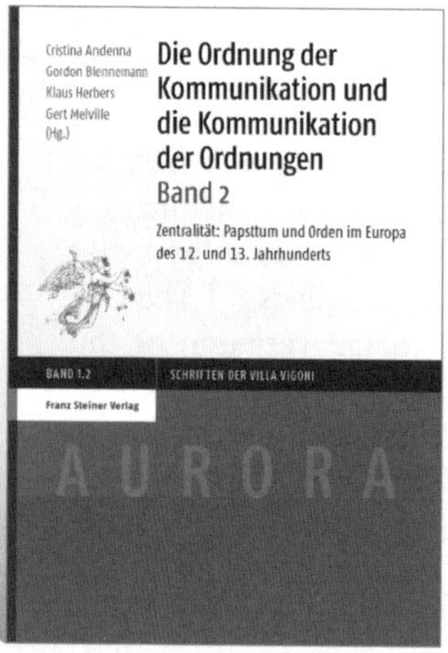

Franz Steiner Verlag

Cristina Andenna /
Gordon Blennemann / Klaus Herbers /
Gert Melville (Hg.)
Die Ordnung der Kommunikation und die Kommunikation der Ordnungen. Band 2

2013.
331 Seiten. Geb.
ISBN 978-3-515-10301-5

Cristina Andenna / Gordon Blennemann / Klaus Herbers / Gert Melville (Hg.)

Die Ordnung der Kommunikation und die Kommunikation der Ordnungen. Band 2

Zentralität: Papsttum und Orden im Europa des 12. und 13. Jahrhunderts

Aurora. Schriften der Villa Vigoni – Band 1.2

Das Papsttum und die *vita religiosa*, die Welt der Klöster und Orden, sind die beiden einzigen institutionellen Lebensformen des Mittelalters, die für sich eine eigene universelle Geltung beanspruchen konnten. Durch die Ausbildung komplexer kommunikativer Strukturen und innovativer Organisationsformen nahmen beide vor allem seit dem 12. und 13. Jahrhundert Anteil an der Grundlegung eines „Kulturraums Europa".
Vor diesem Hintergrund stand der analytische Vergleich von Papsttum und *vita religiosa* als aufeinander bezogene Kommunikationssysteme im Mittelpunkt zweier Tagungen am Deutsch-Italienischen Zentrum für Europäische Exzellenz der Villa Vigoni, deren Ergebnisse nun in einer zweibändigen Publikation vorliegen.
Die Beiträge des zweiten Bandes widmen sich der Rolle der römischen Kurie bei der überregionalen Vermittlung religiöser Normen und kultureller Werte als universal gedachte Ordnungsvorstellungen und fragen zugleich nach dem Anteil der religiösen Orden an diesen Vermittlungsprozessen.

Ebenfalls lieferbar

Cristina Andenna / Klaus Herbers / Gert Melville (Hg.)
Die Ordnung der Kommunikation und die Kommunikation der Ordnungen. Band 1
Netzwerke: Klöster und Orden im Europa des 12. und 13. Jahrhunderts
Aurora. Schriften der Villa Vigoni – Band 1.1

307 Seiten mit 8 Farbtafeln mit 9 Fotos. Kart. € 79,–.
ISBN 978-3-515-09929-5

Franz Steiner Verlag
Birkenwaldstr. 44 · D – 70191 Stuttgart
Telefon: 0711 / 2582 – 0 · Fax: 0711 / 2582 – 390
E-Mail: service@steiner-verlag.de
Internet: www.steiner-verlag.de